LONGMAN ADVANCED GNVQ

TEST AND ASSE...   ...DE

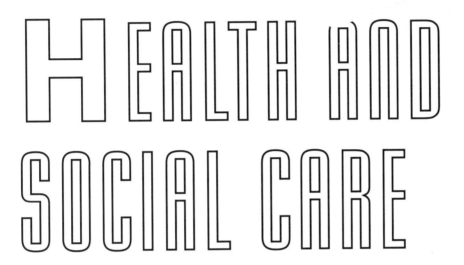

HEALTH AND SOCIAL CARE

Kathryn Lawley and Alan Gardiner

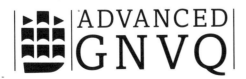

ADVANCED
GNVQ

**Longman Advanced GNVQ
Test and Assessment Guides**

Series Editors:
Geoff Black and Stuart Wall

Titles Available:
Business
Health and Social Care
Leisure and Tourism

Due for publication in 1995:
Construction and the Built Environment
Hospitality and Catering
Science

Longman Group Ltd,
Longman House, Burnt Mill, Harlow,
Essex CM20 2JE, England
and Associated Companies throughout the world.

© Longman Group UK Ltd 1995

First Published 1995

ISBN 0 582 23777 7

British Library Cataloguing-in-Publication Data

A catalogue record for this book is
available from the British Library

Typeset by 19QQ in 9/11pt Sabon
Produced by Longman Singapore Publishers (Pte) Ltd.
Printed in Singapore

Contents

Acknowledgements

The authors would like to thank the following for their invaluable assistance in the writing of this book: Geoff Black and Stuart Wall; Stephen Lawley for his devoted support; Marian Murphy; John Murphy; Stephen Harris; Heather Smith; Julie and Steve Brown. They are also grateful for the co-operation received from staff and students involved in the Advanced GNVQ Health and Social Care course at Weatherhead High School, Wallasey.

Kathryn Lawley and Alan Gardiner

Using this book

The first eight units provide you with the vital information and knowledge needed in each mandatory unit, both for passing the compulsory external tests (in seven of the mandatory units) and for completing the various projects and assignments set on those units. You will find many self-check questions at the end of each Element in the unit, with answers at the end of the unit. You will also find a unit test at the end of each unit of the type you will face in the external test itself, with answers and examiner comments.

After these eight mandatory units there is a major chapter on the 'Portfolio', helping you develop the skills and insights needed to gain a merit or distinction in your Advanced GNVQ. You will be shown the types of evidence you can present in the portfolio. Actual examples of student assignments are provided, together with examiner comments. There is also material in this chapter on what is meant by the core skills in your GNVQ and how these can be demonstrated in your portfolio of evidence.

Introduction: Advanced GNVQ in Health and Social Care

In order to gain your Advanced GNVQ in Health and Social Care, you have to demonstrate to your tutors and teachers that you have been successful in meeting the standards for the various units on the course; in other words you will be *assessed*, in a number of different ways, to show that you have reached the required standard for each unit. The bulk of the assessment you will be asked to do will be in the form of **assignments and projects**, set and marked by the staff who teach on your GNVQ. You will also need to pass the **external tests** that are set by Health and Social Care experts outside your school or college. In the case of Advanced Health and Social Care, there are currently seven external tests that you will need to pass. An important part of the assessment process for GNVQs is the collection of *evidence* to show that you have successfully completed the different parts of the units. This material is gathered together in a **portfolio of evidence**, which is used by your tutors, and other specialists outside of your school or college, to confirm that you have covered all the necessary parts of the units and to agree your overall grade for the GNVQ.

Before we can look in greater detail at the different types of assessment in GNVQs, it is important that you understand clearly how the different parts of a GNVQ fit together. You will also need to get used to a lot of new words and phrases, so it's important that you get to grips with these from the outset.

The structure of the Advanced GNVQ in Health and Social Care

All GNVQs are based on **units**. Advanced GNVQs are made up of 15 units in total, shared out as follows:

- *Eight Mandatory Units* – these cover the fundamental skills, knowledge and understanding related to the study of Health and Social Care. Mandatory means that everybody studying for the Advanced GNVQ in Health and Social Care must complete these units.

- *Four Optional Units* – these complement the mandatory units and give students the chance to look in more depth at a particular topic. The exact options you will be studying will depend on which awarding body your school or college deals with (BTEC, City & Guilds or RSA), the skills and expertise of your tutors and your own particular interests.

- *Three Core Skill Units* – these help you to develop skills that are vital for anybody wishing to work in Health and Social Care or go on to study the subject at a higher level. You will be assessed in *communication, application of number* and *information technology*.

Don't worry if you discover that you are studying more than 15 units on your GNVQ. This is likely to be because your school or college is giving you the chance to develop a broader range of skills or study certain subjects in even greater depth, by offering you *additional units*. Additional units may be necessary for studying certain courses in higher education, at degree or HND level.

Having a number of different units that go to make up the GNVQ award allows greater flexibility in studying. Although most people studying for an Advanced GNVQ will be on a full-time course of study at school or college, some students will want to study on a part-time basis, passing one unit at a time. The way GNVQs are designed allows students to build up credit for individual units over an extended period of time.

What does a unit consist of?

At the beginning of this section, we talked about the need to meet the required **standard** in order to be successful in your GNVQ. The standards for the Advanced GNVQ in Health and Social Care have been developed by specialists in education and in professional practice as a way of defining what has to be done by students to achieve the award. The standards are set out as **units**; for Advanced GNVQs there are the eight mandatory, four optional and three core skill units we mentioned above. Figure A gives a breakdown of a unit (sometimes called a **unit specification**), showing the different parts of a unit and how they link together.

Elements

Each unit in the Advanced GNVQ in Health and Social Care is broken down into a number of different **Elements**, depending on the depth of material included in the unit. In order to be successful in your Advanced GNVQ in Health and Social Care, you will need to produce evidence to show that you have covered *all* the elements in all the units you are studying.

Performance criteria

Each GNVQ element has a number of **performance criteria** related to it. The number will vary between different Elements. The performance criteria help to explain what that particular element is all about, by telling you what areas you need to cover to be able to pass it. In carrying out the different types of assessment for a unit, you can think of the performance criteria as a 'checklist' of evidence that you will need to collect and include in your **portfolio** to demonstrate that you have successfully met the requirements of the element.

In the course of your assessments, you must show that you

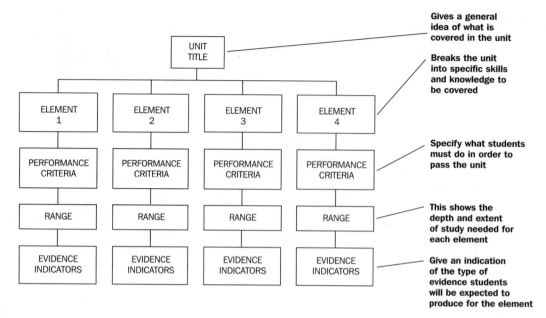

Figure A The component parts of a GNVQ unit

have met the requirements of *all* the performance criteria for each element of your GNVQ.

Range

You will see in Fig. A that, as well as having performance criteria related to it, each Element will identify a **range** associated with it. The range tries to indicate the *boundaries* that each student will need to work within on a particular Element.

To be successful in an element, the evidence that you collect must show that you have covered *all* the range points included in the unit specification.

Evidence indicators

The **evidence indicators** included in the unit specifications give a general idea as to the *sort of evidence* that would be considered suitable for successful completion of the element.

Types of assessment

The **assessment** in your GNVQ concentrates on two main areas:

- External tests
- Continuous assessment

The way in which the two main types of assessment link together is shown in Figure B.

Both types of assessment will produce evidence that can be filed in your **portfolio of evidence** and which will be used when deciding the overall grade that you are given for your GNVQ.

External tests

You will need to sit and pass **external tests**, set by the awarding bodies, before you can be awarded the Advanced GNVQ in Health and Social Care. Seven out of the eight *mandatory units* have external tests; Unit 2 'Interpersonal Interaction' does not have an external test, since it was thought it would be

difficult to ask factual questions on that subject area. You will therefore sit external tests in the following units:

Unit 1: Access, Equal Opportunities and Client Rights
Unit 3: Physical Aspects of Health
Unit 4: Psychological and Social Aspects of Health and Social Health
Unit 5: Health Promotions
Unit 6: Sturcture and Practices in Health and Social Care
Unit 7: Care Plans
Unit 8: Research in Health and Social Care

You will be told the exact dates and times of the tests by your teacher or tutor and will be given the chance to re-sit any tests that you do not pass at the first attempt. Remember, it is essential that you pass all seven external tests in the mandatory units before you can be awarded the Advanced GNVQ.

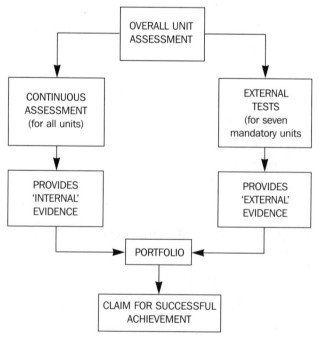

Figure C Unit assessment in the advanced GNVQ in Health and Social Care

Because it is important that you have a good grasp of the basic knowledge and understanding in each unit, the pass mark is set deliberately high at 70%. All the awarding bodies are planning to mark the tests and get the results back to you in the shortest time possible, so as to provide you with early feedback on your performance.

At present, there are no external tests for the optional or additional units, but, as with any new qualification, changes are being made all the time to GNVQs in response to feedback from students and tutors. To be absolutely sure, you should check with your teacher or tutor what the exact position is regarding tests for your particular course.

Although the seven units listed above are the only units with external tests at the moment, you may find that your particular school or college sets their own tests in some units. This is quite acceptable and will provide you with more evidence to include in your portfolio.

Sitting an external test is a way of showing that you have grasped the essential knowledge and understanding for a particular unit. Some people consider that having tests that are externally set and the same right across the country gives GNVQs more credibility than a qualification based entirely on continuous assessment in school or college. Passing a test will show that you understand the basic principles of a particular unit, thus providing a good grounding for working in aspects of Health and Social Care or going on to study the subject at a higher level.

What are the external tests like?

The questions set are *multiple-choice* in character, though of different types. At the end of each mandatory unit in this book for which external tests are set, you can find examples of all the types of question you will face on that unit.

- Each test will have between 30 and 40 questions.
- Each test lasts one hour.
- You will be asked to fill in your answers on a separate answer sheet, not on the test papers themselves. Don't worry if the answer sheet has more spaces than the number of questions on your test; this is because the number of questions varies between 30 and 40 on different test papers.
- You will not be asked to answer the questions by writing sentences, but will select an answer by writing A, B, C or D on the separate answer sheet. Your answers should be written in soft (HB) pencil only, as the answer sheets are marked by machine.
- You will be allowed to use a calculator in the test, but the memory must be wiped clean before you go into the room where the tests are being taken.
- The questions or the test papers are grouped into 'focus areas' (see below).
- The tests use different types of multiple choice questions.
- Tests are taken under secure conditions, on a specified day and at a specified time.

Preparing for the external tests

You will normally take the unit test towards the end of a period of study of one particular unit. This will make sure that the continuous assessment tasks that you have been set will help to provide information and knowledge needed to be able to answer the test questions. You will, however, need to spend some time revising specifically for the tests. Each unit of this book covers the main *content* you need to know when revis-

ing for the test. You may find it helpful to revise with another member of your group, bouncing ideas and questions off each other. Your teachers or tutors may organize revision classes or seminars, which some students find particularly useful. Use the sample tests provided at the end of the mandatory units in this book to practise your test technique, timing yourself to make sure that you are working at the right pace. You are likely to find that there is plenty of time in which to answer all the questions on a test, so rule number one is don't rush!

Once you know the dates of your tests, it is a good idea to draw up a timetable, showing when you will be revising for particular unit tests.

On the day of the test itself, try not to get too worried so that you are able to perform to the best of your ability. Make sure you read each question very carefully before you attempt to answer it and check all answers at the end of the test. If you intend to take a calculator in with you, make sure the batteries will last. Have a spare pencil and rubber with you as well. You shouldn't think of the test as a major hurdle that you have to clear; tests are just one part of the whole assessment process for your GNVQ. Good luck!

Continuous Assessment: The Portfolio

A separate chapter at the end of this book deals with the skills and evidence you need to present for 'the portfolio', with practical examples of students' work and examiner comments.

The bulk of the assessments that you carry out on your GNVQ will fall into the category of *continuous assessment*. It can take many forms, including written assignments, projects, demonstrations, presentations and case studies. You will be given a mixture of assessments that will cover all of the elements of the GNVQ units you are studying. This is important, because you must show that you have met the required standard in *every* unit you are taking before you can be awarded the GNVQ.

An important feature of GNVQ courses is that you will be expected to take responsibility for your own learning and your own assessment. This doesn't mean that you will be setting and marking your own assignments! What it does mean is that your tutors will expect you to come up with good ideas and ways of tackling tasks. They will encourage you to look for information from many different sources, helping you to develop the vital skills that you will need in later life. You probably won't be sitting in classrooms for much of the time that you are studying for your GNVQ. You will often be 'learning by doing' with your tutors providing information, support and advice when needed.

The stages in continuous assessment

Although the exact nature of a piece of assessed work will vary between one school or college and another, there are a number of clearly defined stages that you will go through when carrying out continuous assessment, namely:

Stage 1: Receiving written and/or verbal instructions from your tutor about an assessment that will provide evidence to meet the requirements of a particular element or group of elements.

Stage 2: Discussing the practicalities of carrying out the work with your teacher or tutor and perhaps with other members of your group.

Stage 3: Devising an 'action plan' for the assessment, indicating time deadlines, tasks and sources of information.

Stage 4: Discussing the action plan with your teacher or tutor, who may suggest alterations or improvements to make your task easier.

Stage 5: Carrying out the assessment in line with your action plan.

Stage 6: Having your written and/or oral work checked by your tutor, who will either confirm that it is of the required standard or that more needs to be done to reach the standard.

Stage 7: When completed, claiming credit from your teacher or tutor for the particular element or elements covered, and filing your evidence in your portfolio.

We look at these stages in the 'Portfolio' chapter of the book.

What counts as 'evidence'?

You will quickly learn that collecting and presenting evidence is a crucial part of your GNVQ course; in fact, if you are studying for your GNVQ on a full-time course, by the end of the two years you will have heard the term 'evidence' enough times to last you a lifetime! Most of the evidence that you collect will revolve around the assignments that your tutors give you from time to time, for the different units and elements of the GNVQ; e.g. reports, letters, projects and case studies. Evidence can come from a number of different sources, however, and can be concerned with many different activities, including:

- Questionnaire surveys
- Reports of observations
- Photographs, audio and videotapes
- Computer-generated material
- Role playing
- Organizing an event or service
- Demonstrations and discussions
- Presentations and displays
- Tests set by your tutors
- Notes from lectures or classes
- Activities carried out on work experience
- Records of visits to Health and Social Care organizations
- References and certificates from previous work or study
- Log books and records of achievement

Whatever type of evidence you choose to put forward to claim credit for an element or a unit, you will need to remember a number of important points:

(1) That the evidence is **valid**, ie fit for its purpose. In other words, does the evidence you are submitting *really* satisfy the performance criteria laid down in the element? If not, you will need to change some of the evidence or add to it and re-submit it for assessment. Use the performance criteria as a checklist against which you compile your evidence

(2) That the evidence is **authentic**. Your tutors will check to see that the evidence you submit is genuine and that it is all your own work. This will be especially important when it comes to group work. Working as part of a team is an essential skill that you will need to develop, but you must be able to provide evidence to show that you have played a full part in the working of the group.

(3) That there is **sufficient** evidence to be able to claim full credit for the element or unit. Your tutor will give you guidance on whether or not you have collected enough evidence to satisfy the requirements.

(4) That you have got **permission** to use evidence from other people. There shouldn't be a problem recording and using information that is collected in your school or college, but when you are using data and information from outside sources, you must make sure that you have permission before the evidence is used.

Again, the final chapter of this book will help you develop many of the skills required for the portfolio, giving examples of actual student work with examiner comments.

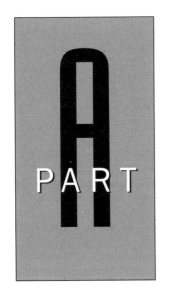

PART A

The Mandatory Units

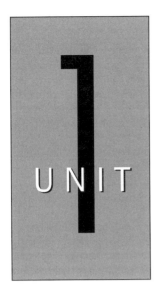

1 UNIT

Access, equal opportunities and client rights

Getting Started

In this unit we will be looking at socialisation, discrimination and equal opportunities.

This unit consists of three Elements:

Element 1 Attitudes and other social influences on behaviour
Element 2 Discrimination and its effects on individuals
Element 3 Equal opportunities

Element 1 explores how attitudes are formed and their influence on social behaviour.

Element 2 investigates discrimination and how it can be reinforced through language, and the effects of discrimination on people.

Element 3 looks at the legislation that exists to maintain equal opportunities and how people can seek redress if they are discriminated against.

Cross references:
Unit 1 Element 1
Unit 2 Element 3
Unit 4 Element 1

Affective Involving emotions or feelings.

Cognitive Involving intellectual thought.

Covert Behaviour which cannot be directly observed.

Discrimination Actions to the disadvantage of others; often based on prejudice against an individual or group.

Extended family Broader kinship group than the nuclear family. Often three or more generations of relations share a house or live near each other.

Gender Male/Female distinction; often refers to the differences in social expectations as to the role of males/females.

Hidden curriculum Informal socialisation which occurs in educational institutions, e.g. via attitudes and ideas, way in which school/college is organised, etc.

Norms Standards of behaviour expected of people within a group.

Nuclear family Parents and children living together

Overt Behaviour which can be observed directly.

Peer group A group consisting of others of a similar age, or who have other characteristics in common.

Primary Socialisation Socialisation within the home and family.

Secondary Socialisation Socialisation outside the home and family; e.g. in schools, workplace, etc.

Social groups Collections of individuals who are involved in some form of patterned interaction with one another.

Socialisation The process which starts at birth and continues throughout life by which an individual learns the values and accepted patterns of behaviour of his/her society.

Stereotyping Assuming that all people who belong to a particular group have the same characteristics.

Essential Principles

1.1   Attitudes and other social influences on behaviour

The socialisation process

Socialisation is explained in relation to the family, culture, group membership and peer group membership.

Socialisation can be viewed simply as the social learning process which teaches an individual the values and accepted patterns of behaviour of their society. It starts at birth and continues throughout life. There are two forms.

- **Primary socialisation**, which is the most important and takes place within the family.
- **Secondary socialisation**, which takes place *outside the home*, in places such as schools, church, the workplace, and via the mass media.

Family

The **family** generally refers to a group of people living together who are related by blood or marriage ties, and who support each other emotionally and economically.

The **nuclear family** is sometimes referred to as a 'conjugal unit'. It is a social unit, typically of two generations, consisting of parents and children living together.

The **extended family** is a broader kinship group to which the nuclear family can belong. It often consists of three or more generations of various relatives, often sharing a household or living near each other.

The following extract looks at how family patterns have been changing in Britain:

The family pattern has been changing in Great Britain

Everyone has an extended family, but they may not keep in touch with the members of it, or may only meet some of its members occasionally. However, the extended family is still an important feature of life in many long-established communities, particularly in the North of England and among ethnic groups that have settled in Britain recently, especially Indian and Pakistani families. There is a growing tendency, however, for the more usual family type to consist of just a husband, wife and their own children living together with no relations near by. This family is called a nuclear family.

Gerard O'Donnell, *Sociology Today*, CUP 1993

There are many different family forms, with the extended family and the nuclear family predominant. The family's role changes as the individual moves through the *life cycle* of the family; e.g., children are born, brought up by their parents, grow up, start their own family and in turn become grandparents themselves.

In most societies the family provides the location in which children are born and reared. Any alternative to the family would have to deal with this task.

It is likely that for most people the family is the first, and the most important, source of *socialisation*. Gender roles, language and morality are 'learned' by the individual within the family unit and are therefore significant results of family socialisation. Children also learn the culture of their society in the family. Their parents act as *role models*. Children are often encouraged to behave appropriately by parental reward and punishment. (see Unit 4, Elements 1 and 2). For example a parent talking to a child might say 'If you tidy your room you can watch television'. In all these ways the child learns within the family those types of behaviour regarded as acceptable by society as a whole.

Families also provide the basis for rules controlling *sexual behaviour*. These may vary between societies and change over time. In most families during the 1950s young people were not expected to sleep together. In the 1990s parents who may not condone this behaviour may accept that it occurs and be involved in giving advice on contraception and the avoidance of AIDS. Many of these rules are often supported by religious beliefs, through celebration and festivals: marriage, christening, etc. We expect married couples to have a sexual relationship and we have rules against incest which prohibit sexual relationships between close family members. Sexual relationships outside of marriage may be disapproved of by certain 'groups', e.g., grandparents, parents, church groups, etc.

The family is an important source of *economic*, as well as *emotional* support for the individual member. In pre-industrial society and in the early days of the industrial revolution men, women and children all worked together in the home. Although rarely the case today, parents still receive Child Benefit and other financial support (e.g. higher education grants) for their children. Equally children often depend on the family for help in times of financial need.

Another view of the family as an *economic unit* is indicated in the box below. Certainly marketing strategists are paying careful attention to the influence of children on the *purchasing habits* of families.

A report reveals that parents are increasingly nagged by their children about what the family should buy.

More parents are also listening to their children, respecting their ideas, trying new products that the children suggest, and increasingly treating them as equals.

The report says that, in all social classes, children have the greatest effect on their parents' shopping from the age of five until about eleven or twelve. 'At this stage children are old enough to be aware of products and of the power they can exert in determining which ones are bought ...'

Adapted from an article in *The Independent*, 1991

A family can offer emotional support to a family member at all stages of that person's life. Such support is especially important in childhood, when it can help the child to develop a stable and confident personality. In later life an individual may turn to his or her family for support when faced by stressful experiences such as illness or bereavement. If this kind of support is lacking, he or she may find it harder to cope and the role of health and social care professionals who may be in contact with the individual becomes especially important.

To sum up it can be said that the main functions of the family involve:

- Socialisation
- Regulating sexual behaviour
- Reproduction
- Economic support
- Emotional support

Culture

Most human behaviour is *learned*; it is not genetically programmed. It is *cultural* rather than biological. Even basic biological behaviours such as eating, sleeping, sexuality and reproduction are influenced by cultural expectations.

Culture involves a way of life, including customs, values, and beliefs and it affects family and other social arrangements. Culture can refer to a way of life of an *entire society* or to a *group* within a society; e.g. a particular ethnic group within a multi-cultural society.

Although we have to eat to live, there are *social rules* concerning what we eat. Muslims and Jewish people do not eat pork for religious reasons; the English try to avoid eating horse meat for sentimental reasons and Russians will make enormous financial sacrifices to eat caviar because of symbolic and traditional associations with the eating of caviar. Other rules of eating influence the timing of meals and perhaps the need for accompanying prayer or ritual.

Culture also influences what kind of sexual behaviour is permissible, with whom and under what circumstances. Homosexuality is a form of behaviour which has long existed in societies. The criminalisation of homosexual activity varies from country to country and at different points in time within a country. Homosexual acts between consenting adults were only made legal in the UK relatively recently.

Biologically there are lower and upper age limits for human reproduction. These do not, however, always coincide with *cultural expectations*. Women in Britain tend to avoid conception for much of their potentially child bearing life. Unmarried women in many societies are not expected to have children; whereas married women are expected to have them (eventually). The age for first time motherhood has actually risen, although biologically girls appear capable of child birth at a younger age than previously.

Culture can be summarised as a *system* of ideas, values and beliefs, knowledge and customs, which is transmitted from generation to generation within a particular group, or broader society. Having knowledge of the appropriate culture enables members to function within that group, and of course is an important part of understanding for carers dealing with 'clients' from that culture.

The power of culture in influencing the expectations and behaviour of girls in a particular close-knit group is illustrated by the following extract.

Sue Sharpe's study of a group of working class girls in London, "Just Like a Girl: How Girls Learn to be Women" (1976), showed that, for many girls, how they looked, dressed and related to boyfriends were more important to them than how they got on at school. They looked forward to leaving school and getting a job to earn money.

The education and class system acted against these particular girls because they were both female and working class. These girls had taken on a self-image that had very little to do with success in school. They had grown up with the view that love, marriage and having children were more important.

Figure 1.1 shows how culture can express itself in certain attitudes, opinions and values, all of which form part of the socialisation process.

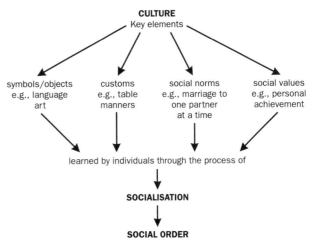

Figure 1.1   Aspects of culture

Institutions can also develop their own culture. Hospitals, for example, are sometimes criticised for creating a culture of dependence, in which patients are encouraged to place all responsibility for their welfare in the hands of professional carers. The nature of the carer/client relationship becomes firmly established and new staff and patients alike soon recognise the kind of behaviour that is expected of them. In recent years, however, there has been a greater emphasis in care settings of giving clients as much independence and freedom of choice as possible (see Unit 2, Element 3).

Group membership

Social groups are aggregates of individuals who are involved in some form of patterned interaction with one another.

Social groups should display three characteristics:

1   The individuals should be involved in regular and patterned (structured) interaction with one another.
2   Each individual should be conscious of being a group member and should be able to identify other people as being either members or non-members of their group.
3   Group members should share similar values.

Groups can be broken into *primary* and *secondary* groups.

- **Primary groups** – are characterised by close face-to-face interaction, such as family groups and school peer groups. The feeling of 'we' arising in primary groups is strong.

- **Secondary groups** – are more formal; here the interaction between the members is less personal, such as a business association. The feeling of 'we' around secondary group members is not as strong.

People's values, beliefs and norms affect the membership of groups; these are briefly reviewed here.

- **Values.** Those aspects of life which an individual considers to be important. A person may, for example, value friendship, honesty and compassion.

- **Beliefs.** These are a special class of attitude which are based more on the ideas held by a person than on a proven fact.

- **Norms.** Groups of people who interact over a period of time are likely to evolve common patterns of behaviour. A norm is an ideal standard of behaviour to which people within the group conform to a greater or lesser extent. Norms can be observed when two or more people interact within the group.

Groups can also take various forms:

- **Religious institutions.** Here religious beliefs, norms and values dominate socialisation; e.g. in religious schools and places of worship.

- **Educational institutions.** Schools and colleges are important institutions for socialisation. Teachers, lecturers and other pupils all play a role in this process, shaping your understanding of the types of behaviour the institution regards as acceptable.

Much of the socialisation within institutions many be *informal* (i.e. not consciously planned) rather than *formal*. Some aspects of *informal socialisation* in educational institutions are outlined below; this informal socialisation is sometimes called the 'hidden curriculum'.

The hidden curriculum includes:

- *Attitudes and ideas* which are taught informally or found in the way text books are written.

- *Organisation of the school or college.* This may itself be a source of learning for pupils. Most organisations are based on a hierarchy, where people at the top exercise authority over those below.

- *Rules.* Teachers are seen to control both time and space. Pupils may not be allowed to pass time unless it is on an approved activity. Teachers may refer to classrooms as "my room" and many spaces are denied to pupils altogether. Toilets are often seen by pupils as a refuge from teacher authority but even this space is open to teacher inspection. There may also be rules about students' appearance and conduct out of school as well as in school.

- *The relationships between teachers and pupils*, and between pupils themselves. As described above, these may reinforce attitudes on gender and race.

- *Competition.* In both academic and sports activities, competition may be seen as part of a hidden curriculum. Of course in some cases competition may be discussed openly and become part of the official curriculum.

- **Mass media.** The newspaper a person reads may help to 'group' people into different categories, and they tend to 'feel' part of that group; e.g. the Sun reader/ the Guardian reader. People tend to buy newspapers that in general reflect their own thinking. However the ideas and values transmitted by the mass media, especially television, exert influence over watchers, listeners and readers. It is a two-way process.

Table 1.1 shows a few of the many ways in which people might be grouped and examples of the membership of each group.

Group	Membership
By region	Liverpudlians, East Enders
Age	Under 5s, over 65s, teenagers
Type of school	Pupils of grammar/comprehensive/public schools
Patient types	Maternity, Geriatrics
Sport	Athletes, footballers, cricketers
Hospital staff	Nurses, Doctors, Consultants

Table 1.1 Examples of groups and group membership

Peer group membership

The word **peer** means equal; in practice the terms refers to a group consisting of members of a similar age, or who have other social characteristics in common. **Peer groups** play an important part in the socialisation process. Peer groups have characteristics typical of other small groups, such as a system of norms maintained by sanctions against a deviant member. The young quickly learn how to interact with youngsters of a similar age who are not family members. A youngster's peers include the other children of similar age at school or college, or in a neighbourhood grouping (e.g. gang).

Role of attitudes and attitude formation

Here we look at the role of attitudes and attitude formation in influencing behaviour

An **attitude** is a disposition towards a person, idea or object. An attitude can be *positive* or *negative*; a *neutral* attitude is in fact the same as having no attitude to the situation. Attitudes are influenced by the whole process of socialisation we have already outlined.

Attitudes, beliefs, values and behaviour overlap. Attitudes are internal states that influence external factors such as our choices and actions.

In Figure 1.2 we can see that two important components of attitudes are:

- cognitive, i.e., thinking, often based on our beliefs
- affective, i.e., feelings and emotions, often based on our values

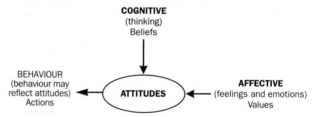

Figure 1.2 Development of attitudes

Let us look at these components in a little more detail.

Cognitive component
This refers to intellectual thought. A person's *beliefs* suggest that what s/he thinks is true. Beliefs involve making assumptions that things exist; e.g. that a person can catch a sexually transmitted disease (STD) by engaging in a sex act. In this case the belief can be reinforced by medical knowledge and tests. Such a belief may then affect the attitude of the person to casual or unprotected sex, for example.

Affective component
This involves emotions or feelings, like anger, fear or love. If someone smokes in your home, and you have strong feelings regarding smoking, this may cause you to have a negative attitude towards the person smoking.

- **Behaviour.** This is often an *outcome* of our attitudes and can result in action being taken. If your beliefs and emotions are negative towards cigarette smoking and smokers, this may result in your not buying shares in companies linked to the smoking industry. Of course behaviour may not always reflect one's attitude: a person may be anti-pollution but may still use leaded petrol.

Attitude formation

This may be the result of the following **interactions**:

- *Child rearing* – Parents are very influential in the formation of their children's attitudes. Children often adopt similar attitudes to those of their parents. This may range from political attitudes, to family attitudes influencing how they bring up their own children.

- *Interaction with others/group members.* If we hold people in high regard then they can become a potentially strong influence on our attitude development; e.g. we can form a negative attitude towards another person simply based on the gossip of our peer group.

- *Chance conditioning/Direct contact* – we can develop attitudes towards a group, e.g. an ethnic group, doctors, dentists, etc. on the basis of one or two good or bad experiences.

- *Mass media* – This can shape a person's attitude. People who have never been in a hospital may obtain all their information about hospitals from hospital serial programmes on television.

Function of attitude

Attitudes can fulfil a number of different *functions*.

- **Instructional function** – linked to social learning theory. The suggestion here is that attitudes play a part in obtaining rewards and avoiding punishment. In a work situation a person who adopts appropriate attitudes and is liked by his colleagues is more likely to be accepted as part of the group and receive promotion in due course.

- **Value expressive function** – an individual receives satisfaction from expressing attitudes appropriate to his or her personal values. An example would be a nurse expressing openly a humane attitude towards terminally ill patients.

- **Knowledge function** – people need to make sense of the universe, and therefore need adequate theoretical structures which will provide them with the basis for interpreting what is observed. We learn many things in theory and may go on to develop attitudes based on that theory which can be positive or negative. These attitudes can, of course, change once the theory is put into practice. Like a doctor learning a particular procedure and being favourably disposed to that procedure until it comes to the point of putting the theory into practice!

- **Ego – defensive function** – attitudes may help to defend one's self image, as when medical staff adopt particular clinical attitudes as defensive techniques to distance themselves from their patients in order to protect themselves from the pain of suffering.

Influence of social context

The part played by **social context** in influencing behaviour is described in relation to the following three settings:

- public setting
- private setting
- care setting

Within public, private and care settings, people have certain **roles**. All individuals hold various positions in the group of which they are members. These positions are *ascribed* (given) or *achieved*, or may be a combination of both.

A role is the *pattern of behaviour* associated with a position. Such a role is common to all who fill similar positions and is not unique to particular individuals. Nevertheless a role is not absolute or rigid, there is always some room for interpretation. Here are some useful terms and definitions involving the idea of 'role'.

> **Role expectations** – expected or desirable behaviour linked to a position, not actual behaviour.
>
> **Role play** – when in a role, people 'act out' that role; like actors taking a specific part in a play.
>
> **Role set** – involves all those (including the individual) who hold common expectations of a person in a given position.
>
> **Role strain** – occurs when there is a difficulty in fulfilling expectations associated with a particular position.
>
> **Role conflict** – occurs when a person is faced with mutually contradictory and competing role expectations, often resulting from membership of different groups. Conflict arises as the different expected behaviour styles inevitably clash.

The relationship between the roles we play and who we really are is a complicated one. Roles can influence our nature through **self-fulfilling prophecy**, i.e. when a belief that something is going to happen causes it to happen. If people are given a role, they are likely to act up to it. Also, once people accept a definition of themselves, this influences how they think about themselves and consequently influences their behaviour. Through socialisation we learn such roles as conjugal roles (man – wife), gender roles, parent/ child roles, work roles, teacher/pupil roles, etc.

Public setting

All types of employment in a public setting have acceptable and unacceptable behaviour patterns. Certain formal public behaviour is associated with various professions, including in some cases the wearing of uniforms. Uniforms are used so that a stranger can quickly distinguish the role a person is seeking to fulfil.

Private settings

In private settings, such as at home, one can drop the public role. Many people immediately take off their uniform, even informal uniforms. Most people who wear suits to work change into casual wear as soon as they get home. In private settings other, less formal, roles are immediately entered into:

- father
- parent
- tired worker
- sports person
- gardener
- house worker

Care settings

The care setting has its own set of predetermined values, attitudes and behavioural patterns. For example, certain employees (such as doctors and nurses) will be expected to wear a uniform, while others (e.g. consultants) may not. Both uniformed and non-uniformed staff will be expected to conform to the norms of behaviour appropriate to the positions they hold. No one would be too surprised if a student nurse repeatedly sought guidance from more senior staff, but similar behaviour by a staff nurse would be less acceptable.

In the patient–doctor relationship, each has their own expectation of behaviour *before* the two meet. The nature of the interaction could be:

* agreeable
* confrontational
* one of negotiation
* one sided
* a service relationship (give advice/ receive advice)

Staff working in the caring professions must be aware of their own attitudes, both as individuals and as part of a particular group, such as midwives, casualty staff, and ward based staff. It is a good idea to discuss individual and group attitudes at all levels on a regular basis.

It is important to be aware of the different attitudes, such as cultural, social and sexual attitudes, held by specific groups. Inappropriate attitudes can affect the quality of health care. For example, some casualty staff may have a judgemental attitude towards patients who have tried to commit suicide, because of having to spend scarce available time and resources carrying out stomach pump procedures. These attitudes could make it more difficult for the nurse to assess that patient's needs and the underlying causes behind the attempted suicide, making it less likely that she will provide the most suitable immediate after-care provision. It is also important for medical staff to assess the attitudes of their clients and their families.

The key aim for staff is to develop an *attitude* which will help them to deliver the appropriate care. It will help if staff can also promote appropriate attitudes in patients and their families to help them maximise the benefits of any care provided.

An example of a role in the care setting is the nurse role in the nurse-patient relationship. The box outlines the six roles associated with the stages of the nurse-patient relationship.

> * **Stranger** – this is the first role. The patient and nurse meet as strangers. The nurse has to practise social skills and establish an atmosphere of acceptance.
>
> * **Resource** – the nurse offers information. S/he clarifies and encourages the patient's involvement in and under-standing of, the treatment offered.
>
> * **Teacher** – the nurse gives information, s/he answers queries and facilitates.
>
> * **Leader** – the nurse leads the process of identification and goal setting.
>
> * **Surrogate** – the nurse stands as representative of other people relevant to the patient to help the patient recall feelings and experiences.
>
> * **Counsellor** – the nurse can help the patient to reflect, recognise, accept and come to terms with the various aspects of experience and feeling commonly involved in a particular treatment.

Power and other social roles

Power does not exist in the context of an isolated individual. You cannot have 'power' unless it is in relation to another person or group. Power involves the ability to offer or withhold what someone else desires or needs. Power should be viewed in terms of *balances* (equal or unequal) which are constantly fluctuating or are relatively stable. A simple definition of power is being able to get one's own way, or being able to get someone else to do what you want.

Power within society can have a variety of sources. A few are listed below.

Political power – wielded by politicians, and those in a position to influence politicians (e.g. pressure groups, newspaper editors)

Economic power – based upon wealth or control/ownership of business

Social class – membership of the higher social classes may give an individual greater status, and as a result greater power and influence within society

Within smaller social groups, other sources of power exist. Within a family, for example, grandparents may be shown special respect and consideration because of their age. In a care context, it is important for the health and social care professional to be aware of the power he or she exercises over clients. In extreme cases this can include legal powers of detention (as when a person is detained under the Mental Health Acts). More commonly, the power is less absolute but is nevertheless real, and exists because the client is vulnerable and in need of help. A care worker should never exploit this vulnerability by adopting an authoritarian or dictatorial approach. Rather the carer should seek to **empower** the client. This means giving clients power by involving them as much as possible in all aspects of the care they are receiving.

It has been said that 'knowledge is power' and sharing **knowledge** with clients is one way of increasing their control over their lives. They need to be given information and encouraged to participate in the making of decisions about their own care. (For more on this aspect of care work see Unit 2, Element 3).

Authority is *legitimate* power. Authority is a type of power when people give their *consent* to the person who orders them to do something. They give their consent because they see the power of their leader, boss, teacher, father, etc. as *legitimate* (or justified).

There are different reasons why people see power as legitimate. In a public setting power/authority can be viewed as:

* *Traditional* – based on habit and an acceptance of the informal social order.

* *Rational* – based on a formal set of rules establishing a particular 'office' or position. Such a set of rules is regarded as 'making sense' to members of the group or organisation.

* *Charismatic* – based on a devotion to the leader and the personal qualities the leader displays.

Status is based on honour, prestige, occupation and/or birth. Status groups share the same lifestyles, schooling, education, etc. and often consume similar items.

The **management role** involves some, or all, of the following aspects:

* wearing a suit
* getting to work on time
* being the team leader
* delegating to staff
* reporting to senior management on progress of work
* liaison with fellow managers/staff nurses etc.
* being proactive (i.e. initiating change)
* forecasting for the future
* knowledge of the present situation

Self Check ✓   Element 1

1. What is the difference between primary and secondary socialisation?

2. What is the difference between values, beliefs and norms?

3. Extend the list in Table 1.1 with an additional three types of groups, with examples of the membership of each new group.

4. Give examples of professions that have uniforms. Extend the list with less orthodox workers who have a uniform.

5. What 'uniform' do social workers have and why?

6. What roles do you play in your private setting? Is there conflict with your public role(s)?

7. Can you think of examples where money relates to status?

8. Is a doctor or consultant viewed in society as having a 'higher' status than a student nurse? Why? What about a low-paid priest and a high-paid prostitute?

9. Can you think of roles that a good manager needs to play? (include roles not included in the list on p 6)

10. What are the main advantages/disadvantages of 'keeping' knowledge from colleagues?

11. What is meant by a culture of dependence?

12. Name 3 sources of power within a society.

1.2 Discrimination and its effects on individuals

Discrimination is when we act on the basis of a *prejudice*, to the advantage of some individuals or groups and to the disadvantage of others. Prejudice is very likely to lead to discrimination. **Prejudice** is a particular form of attitude involving a relatively permanent disposition towards something which does not take any evidence into account, that is, you have decided in advance what you are going to think of someone or something.

Types of discrimination
Discrimination may involve *overt* or *covert* behaviour towards an individual or group.

*   **overt** – behaviour which is observable
*   **covert** – behaviour which cannot be directly observed

As we have seen, discrimination may be based on prejudice.

Prejudice is an attitude, which is usually hostile, towards a group of people. It exists in people's minds and therefore cannot be *directly observed*. Prejudice may or may not lead to discrimination. An example of **racial prejudice** is thinking that people are inferior in ability or morality because of their race. **Racial discrimination** takes that negative attitude one stage further, into action itself. It is the treatment of an individual or a group on less favourable grounds than another because of 'racial' differences, such as skin colour. For example, denying people from certain ethnic groups equal opportunities to get a job. There is, however, the possibility of *positive* discrimination by trying to help people from disadvantaged groups have a better chance than those from advantaged groups.

Stereotyping – involves the act of assuming that all people who belong to a particular group have the same characteristics.

The extract below looks at a common stereotype of teenage mothers as producing delinquent children and wanting babies to gain access to welfare benefits. Often the facts *do not* support such stereotypes.

Ann Phoenix, with a team from the Thomas Coram Research Institute, has made a detailed longitudinal study of 79 young women who gave birth while still in their teens. The sample included young women who were married, cohabiting and single.

The two most common stereotypes of teenage mothers are: firstly, that they are likely to produce delinquent children and secondly, that they have babies because they want council housing and welfare benefits. Phoenix found no evidence of these two stereotypes in her study. Even among those who had planned their pregnancies, no-one reported that she wished to get pregnant in order to receive housing or benefits. There was no evidence that children born to teenage mothers (married or not) developed less well than those born to older women. Nor was there any evidence that early motherhood caused poverty. If anything, motherhood acted as a spur to seek education and training, so that they could earn a living in the future. However, almost all women had low expectations of paid employment. They felt, as a result, that motherhood would be the most significant and fulfilling development in their lives.

Source: A. Coote's review of A. Phoenix's study 'Young Mothers?' in *New Society* 11 December 1990

Stereotyping is often undertaken by one ethnic group against another, usually by a majority group against minorities in a society. However stereotyping can work in both directions.

Western ways are bad

The following extract shows that it is not only the lives of minorities which are subject to stereotypes:

... South Asians perceived English family life as cold and insecure, lacking in affection and in respect for the older generation. Families were small, young adults left home to make their own way, old people lived alone or were put into homes without good reason; marital breakdowns and sexual licence were rife. By Asian standards it all seemed outrageously immoral and inhumane.

J. E. Goldthorpe, *Family life in Western Societies* (CUP 1987)

Bases of discrimination

Different bases for discrimination include:

*   race
*   gender
*   age
*   physical ability
*   cognitive ability

Each are discussed in turn.

Race
There is no universally accepted meaning of the word race. Attempts have been made to identify distinct groups on the basis of biological and physiological characteristics which are then often related to skin colour; white, brown, black, yellow – skinned people. It was once widely believed, mainly by whites, that there were important mental, physical, moral

and intellectual differences between different skin – colour groups. Modern genetics has destroyed such a simplistic view.

Race discrimination is where someone acts differently towards an individual on grounds of race. *Racism* is prejudice or discrimination which is determined by the belief that one race is superior to other races. Racial discrimination occurs when a *racist idea* becomes a *racist action*.

Many statistics have been used to illustrate (alleged) racial discrimination in the labour market. In Fig 1.3 we can see that the rate of unemployment in specific ethnic minority groups was higher than in the *total* population in the UK in the early 1990s.

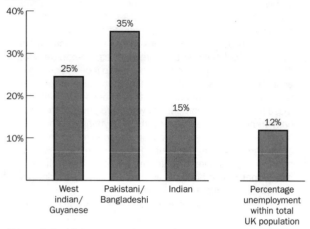

Figure 1.3 Higher unemployment for ethnic minorities

Expressions of racism, until 1994, have even been observed in the sign language used by the deaf. New, less offensive, signs have been designed which will now be taught to the 500,000 deaf people in Britain.

Racist examples involving sign language (replaced in 1994)

• Chinese people – slanting of the eyes; now replaced by drawing a hand across the chest.

• Black people – flattening of the nose; now replaced by a stroke of the cheek suggesting colour.

• Jewish people – make a large nose from the fist; now replaced by a sign of an imaginary beard.

Did You Know ?

Direct discrimination occurs where a person is treated less favourably for training, promotion, transfer or other benefit than another person on the grounds of race. *Indirect discrimination* arises as a result of applying a condition or requirement to all employees but which has the effect of preventing the majority of one racial group being able to comply. Thus a requirement for a 'good command of English' may be indirect discrimination if this is not essential to carrying out the job properly.

Gender

The term **sex** refers to the *biological differences* between males and females. The term **gender** refers to the differences in *social expectations/roles* between males and females.

Discrimination occurs between males and females. Some people use traditional ideas of masculinity and femininity to pre-judge the abilities of women and thereby to argue that women should not be given equal opportunities with men.

The *traditional view* of the male/ female roles has meant that certain jobs have been seen as suitable exclusively for men. These jobs have included miners, firemen, doctors, chefs, MP's, policemen, businessmen, engineers. Even women themselves have often been socialised into accepting such views, as can be seen below.

A sample of men and women was asked whether they felt that particular types of job were more suitable for men or for women, or were equally suitable for both sexes. Table 1.2 on page 9 summarises their answers. Clearly men have a less favourable view than do women themselves, as to which jobs are 'equally suitable' to men or women

The traditionalist view also sets out various female only jobs. Remember all the Cs – Cooking, Cleaning, Caring, Clerical. In practice such jobs would include cooks (not chefs who are predominately male), part time workers, e.g. in cleaning and the clothing industry, education, health and welfare, clerical work, and home working.

Did You Know ?

Until the mid 1970s men could not become nurses in Australia (it was designated as women's work).

In a survey (New Earnings Survey) 70% of full time women workers were concentrated in only three types of work

1. Clerical (70% women)
2. Education, health and welfare (70% women)
3. Personal services (76% women)

Full time women earned, on average, only 64% of male hourly earnings in 1970; by 1993 this figure had risen only by 10% to 74% of male hourly earnings. Despite some improvements, there is clearly still considerable gender discrimination in the labour market.

Did You Know ?

The roots of labour market discrimination can begin early! "...teachers gave 65% of their attention to the boys and 35% to the girls. Moreover, when teachers attempted to redresss the balance, they only succeeded in giving the girls 40% of their attention and when this happened the boys complained".

Source: Economics and Business Education (1994)

Age

Discrimination by age is also common. It can occur at any part of the age spectrum. The following is a typical example in the area of appointments.

'Applications for the appointment of executive officer must be no older than 48 years.'

Advertisements of this type were held to discriminate against people on the grounds of age. This concept of 'older' employee has changed dramatically in recent years. In certain new fields such as the computer industry, 'old' can even be used of persons in their late 20s or early 30s.

At the other end of the scale some employers will not employ teenagers, because they do not have the experience to do the job.

	Men's answers			Women's answers		
	Suitable for men only	Suitable for women only	Equally suitable	Suitable for men only	Suitable for women only	Equally suitable
Type of job	%	%	%	%	%	%
Car mechanic	73	–	26	62	1	36
Bank manager	31	–	68	26	1	72
Secretary	1	59	39	1	50	49
Nurse	–	41	59	1	23	75
Member of Parliament	11	1	88	8	–	91
Computer programmer	5	3	91	3	1	95
Social worker	1	15	83	1	15	83

Source: Adapted from *British Social Attitudes Survey* Social and Community Planning Research

Table 1.2   Male and Female attitudes to types of job

Certainly the elderly are disproportionately represented in the lower income groups. Over 40% of households over 60 years of age have incomes *less than half* the UK average.

The situation of the old in simple, pre-industrial societies is often very different to that of the old in modern societies, such as Britain.

In simple, pre-industrial societies:

- The old have high status.
- They are the heads of family and kin groups.
- Their knowledge and skills do not become obsolete as technological change is slow.
- Knowledge comes from memory, tradition and wisdom.
- The old continue to contribute to valued activities.

In modern industrial societies, such as Britain:

- The old may have low status.
- The old tend not to head the family.
- Families are usually nuclear and kin live in separate households. The old frequently live alone, with their partners, with only one of their children or in institutions.
- The knowledge and skills of the old, and everyone else, becomes quickly outdated.
- Knowledge and skills come mainly from education and training rather than experience.
- There tends to be a formal, and often compulsory, retirement age which may force dependency onto the old. The Civil Service introduced compulsory retirement at 60 in 1959 because the workers' "bodily and mental vigour began to decline".

The UK is experiencing the growth of an ageing population which is a key factor in health care provision. Even here there are sometimes accusations of discrimination. For example, in April 1994 there were allegations that people above the age of 65 were being refused physiotherapy treatment by the National Health Service in certain regions.

Causes of an ageing population

An ageing population means that the average age of the population rises, so that the proportion of old people in the total population rises. By the year 2021, nearly one in five of the population will be over 65 – compared to only one in ten in 1951. The following factors have played a part in this trend.

1   *Lower birth rates*. Birth rates have generally fallen this century although there have been baby booms. This means a reduction in the number and proportion of young people.

2   *Longer life expectancy*. More people survive to old age than was previously the case and the old now tend to live longer. Even during this century, 25 years has been added to life expectancy because of improvements in living standards and to a lesser extent in health care.

3   *Immigration control*. Immigrants tend to be young and of child bearing age, and there is a tendency for some immigrants to have larger families in the first generation. However, compared to the 1950s and 1960s there is now virtually no immigration to the UK and this has taken away one of the factors producing a younger population. It is also the young who are most likely to emigrate.

Physical ability

Discrimination against people with a **physical disability** is very common. Larger organisations must employ a minimum percentage of registered disabled personnel (3%).

Discrimination on the basis of physical disability can take many forms:

- The "Does he take sugar" syndrome! This is an example of talking as if the person is not there or cannot hear, talking to the person who is *accompanying* a wheelchair bound person, rather than the disabled person him/herself.
- Physically talking across the person/ above their heads etc.
- Where institutions (e.g. offices/ shops) fail to provide access and other facilities for disabled people to give them the opportunity of involvement in an activity.

Cognitive (intellectual) ability

Discrimination against people who are intellectually impaired is common. This may involve retarded people with learning problems and those with other special needs.

Did You Know **?**

Other types of discrimination can occur, e.g. against ex-offenders. There is a right of the ex-offender not to disclose past convictions after a rehabilitation period if no further offences have been committed. *The rehabilitation period* – after which the conviction is said to be 'spent'– depends upon the severity of the offence and is calculated as follows:

Sentence	Rehabilitation period
Probation	1 year
Fine	5 years
Under 6 months' imprisonment	7 years
Under 18 months' imprisonment	10 years

For juvenile offenders these periods are halved. However, for some occupations the conviction is never 'spent' and there is a requirement to reveal details of any convictions. Workers coming into this category include doctors, policemen and teachers.

Reinforcement of discrimination

Discrimination can be **reinforced** by a variety of verbal and non-verbal signals and mechanisms. These are considered in detail in Unit 2, pages 19 – 23.

There is one more exception to the laws involving racial (or gender) discrimination at work. This exception applies to genuine occupational qualifications (GOQ) where certain types of person would genuinely be unable to perform the functions of that occupation, such as modelling, acting, dancing and singing. Racial or gender discrimination is also permitted in certain types of prisons (single sex establishments), and night work (single sex establishments).

The above are all examples where employees have the legal right to employ people of a particular racial or sexual group for particular purposes. However GOQ cannot be used in relation to married people.

Effects of Discrimination

Here we consider the potential effects of discrimination on the individual in different contexts.

Self esteem/self confidence

Self – esteem is the judgement or evaluation of one's own self-worth. This judgement may be in relation to an individual's perception of an 'ideal' self and/ or to the observed performance of others. If a person is discriminated against in anyway, it can affect their self esteem/ self confidence, undermining them and making them feel worthless or helpless. In order to protect themselves against further loss of self esteem they may then present an aggressive or very assertive front.

Access to services and opportunities

Discrimination can cause a reduction in the access of groups of people to the services they are entitled to. This could be overt or covert discrimination. A typical example of covert discrimination is by not informing people in a language that they can understand, for example using English for non-English speakers. Covert discrimination might also involve making the system so complicated for certain groups of people that they give up trying to obtain a service, thereby reducing opportunities for those groups.

For example: a single mother with three children who is asked to complete a five page form and then attend a surgery in order to receive certain benefits may be put off by such a bureaucratic system.

How services are marketed could also be discriminating. For example a new children's nursery being advertised in a newspaper read predominately by non-ethnic groups, could be viewed as unfair to the ethnic minorities.

Self Check ✓ **Element 2**

13. Define discrimination. How is prejudice related to discrimination?

14. Show how prejudice and discrimination might affect the life chances of ethnic minority groups.

15. Can you think of three bases for discrimination?

16. Distinguish between overt and covert discrimination.

17. Identify three causes of an ageing population

18. List some health care problems linked to an ageing population.

19. Provide some evidence for gender discrimination.

20. List some words/terms that traditionalists often apply to the expected characteristics and roles of a) males, b) females.

1.3 How equal opportunities are maintained

This element will look at the following four areas:

1. legislation to maintain equal opportunities
2. the purpose of legislation
3. sources of literature
4 systems of redress

Legislation to maintain equal opportunities

This section identifies legislation to maintain equal opportunities. We examine legislation involving race equality, gender equality and disability equality, and we consider the purposes of this legislation.

The last twenty years or more have seen many changes in legislation intended to provide a fairer and more equal treatment of people, whether they are members of an ethnic minority, male or female, able bodied or disabled.

Race equality

A major piece of legislation in this area is the *Race Relations Act of 1965*. This made it illegal to discriminate on the basis of race in the provision of goods or services to the public, or in the areas of employment and housing. It also became illegal to incite racial hatred. Further parts followed in 1968 and 1976. In practice employers must not discriminate in selection procedures, promotion, training or any other benefits. Likewise an employer may not dismiss, or impose any other penalty on racial grounds. The Acts are enforced by the **Commission of Racial Equality** (CRE) who can assist individuals in bringing an action against anyone thought to be violating the Acts. The CRE was established in the 1976 Act and had more power than the earlier Race Relations Board. The CRE can bring cases to court for indirect discrimination, e.g. only allowing certain types of headgear in a certain occupation which then discriminates indirectly against Sikhs who must wear turbans.

Racially offensive language (at work)
Under the above Acts the receiver of abusive language must be shown to have suffered a detriment before a claim for compensation can be made. In other words s/he must demonstrate some concrete disadvantage arising from the offensive language.

Public Order Act 1986
The Public Order Act of 1986 is also relevant to the promotion of race equality. It is an offence to incite racial hatred by threatening, abusive or insulting words or behaviour intended to stir up racial hatred. This includes broadcasting material, by word of mouth or in writing, by videos, cassette tapes, etc. It is an offence to possess any such material. The police have the power to search and seize such material.

Gender equality
The key pieces of legislation involving gender are *The Equal Pay Act, 1970*, *The Employment Protection Act 1975* and *The Sex Discrimination Acts 1975 and 1986*.

- **The Equal Pay Act 1970** – Men and women, both full-time and part-time, are entitled to equal treatment in their terms and conditions of employment where they do similar work or work of equal value.

- **The Employment Protection Act 1975** – This gave women the right to have paid maternity leave.

- **Sex Discrimination Acts 1975 and 1986** – These acts apply to both men and women. It is unlawful to discriminate on the grounds of sex, in the recruitment, training or promotion of both full-time and part-time staff. Both direct and indirect discrimination (as discussed earlier) are unlawful.

The following cases have established precedents which must be taken into account by UK courts.

1. To refuse a woman employment because of her family commitments is held to be discriminatory. (Thorndyke v. Bell 1979)
2. The assumption that the man is the breadwinner is held to be discriminatory. (Skyrail VS Coleman 1980)
3. Dismissal because of pregnancy is, in principle, discriminatory. (Hayes VS Malleble W.M.C. 1985)
4. Asking women to wear skirts and men trousers is NOT discriminatory as long as the request is 'reasonable' by the employer. (Schmidt V. Austick 1977)
5. Dirty jobs are not a male preserve. (Ministry of Defence V Jeremiah 1979)

Disability equality
The key pieces of legislation here are the *Disabled Persons (Employment) Acts 1944 and 1958*.

These Acts state that employers with more than 20 regular workers must employ a quota of registered disabled workers. This is approximately 3% at present. However it is very rare that prosecutions (in the form of fines) are applied.

The purposes of legislation
Legislation involves Acts of Parliament and an Act is a law passed by the House of Commons and the House of Lords and signed by the Queen. Definitive interpretations of the provisions of an Act can be given only by the *Courts of Law*, by any *Industrial Tribunals*, to which disputes arising under an Act involving individuals may be referred, and by the *Central Arbitration Committee*.

The purpose of these Acts is for Government to set out (for certain areas of activity) minimum acceptable standards of behaviour in society. Any failure to reach these minimum standards then gives an individual, an organisation or the state itself the right to penalise the offending parties. In relation to employers and employees, particular legislation is available covering various aspects such as redundancy, contracts of employment, unfair dismissal, health and safety, and discrimination.

European law
UK law is subject to European rules on equal pay and opportunities, as contained in article 119 of the treaty of Rome

Sources of literature
This section will identify the *sources* of information and literature on equal opportunities policies.

Codes of practice explain in detail how to avoid discrimination in employment. They are also available from the sources outlined below.

Employment
ACAS can provide information about the Sex Discrimination Acts and its application to employment (and health) issues. ACAS produces advisory booklets series, including no. 15 Health and Employment. 'This is ACAS' is also a useful booklet as are many leaflets and booklets on individual employment rights. The address below is the head office, but other offices are available across the UK.

ACAS – Advisory, Conciliation and Arbitration Service.
11/12 St. James Square
London
SW1Y 4LA
(071) 214 6000 (telephone)
Address mail to the director.

Health and Social Services
Advice on equal opportunities is widely available at the national level from:

- Department of Health
- Department of Social Services

or at the local level from:

- Unemployment benefit offices

- Social Services departments
- Citizens Advice Bureau
- Various rights groups
- HMSO – Her Majesty Stationery Office

Commission for Racial Equality (CRE)

For useful literature a full list is available from the CRE Publications Mail Order list. Case studies on alleged racial discrimination on a 'formal investigation report' basis are also available. Literature includes:

A guide to the Race Relations Act 1976
Racial Equality Councils
Your Guide to Equal Treatment under the Race Relations Act 1976

The Commission for Racial Equality (CRE) can be contacted as follows

Commission for Racial Equality
Ellist House
10/12 Allington Street
London
SW1E 5EH
(071) 828 7022 (telephone)

Equal Opportunities Commission

The Equal Opportunities Commission has its headquarters in Manchester, and has other offices in Wales (Cardiff) and Scotland (Glasgow). It is a public body and was set up under the Sex Discrimination Act. It has the following duties:

- to work towards the elimination of discrimination
- to promote equality of opportunity between men and women generally.
- to review the above act and related acts

The Equal Opportunities Commission can be contacted as follows:

Equal Opportunities Commission
Head Office
Overseas House
Quay Street
Manchester
M3 3HN
(061) 833 9244 (telephone)

Systems of redress

This section will identify *systems of redress* available to those discriminated against. We consider both internal policies and procedures and legal rights.

Going to law should only be the final resort if all else fails. This is so for a variety of reasons, including the facts that going to law can be

- expensive
- time consuming
- a process whereby individuals are not in control
- frustrating

All in all, going to law should only be used after all other more informal approaches have failed.

Internal policies and procedures

Various *procedures* may be followed in different situations to give the best chance of preventing the discrimination continuing or otherwise obtaining redress (e.g. compensation).

- keep a diary; record all the instances and situations when discrimination occurred
- include time, date, situation
- discuss the problem with other work colleagues
- go to the union for advice; if the company do not have a union then other routes need to be followed
- legal protection exists under the Employment Protection Act (1978) and the Sexual Discrimination Act (1975)

Legal Rights

If the more informal route of internal policies and procedures is ineffective, then legal rights might be enforced in the courts. Here we look at employee rights. Any failure to provide for these rights in the case of a particular individual or group of individuals might be the basis for a claim of discrimination.

- **Redundancy** – This is when a person is dismissed because there is no work, either generally or in a particular job or in a particular area. Under the 1978 Employment Protection (Consolidation) Act redundancy can only occur in certain clearly defined circumstances.

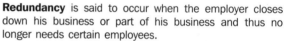

Did You Know ?

Redundancy is said to occur when the employer closes down his business or part of his business and thus no longer needs certain employees.

For the employer to avoid a claim for unfair dismissal he must consult with the employees affected, or their representatives. Where ten or more employees belonging to a recognised union are involved a minimum of 30 days' notice must be given. Where over 100 employees are to be made redundant within a three month period 90 days' advance notice must be given. Employees affected by redundancy are also entitled to reasonable time off with pay during the notice period to seek other work.

- **Termination of contract of employment** – A contract of employment is terminated automatically at the end of a fixed period. If no fixed period has been agreed, then the contract may be terminated by either party after giving 'reasonable' notice. The Employment Protection (Consolidation Act) of 1978 lays down *minimum* periods of notice.

- **Unfair dismissal** – Although an employer can terminate a contract of employment by giving reasonable notice, there are certain circumstance when employers will have to pay compensation. Action for *unfair dismissal* can be brought before an Industrial Tribunal. The Act lists reasons which will be regarded as 'fair' if they can be proved by the employer.

1. The employee's poor performance at his job.
2. The employee's poor qualifications.
3. The employee's bad conduct.
4. Redundancy (see above).
5. It is contrary to law to continue the employment.
6. Any other reason which the employer is able to convince the tribunal is fair.

The Industrial Tribunal will normally award compensation to the employee if it finds that s/he has been *unfairly* dismissed.

- **Industrial injuries compensation.** A person injured in the course of their work or who contracts a disease in the course of that work can claim an industrial injuries benefit.

- **The right to equal pay**
  Before 1970 women could be paid less than men for undertaking the same work. Today, the law (Equal Pay Act 1970) requires that men and women are treated equally. The Equal Pay Act stipulates that where women are employed on

- 'like work'
- 'work rated as equivalent' under a job evaluation scheme

the terms and conditions offered should be equal.

However, in 1983 an amendment to the act meant that women could claim equal pay for work of 'equal value'. Thus in one printing industry case a woman received an increase of over £100 per week by successfully claiming that her work as a VDU operator was of equal value to that of a male typesetter.

Unit Test   Answer all the questions. Time 1 hour

Question 1
Socialisation can be defined as:

A   The process of learning to socialise with other people
B   The social learning which teaches an individual the culture of his or her society
C   The transition from adolescence to adulthood
D   The movement from one social group to another

Question 2
Decide whether each of these statements is True (T) or False (F).

(i)   Primary socialisation takes place within the family
(ii) Secondary socialisation takes place after marriage

Which option best describes the two statements?

A   (i)   T   (ii)   T
B   (i)   T   (ii)   F
C   (i)   F   (ii)   T
D   (i)   F   (ii)   F

Questions 3-5 share answer options A to D
The functions of the family include:

A   Socialisation
B   Reproduction
C   Economic support
D   Emotional support

Which of these functions are illustrated by the following examples?

Question 3
A mother comforts her son when his pet rabbit dies.

Question 4
A daughter who lives with her parents gives them some of her wages each week.

Question 5
A father emphasizes to his son that success is only achieved through hard work.

Question 6
Which of the following best describes an extended family?

A   A family whose members are spread over a wide geographical area
B   Three or more generations of a family living with or near each other
C   A family in which one or both parents has remarried
D   A family in which one or more of the children has been adopted

Question 7
Which of the following best describes a nuclear family?

A   A family of two generations – parents and children living together
B   A single parent family
C   A family whose members were all born after 1945
D   A married couple with no children

Question 8
Decide whether each of these statements is True (T) or False (F).

(i)   The culture of a society can be transmitted from generation to generation.

(ii) Television soap operas cannot be considered a part of our culture.

Which option best describes the two statements?

A   (i)   T   (ii)   T
B   (i)   T   (ii)   F
C   (i)   F   (ii)   T
D   (i)   F   (ii)   F

Question 9
A culture of dependency is most likely to be found in which one of the following?

A   The Department of Health and Social Security
B   A hospital
C   A hospital management team
D   A neighbourhood community centre

Question 10
Norms are:

A   Standard rates of pay for particular jobs
B   Opinions held by the majority of people
C   Standards of behaviour to which members of a group usually conform
D   The particular characteristics which distinguish one group from another

Question 11
The mass media are an example of:

A   Primary socialisation
B   Secondary socialisation
C   Peer groups
D   Primary groups

Questions 12-15 share answer options A-D
Within a school, the following all contribute to the process of socialisation:

A   Peer groups
B   The hidden curriculum
C   Lessons
D   Rules

Which of the above options are illustrated by the following?

Question 12
A storybook in which the central male character has a paid job and the central female character is a housewife.

Question 13
A school forbids running in the corridors

Question 14
Children are taught the main features of the British electoral system.

Question 15
A boy begins smoking because his closest friends all smoke.

Question 16
Which of the following best defines the term 'role'?

A   Behaviour which imitates others
B   Behaviour which is false
C   The power and influence which a person has
D   The patterns of behaviour associated with a position within a group

Question 17
Decide whether each of these statements is True (T) or False (F)

(i) A care worker is potentially in a position of power over a client
(ii) Empowerment means seeking to limit the power that others have

Which option best describes the two statements?

A (i) T (ii) T
B (i) T (ii) F
C (i) F (ii) T
D (i) F (ii) F

Question 18
Overt discrimination is:

A Open and observable
B Hidden and indirect
C Spread over a long time
D Temporary

Question 19
Decide whether each of these statements is True (T) or False (F)

(i) The term *sex* refers to the biological differences between males and females
(ii) The term *gender* refers to the differences in social expectations/roles between males and females

Which option best describes the two statements?

A (i) T (ii) T
B (i) T (ii) F
C (i) F (ii) T
D (i) F (ii) F

Question 20-23 share answer options A to D
Different bases for discrimination include:

A Race
B Gender
C Age
D Cognitive ability

Which of these kinds of discrimination are illustrated by the following?

Question 20
A mentally handicapped person is refused service in a restaurant.

Question 21
The menu at a hospital in a multi-cultural community only lists Western dishes.

Question 22
A nurse loses her temper and calls a patient a 'silly old fool'.

Question 23
A private hospital advertising a vacancy for a nurse decides before receiving any applications that it will only interview female applicants.

Question 24
Prejudice.

A has nothing to do with discrimination
B may lead to discrimination
C is unlikely to lead to discrimination
D always leads to discrimination

Question 25
Decide whether each of these statements is True (T) or False (F).

(i) The law can remove people's prejudices
(ii) Discrimination can be reinforced through language
Which option best describes the two statements?

A (i) T (ii) T
B (i) T (ii) F
C (i) F (ii) T
D (i) F (ii) F

Question 26
A hospital organises a 'Friends and Neighbours' scheme which provides free transport for its outpatients. The application form for receiving assistance under this scheme is however so complicated that few patients for whom English is a second language apply. Is this:

A Covert discrimination
B Gender discrimination
C Harassment
D Positive discrimination

Question 27
Decide whether each of these statements is True (T) or False (F)

(i) Britain has an ageing population
(ii) Over the last thirty years the number of immigrants entering the UK has steadily increased

Which option best describes the two statements?

A (i) T (ii) T
B (i) T (ii) F
C (i) F (ii) T
D (i) F (ii) F

Question 28
The Public Order Act 1986 is relevant to the issue of:

A Race equality
B Gender equality
C Age discrimination
D Discrimination against the disabled

Question 29
Discrimination can damage a person's self esteem. Is self esteem:

A A person's degree of independence
B The evaluation of one's own self-worth
C A person's ability to form relationships
D The feedback about oneself received from others

Questions 30-33 share answer options A to D
Listed below are four important bodies:

A Advisory, Conciliation and Arbitration Services (ACAS)
B Commission for Racial Equality
C Equal Opportunities Commission
D Department of Health

Which of these bodies might be of most use in the following instances?

Question 30
A female employee feels she has been denied promotion because she is a woman.

Question 31
A male employee feels he is being unfairly treated by management because he is black.

Question 32
A student needs advice and information for a project on AIDS.

Question 33

A union in dispute with an employer is about to call a strike.

Question 34

A colleague feels she is the victim of racial discrimination.

Which of the following courses of action would you advise?

A   Begin legal proceedings immediately
B   Follow internal policies and procedures
C   Press her union to call a strike
D   Do nothing and see if the problem continues

Answers to Self-check Questions

1. See the definitions on page 2 of the Unit: Primary – within the family; secondary – outside the home.

2. See the definitions on page 3 of the Unit

3. *Group*   *Membership*
    Political   Labour/Conservative voters
    Gender   Males, Females
    Educational   University students, primary school pupils
                        (many other answers are possible)

4. Many possible answers: postmen/women; policemen/women; fireman/women; doctors; nurses, even business-men/women may feel they need to adopt 'normal dress'(e.g. suits) to conform to expectations.

5. Social workers' 'uniform' is normally casual clothes because, historically, social workers have wanted to avoid putting a barrier between themselves and their clients.

6. Many possible answers to private roles: dutiful son/daughter; 'livewire' at parties; responsible member of local football/tennis team; etc. Public roles are more formal: e.g. prefect; captain of school/college football/ netball team; leader of scout/girl guide group; etc. Conflicts may arise between private and public roles: e.g. may need to be stern and serious as captain of team with people you were relaxed with in a social setting the previous day. Scarcity of time available for different roles may also cause conflict.

7. Many possible examples: purchase of expensive cars (Rolls Royce), houses, clothes, etc.

8. The lengthy education, training and experience needed to be a doctor or consultant, give them higher status over, say, a student nurse. So too does their greater authority over resources/decisions etc. The low-paid priest may earn less than a high-paid prostitute, but his position in society may command greater status. It is important to remember that money is not the only criterion used to determine status.

9. Other managerial roles might include those of negotiator, representative, communicator, listener, carer, etc.

10. Knowledge can be power. Having access to knowledge that someone else does not have, can increase influence and authority. On the other hand, sharing knowledge can be a help to team-building, improving effectiveness of decision making, etc.

11. This exists when members of a group are socialised into a state of dependence upon other members of the group. The term is sometimes applied to hospitals and other care institutions (see page 3)

12. Political power; economic power; social class.

13. See page 7. Prejudice is an *attitude* based on negative assumptions about an individual or group. Discrimination is *behaviour* that results from prejudice.

14. The employers may be reluctant to interview, or offer the positions to, members of ethnic minority groups. Those employed may find it more difficult to gain promotion. Of course earlier prejudice and discrimination may occur, e.g. at school if some teachers give less attention to children from ethnic minority backgrounds; etc.

15. Any three from race; gender; age; physical ability; cognitive ability; etc.

16. Overt discrimination is open, direct and observable. Covert discrimination is hidden and indirect.

17. See page 9

18. Higher incidence of illness; more resources needed for health service; less working people to support (via taxes) health care; changing *pattern* of illness e.g. more need for geriatric provision; etc.

19. See page 8.

20. Words which traditionalists might associate with males or females could include:

Males	*Females*
Strong	Weak
Aggressive	Passive
Breadwinner	Home-keeper
Unemotional	Emotional
Brave	Timid

21. Exemptions from gender or racial discrimination involving 'genuine occupational qualifications', such that certain types of person would genuinely be unable to perform the functions associated with that occupation.

22. Modelling; acting; dancing; singing; nightwork (single-sex establishments); etc.

23. Promotion, training, housing, incitement of racial hatred, etc.

24. 3% of 500 is 15 people

25. Commission for Racial Equality

26. Any one from:
    The Equal Pay Act 1970; the Employment Protection Act 1975; the Sex Discrimination Acts 1975 and 1986.

Answers to Unit Test

Question	Answer	Question	Answer	Question	Answer	Question	Answer	Question	Answer
1.	B	8.	B	15.	A	22.	C	29.	B
2.	B	9.	B	16.	D	23.	B	30.	C
3.	D	10.	C	17.	B	24.	B	31.	B
4.	C	11.	B	18.	A	25.	C	32.	D
5.	A	12.	B	19.	A	26.	A	33.	A
6.	B	13.	D	20.	D	27.	B	34.	B
7.	A	14.	C	21.	A	28.	A		

Unit Test Comments (selected questions)

Q2. Answer is B.
Secondary socialisation takes place outside the family.

Q5. Answer is A.
Here the father is passing on to his son an attitude that is widely held in society as a whole.

Q8. Answer is B.
The mass media are an important part of our culture.

Q9. Answer is B.
(Although, as explained in the Unit, in recent years increasing efforts have been made to remove the culture of dependency that exists in some hospitals.)

Q11. Answer is B.
(Secondary socialisation occurs outside the family)

Q12. Answer is B.
The book *implies* that males and females should have stereotyped roles. This is therefore a 'hidden' message of the book

Q17. Answer is B.
Empowerment means *giving* power to others rather than taking it away.

Q18. Answer is A.
(B is a definition of covert discrimination.)

Q25. Answer is C.
The law cannot dictate how people think (though it may *influence* our thinking)

Q34. Answer is B.
A and C are drastic, last resort measures. However, she should do something and her initial course of action should be to make use of internal policies and procedures.

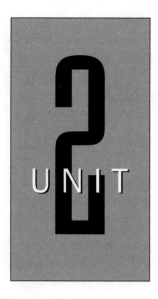

Interpersonal Interaction

Getting Started

This Unit is concerned with **interpersonal interaction** – that is, with the different kinds of contact that may take place between people in a health and social care context. The aim of the first two Elements is to increase your understanding of the ways people communicate, on a one-to-one basis (Element 1) and within groups (Element 2). We shall examine both **verbal communication** (communicating through the use of words) and **non-verbal communication** (communicating by other means, such as gesture, touch and so on). Another aim of these Elements is to improve your own communication skills, especially those that you may need to employ with clients. The third Element is intended to give you an understanding of clients' rights in interpersonal situations, and of the ways that these can be safeguarded. It covers such topics as confidentiality, freedom of choice and freedom from discrimination.

This Unit is different from others in that you will not need to take a Unit Test for it. This is not because it is less important than other Units, but because a Unit Test is considered an inappropriate form of assessment for the knowledge and skills with which the Unit is concerned. You will however need to provide evidence in your portfolio that you have satisfied the performance criteria for the Unit.

In this Unit a number of interpersonal skills are examined, including for example listening, talking, asking questions and showing support and understanding. Although these skills are discussed separately, in practice a successful interaction will probably involve employing several of these skills at once. This may sound daunting: being asked to concentrate carefully on what another person is saying and then think of a suitable response, while simultaneously observing that person's non-verbal communication and making sure that your own non-verbal communication is appropriate, seems a tall order! In fact, you almost certainly already possess many of these skills to some degree, and practise them without thinking. This Unit should help you to develop these skills further,

and may help you to acquire some new ones. Proficiency in interpersonal communication is achieved through experience: the regular use of these interpersonal skills will enable you to master them. When you apply these techniques in practice, try to avoid giving the impression that your speech and behaviour are artificial and contrived. This may be difficult when you are using a skill for the first time, but the more you use the skill the easier you will find it to be natural and spontaneous.

Dealing effectively with others, and being able to demonstrate such qualities as warmth, understanding and sympathy, is self-evidently a vital part of health and social care. In this Unit we shall look more closely at why these skills are so important and examine ways in which they can be learned and developed.

Autocratic (leadership) authoritarian, perhaps even dictatorial.

Covert (discrimination) hidden and subtle.

Democratic leadership brings others into the process.

Empathy entering into the perceptual world of another person.

Group three or more people sharing in a common purpose or goal.

Laissez-faire leave well alone.

Overt (discrimination) open and direct.

Paralanguage extra information conveyed in a spoken message by the *way* in which it is delivered.

Essential Principles

In this first Element we shall be looking at the following important aspects of communication between individuals: Non-Verbal Communication; Verbal Communication; Listening. Finally we shall consider some factors which can prevent effective communication taking place.

Non-verbal communication

What is non-verbal communication and why is it important?

Non-verbal communication is a broad term which refers to all the ways in which one individual might communicate with another, excluding the actual words that the individual uses. It includes not only 'body language' (gestures, facial expression, posture and so on), but also the way in which words are spoken (tone and speed of voice, for example).

Research has indicated that a remarkably high proportion of what we communicate to others is conveyed by non-verbal means. Indeed, one authority on non-verbal communication, J. Birdwhistell, has claimed that the average person speaks only for a total of ten to eleven minutes a day, and that even then only around a third of the meaning of each conversation is conveyed by words alone.

Non-verbal communication has three main functions:

- **It can take the place of speech.** Someone who has just taken a driving test may give a thumbs-up sign to a waiting friend to indicate that he has passed; at a party, a smile across a crowded room, accompanied by a look of recognition, can be used to greet someone you know. Sign language is of course especially important in helping those with impaired speech or hearing to communicate.

- **It can consciously reinforce or supplement what we say.** Strong expressions of agreement or disagreement are often emphasised by a vigorous nodding or shaking of the head. At a noisy meeting the chairman may seek to increase the effectiveness of his calls for order by raising his voice and by banging his fist on the table.

- **It can reveal or suggest attitudes and emotions without our conscious knowledge.** Often what is conveyed non-verbally is consistent with the spoken message: a person may tremble involuntarily when recalling a frightening experience. Sometimes, however, non-verbal behaviour contradicts the spoken message, suggesting to others what is truly thought or felt. Students may claim to have great interest in a lesson, but the glazed look in their eyes may suggest otherwise!

It is important for those who work in the field of health and social care to be both receptive to the non-verbal communication of others and aware of what is conveyed by their own non-verbal behaviour. For example, an elderly lady in hospital may be worried about some aspect of her treatment but afraid to speak openly of her concern; a skilled nurse is likely to notice signs of anxiety and respond in an appropriate way. A social worker dealing with a distressed client knows that casting continual glances at the clock will suggest that she has little interest in the client's problems.

We shall now look in more detail at the components of non-verbal communication and at their particular relevance to health and social care.

Paralanguage

Paralanguage is a term used for the additional information conveyed in a spoken message by the way in which the speech is delivered. Aspects of paralanguage include:

- **Volume** For example, if 'Pass the salt, please' is said quietly it is likely to be a polite request; shouted loudly it will sound more like an angry demand.

- **Emphasis** Note in the following sentence how placing the emphasis on a different word each time significantly alters the meaning that is conveyed:

  HE gave the money to me.
  He GAVE the money to me.
  He gave the money to ME.

- **Tone** This can also alter meaning. 'Well done!' can be made to sound like sarcasm or genuine praise. Variation of tone enlivens our speech, making different shades of meaning or emotion more distinct and helping to retain a listener's attention. Contrastingly, a flat monotone will not engage the listener and will lessen the listener's ability to comprehend fully what is being said.

- **Speed of delivery** Slow, measured speech can convey calmness and reassurance, while interest or enthusiasm are often reflected in more rapid delivery. Fast, muddled speech may be the result of anxiety or panic.

- **Distribution of pauses** Pauses in a conversation may reflect awkwardness between the participants and can even have a menacing effect, but they can also be relaxed and tension-free. Hesitation in speech may be an indication of uncertainty, stress or fatigue.

A care worker needs to be conscious of his or her own paralanguage, and aware of the paralanguage of clients. As a general rule, you should try to ensure that your paralanguage confirms and reinforces the verbal meaning of your speech. In other words, expressions of concern, interest and support should *sound* concerned, interested and supportive. If you sound bored or impatient you are unlikely to win the client's confidence and trust. Sensitivity to a client's paralanguage involves attending closely to tone, emphasis and so on as well as to the explicit meaning of what is being said. If a normally fluent speaker becomes hesitant it may be a sign that the matter being discussed is a source of anxiety and needs to be addressed with particular tact and delicacy.

Activity

An experiment carried out by J.R. and L.J. Davitz in 1959 demonstrated the power of paralanguage as a means of communication. Eight people were asked to recite part of the alphabet ten times, on each occasion attempting to convey a different emotion. They were heard by a group of students, who had to decide which emotion was being expressed on each occasion. The experiment showed that for each emotion the rate of identification was far higher than could have been achieved by random guessing.

A variation of this experiment is to write the ten emotions used by Davitz and Davitz on separate pieces of paper and distribute them randomly to ten people you know or to members of your class or group (if fewer than ten people are present, give each person more than one piece of paper). Each person must then recite the first dozen or so letters of the alphabet, trying by means of their voice alone to convey the emotion designated to them. The rest of the group must attempt to identify which emotion has been expressed by each group member. Record the number of correct identifications each emotion receives. The ten emotions are: anger; fear; happiness; jealousy; love; nervousness; pride; sadness; satisfaction; sympathy.

Davitz and Davitz found that anger and nervousness were the emotions most easy to identify, pride and jealousy the most difficult. How do your findings compare? You might want to write a report on the experiment for inclusion in your portfolio. Later, when you have studied the other components of non-verbal communication discussed in this Unit, you may find it interesting to repeat the experiment, this time employing some of these other components (gestures, facial expressions etc.) as well as paralanguage. You should find that the number of correct identifications increases still further.

Posture/Body position

Moods, emotions and attitudes are often reflected in a person's **body position**. For example, a slouched position may indicate depression, while tightly clenched hands and a tense, upright position may show anxiety. Noting body position can therefore help us to gauge a client's mental and emotional state.

At the same time, it is important for care workers to be conscious of the messages that their own body language conveys. Generally, you should seek to show that you are relaxed, accessible and attentive. Experts suggest that this is achieved when standing by allowing the arms and hands to hang loosely along the sides, and when sitting by resting the hands loosely in the lap. Folded arms are seen as a defensive gesture that inhibits free and open communication. If the body position is too relaxed (feet up on an adjacent chair!) this is likely to suggest laziness or inattention, though deliberately informal positions are sometimes appropriate (for example, you may sit on the floor to talk or play with a child).

If you are *seated*, leaning forward towards a client can be an appropriate way of communicating interest and concern, especially if the client is anxious or distressed. Sensitivity is needed here, however, as some clients may be unsettled by this and consider it intrusive. Seating positions should also be considered. Sitting directly opposite another (especially on either side of a table) can imply competition and may cause a client to feel intimidated. Sitting side-by-side implies co-operation: students working together on a project, for example, will often sit like

this. The position often favoured by health and social care professionals when meeting clients is to sit at an angle (roughly ninety degrees) to the other person. Research suggests that this makes conversation easier, and it also enables the client to look at or away from the care worker as desired.

Physical proximity can also affect the client's perception of the care worker. Standing or sitting too far away can appear cold and impersonal and is likely to inhibit the client's conversation. On the other hand, standing or sitting too close can have the same effect as the client may see it as an invasion of privacy. As with all aspects of health and social care, you need to be sensitive to the individual client's needs and reactions and to respond accordingly.

Did You Know ?

Heads of state tend to face each other across a table when negotiating a treaty, but pose side by side for the cameras when the treaty has been agreed. This non-verbal behaviour suggests a progression from opposition to co-operation.

Eye contact

Eye contact is usually a sign of friendliness and a willingness to communicate. It helps to initiate a conversation and regular eye contact during the course of the conversation is a way of showing attention and interest. Too much eye contact, however, can appear hostile or intrusive; a person who is stared at is likely to feel uneasy, angry or embarrassed.

Health and social care professionals generally make quite frequent eye contact with their clients (showing their interest and concern), but not to the point that the client is unsettled or intimidated. Again the needs and preferences of each individual client need to be considered – some will wish for more eye contact than others. It is also important not to force eye contact on an unwilling client, especially at the beginning of an encounter. A person who is distressed or embarrassed may wish to look away, and their need to do this should be respected.

Facial expression/movement of the head

The **face** is the most expressive part of the body. It is capable of suggesting an enormous range of emotions but is also on occasion used to disguise how we truly feel. Changes in facial expression may be voluntary or (as in the case of blushing) involuntary. Research suggests that when a person's facial expression contradicts what he or she is saying, others (especially children) are likely to believe what they see rather than what they hear. This has important implications for those who

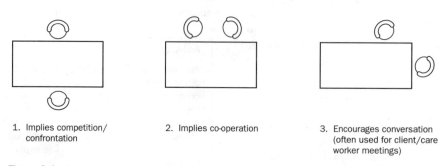

1. Implies competition/ confrontation

2. Implies co-operation

3. Encourages conversation (often used for client/care worker meetings)

Figure 2.1 Importance of seating positions, summarising the attitudes and behaviour that can be implied or encouraged when two people sit as illustrated at a table

work in health and social care, and emphasises again that what is said to a client should be accompanied by non-verbal signals that are consistent with the verbal message. More positively, appropriate facial expressions can support and reinforce what is said: a smile can help to reassure an anxious client.

Facial expressions and movement – especially smiles and nods of the head – are also important in sustaining conversation. Smiling and nodding during a conversation usually indicates agreement and understanding, and can be used to encourage a client to continue speaking. A rapid succession of nods can indicate especially vigorous agreement but is also often a sign that the person nodding now wishes to speak.

Did You Know ?

A great number of different meanings can be conveyed by facial expressions. It has been estimated that there are at least eight different positions of the eyebrows and forehead, each with its own meaning; eight more of the eyes and eyelids, and at least ten for the lower part of the face. The range of possible expressions is even greater when you consider the different combinations of these that can be employed!

Gestures
Gestures may be used to replace speech (as in sign language) or may serve to clarify or emphasise what is said (as when the words 'I don't know' are accompanied by a shrugging of the shoulders). Many gestures are spontaneous and involuntary, and they may help to indicate a client's emotional state. Nailbiting, for example, might suggest nervousness and a hand over the mouth when speaking might be a sign of embarrassment. Correspondingly, the care worker should be aware of what might be conveyed by his or her own gestures. Drumming one's fingers on a table during an interview, for example, is bound to suggest impatience. Some gestures (scratching the nose, pulling on the ear) can be a distraction and may therefore inhibit conversation.

Touch
In a caring context **touch** is an important means of expressing warmth, reassurance and compassion. A touch on the arm, a pat on the shoulder or a squeeze of the hand can be very effective ways of showing support and understanding, and can give a client a sense of being valued. Such gestures are often especially appreciated by children and the elderly, but again individual needs and preferences must be respected. Some people will respond positively to touch, but others may be embarrassed by it or find it intrusive. One elderly hospital patient may be greatly comforted by an arm around the shoulder, but another may consider it a patronising gesture. Sensitivity to such individual differences is, as always, essential.

Interpreting non-verbal communication
A final point about non-verbal communication which cannot be emphasised too strongly is that it should not lead us to make snap judgements about others. The precise significance of particular non-verbal signals will depend on a number of variables, including for example an individual's personality and cultural background. Non-verbal behaviour can suggest much about a client's state of mind, but what is suggested

must be confirmed before it is assumed to be true. If possible observe clients over an extended period and consider their non-verbal behaviour in the light of other information you have gathered about them. Often the best approach is to ask clients to clarify their own feelings for you. Imagine for example that a client claims to be amused by something while his non-verbal behaviour suggests that he is actually quite anxious about it. A care worker might ask him:

'I can see this has a funny side to it, but isn't it pretty worrying as well?'

Note how the care worker does not presume to know how the client feels, but at the same time gives him an opportunity to share any anxiety that he might have.

Verbal communication

We shall now look at some important aspects of **verbal communication**, seeking in particular to identify those which are most conducive to effective communication between individuals.

Environmental factors
Successful communication is helped by an **environment** which is comfortable and free of distractions. Hospitals, offices and clinics can sometimes appear cold, forbidding places to clients and an effort should always be made to create as warm and pleasant an atmosphere as possible. Clients who are physically ill at ease will find it hard to relax; a comfortable chair and a welcoming cup of coffee can do much to make a particularly stressful encounter more congenial. Of course, extraneous noise from radios, television, other people's conversations and so on should be reduced to a minimum. This is sometimes outside the care worker's control but it may well be possible to move to a quieter part of the room or building.

Clarity
For effective communication to take place it is essential that each participant in a conversation has a **clear understanding** of what the other person is saying. You therefore need to ensure both that you have not misunderstood the client and that the client has not misunderstood you. There is no harm in asking the client to repeat or clarify what they have just said, by means of such responses as 'I'm sorry, I didn't quite catch that last part' or 'Can you tell me a bit more about that?'. Try to make sure that your own speech is not hurried, confused or ambiguous. In particular take care when using technical terms or jargon with which the client may be unfamiliar. In a hospital, for example, a patient may be unnerved to be told that she is to undergo 'tests', and a fuller explanation may be necessary to reassure her.

Empathy, warmth and sincerity
The American psychotherapist Carl Rogers (1902–87) first emphasized the importance of **empathy** to carer-client relationships. He defined it as 'entering into the perceptual world of the other and becoming thoroughly at home in it'. It means understanding what the client is experiencing and recognising why the client sees things in the way that he does. This involves an acceptance of human differences – a client's appearance, attitudes and behaviour may be very different from your own but you should not react to this with irritation

or disapproval. Demonstrating empathy entails showing clients that you can understand their point of view and that you are aware of their needs and concerns – that you are on their 'wavelength'. For example, if a client is seriously concerned about an apparently trivial matter, you should not simply dismiss the client's concern as irrational. Rather, you should begin by showing that you recognise the concern to be real. (You would then seek to discover the exact cause of the concern.) In a conversation, empathy is often shown by *reflection*. This means repeating, paraphrasing or summing up what the client has said to you, as in the following exchange:

| Client | I'm also finding it difficult to cope at work. Two people left last month and the boss seems to think I should do their jobs as well. |
| Care worker | You feel too much is being expected of you. |

Reflection is an important aspect of interpersonal communication and will be discussed more fully later in this Unit.

Empathy shows warmth towards the client and helps to convince the client that the care worker is sincere – it indicates that the care worker is genuinely concerned and has a positive regard for the client's feelings, beliefs and attitudes. Sincerity in conversation also involves avoiding too many rehearsed phrases and responses. Inevitably, similar situations often require similar reactions but it is important not to lose sight of the individuality of the client. Too standardised a response will appear unfeeling and mechanical. Clients will be reassured if you seem knowledgeable and competent, but they will also want you to be a human being.

Self-disclosure

Self-disclosure is the deliberate revealing of personal information to another. The information may be of a simple factual kind (revealing which primary school you attended, for example) or intimate and emotional (explaining how you felt when a loved one died). Much of this Unit is concerned with ways of encouraging self-disclosure by clients, but self-disclosure by the care worker is sometimes helpful also.

Firstly, it may encourage the client to disclose, or to disclose more. If people are open with us, we in turn are more likely to speak freely to them. Secondly, it can be a way of offering reassurance to a client and making them feel less isolated. If a client is worried about starting a new job, for example, a care worker might say:

'It's very common for people to feel like that when they're beginning a new job. I was nervous myself when I first started working here – but things improved once I got used to the place and got to know the other staff.'

Thirdly, it helps to show that the care worker is an ordinary human being and not some remote, impersonal figure. Finally, hearing of another's experience may help the client to take a wider, more balanced view of his own situation.

It must never be forgotten that the purpose of the self-disclosure is to assist the client; if it is not likely to achieve this it should not take place. Lengthy personal recollections are to be avoided and we should not burden clients with our own troubles. Self-disclosure when it occurs should therefore be brief and clearly relevant to the help we are seeking to give to the client.

Questions

Asking **questions** can help to facilitate effective communication in a number of ways. In the field of health and social care the main purposes served by asking questions of a client include:

- Obtaining specific information ('How old are your children?')
- Clarifying what has been said / Checking that you have understood correctly ('You mean you find it harder to relax now?').
- Discovering more about the client's thoughts, feelings and attitudes.
- Encouraging clients to speak and showing that you are interested in what they have to say.

There are also different types of question that are commonly used. The main ones include:

- **Closed questions** These invite a short, limited response and can often be answered with a simple 'yes' or 'no'. The following are examples of closed questions:

  'Have you got enough medicine?'
  'Do you enjoy going to school?'
  'How old are you?'

  They can be useful if you wish to obtain specific information quickly. They can also help to reduce tension at the beginning of a conversation – answering a few short, simple questions may help a client to relax. However, too many closed questions can turn a conversation into an interrogation. Another drawback of closed questions is that they limit the amount of true communication that takes place. If you wish to explore a situation more fully, or to encourage a client to elaborate, closed questions are inappropriate.

- **Open questions** These allow for a less restricted response. They often begin with the words 'What', 'Why' or 'How' and they encourage clients to talk freely about their feelings and attitudes. These are examples of open questions:

  'What's it like now that your children have left home?'
  'Why don't you enjoy coming to the day centre as much as you used to?'
  'How did you feel about that?'

  Open questions can be very helpful if you wish to encourage a client to speak at greater length, or if you want to explore more fully how a client feels. Disadvantages of open questions are that they can be time-consuming and the answers to them may contain a great deal of irrelevant information – though answers can sometimes be unexpectedly informative, revealing more than had been anticipated. Too many open questions may make a client feel uncomfortable and under pressure.

- **Probing questions** These enable the questioner to explore more fully something that has been said. A probing question may ask for clarification ('Do you mean...?') or elaboration ('What happened next?'), or it may be a way of looking into something more deeply ('What do you think made you feel so upset?').

- **Leading questions** These steer the client towards an expected reply ('Surely you wouldn't want to do that?')

or contain built-in assumptions which the person being questioned is forced to accept, as in the oft-quoted example 'When did you stop beating your wife?'. Generally, leading questions are to be avoided, because they may entail unjustified assumptions and because they put pressure on the client to agree with the questioner. No harm is caused however by questions which accurately reflect a client's views ('Isn't that a lovely photograph of your daughter?').

A skilled professional will employ a variety of questioning. Note though that a long series of questions can make a client feel defensive and ill-at-ease. An alternative to direct questioning is to make statements which invite a response of some kind from the client.

'I'm not entirely clear what you mean by that.'
'I can't quite see how that connects with what you were telling me earlier.'

A client can also be encouraged to continue talking by simple verbal prompts ('yes', 'of course', 'I see'), by nods of the head and by such oral signals as 'hmmm' and 'ah'.

Reflection
Reflection occurs when one person in a conversation echoes, or reflects back, what the other has said. The simplest kind of reflection is a *repetition* of the last few words spoken by the other person:

Client	When I moved house I left all my friends behind and I realised then how much they'd meant to me. I just sat in the house by myself all day. Nobody called, I hardly ever went out and I felt thoroughly miserable.
Care worker	You felt miserable.

Like other forms of reflection, this kind of response shows the client that the care worker is listening, and encourages the client to continue. However, continual use of this technique soon becomes irritating and tedious. It is generally more effective to *paraphrase* what the other person has said. This means grasping the essence of what has been said and putting it in your own words. In the above example the care worker might have paraphrased the client's words by saying:

'After you moved you felt very lonely and you missed your old friends.'

This does more than show that the care worker has been listening – it shows that the client has been understood, and as we saw earlier this kind of empathy is an important element in a successful client-care worker relationship. Another advantage of paraphrase is that it may help the client to see his own situation more clearly. Hearing what he has been saying expressed in a different way may encourage him to see things afresh, and give him a better understanding of his own thoughts and feelings.

Summarising what the client has said can serve similar purposes. It again demonstrates understanding and, by bringing together the main points made by the client, clarifies what has emerged from the conversation. Summarising is often a sensible way to end a conversation (see 'Closing a conversation' below), but it can also take place during a conversation. Pausing occasionally to 'take stock' helps to ensure that the conversation has a coherent structure, that it does not drift into irrelevancy and that both client and care worker have a clear understanding of what has been said.

Opening a conversation
The **beginning of a conversation** is important because it sets a mood or atmosphere for the ensuing interaction and gives the client expectations about what is to follow. Before you begin to tackle the more serious matters you may have to deal with in the conversation you should try to create an atmosphere that is friendly and relaxed. Non-verbal signals are a customary way of showing friendliness at this stage of an encounter: eye contact, a smile, a handshake. It can also help to begin by talking about something unrelated to your professional role ('How was your holiday?' 'What a lovely day!'). Use of the client's name early in the conversation is another sign of friendliness and demonstrates a personal interest in the client. It may also be appropriate to introduce yourself and to give an outline of your professional responsibilities. This ensures that the client knows what to expect (and what not to expect) from you, but may be delayed until the initial 'ice-breaking' has taken place.

Closing a conversation
The last impression that a person is left with at the **end of a conversation** is important and may well determine the person's feelings about the conversation as a whole. For example, a client who is told 'I must go now, I've got a lot of other people to see' may well find such a remark hurtful; it suggests that the client has been delaying the care worker and emphasises that the amount of attention and interest the care worker can give to the client is limited.

At the close of a conversation the impression of friendliness and warmth you have been seeking to create should be reinforced. As at the beginning of a conversation, this may be achieved by stepping outside your professional role and chatting informally for a minute or two ('Are you going to watch the football on television tonight?').

This informal close may well be preceded by a more purposeful summary of what has been established and agreed during the conversation. A summary ensures that both parties have a clear understanding of what has been said and can be used to confirm any decisions or arrangements that have been made. If the conversation has been a fruitful one you can give encouragement to the client by emphasising what has been achieved and by comments such as 'I understand much more clearly now what's been worrying you.' If you are going to meet again, it is appropriate to mention this, and to indicate that you are looking forward to the meeting.

Listening

Listening is a complex process that entails much more than passively receiving another's verbal message; for effective communication to take place there must be *active listening*. This means:

- registering the other person's non-verbal behaviour as well as what he says;
- understanding these verbal and non-verbal messages;
- giving our full attention to the person being listened to;
- demonstrating this understanding and attention by responding appropriately.

Several of the skills that have already been discussed in this Unit are associated with active listening: interpreting non-verbal communication; showing empathy; reflection; responding to what has been said by asking questions. We shall now look at some other characteristics of listening and at ways of ensuring that effective listening does take place.

An appropriate *environment* is an aid to effective listening. A location that is private, quiet and comfortable is clearly more conducive to successful communication than one that is lacking in privacy, noisy and uncomfortable.

It also helps if we adopt an appropriate *body position*. Attention can be shown by regular (though not continuous) eye contact, facial expressions of interest and concern, a relaxed, open posture and, if seated, by leaning slightly towards the person speaking. Correspondingly, you should avoid body movements that imply inattention (staring out of the window, for example, or looking at somebody other than the person speaking).

A good listener *allows the other person to speak*. In everyday conversation with family or friends we may well interrupt, or talk over each other; in a client–care worker conversation such behaviour would be inappropriate. There is also the danger that a care worker who is more confident or knowledgeable than the client will dominate the conversation, and you should be careful not to do this.

To listen effectively we must *concentrate fully* on what the other person is saying. This may sound obvious but it is often very difficult to do! Apart from personal concerns which may be preoccupying us and which we must try to push aside, thinking about how we are going to respond when the other person finishes speaking can also cause us to lose attention. It is extremely difficult to clear our minds completely so that we are able to focus exclusively on what is being said to us, but a conscientious care worker will strive to achieve this.

During the conversation we should show that we are listening by *acknowledging* what the other person is saying. The acknowledgement may be non-verbal – a smile and a nod, for example. Other forms of acknowledgement include oral signals such as 'Mmm' and 'ah' and brief spoken responses ('Yes', 'Fancy that!', 'Really?').

Such acknowledgements not only confirm to the speaker that we are paying attention, they also *encourage* him to continue. Encouragement is especially helpful when a person is embarrassed or distressed and because of this is finding it difficult to speak. Here a simple 'Yes, I see' or 'Please go on' can offer support to clients and make it easier for them to continue.

Factors which prevent effective communication

Effective communication is achieved not only through an awareness of the kind of behaviour that characterises successful interaction but also through knowing what *not* to do. If we understand the factors that commonly *inhibit* successful communication between individuals we are more likely to avoid them. Listed below are some of the main barriers to effective communication.

Environmental factors As we have seen, the right kind of environment can make conversation easier. Successful interaction is less likely to take place in a location which is noisy, unattractive, or too hot or cold. If the environment is bleak and impersonal a client may feel intimidated.

Distractions Common distractions include: other activity taking place in the same room; attempting to carry on two conversations at once; thinking about something else rather than giving full attention to the other person.

Preconceived ideas/Bias Dress or appearance may cause you to pre-judge a person before he or she begins speaking – assuming that someone who looks untidy is lazy, for example. Ignorance of another person's culture can also lead to incorrect assumptions (for more on this see 'Respect for others and awareness of individual needs' later in the Unit). If you are working in a health and social care context your attitudes may be influenced by previous encounters with other clients. Drawing on what past experience has taught them is of course something all professional care workers do, but you must remember to treat each client as an individual and to avoid beginning a conversation with set ideas and assumptions.

Jumping to conclusions Avoid arriving at conclusions too early in the course of a conversation. This is especially likely to happen if you are in too much of a hurry. Jumping to conclusions can cause you to ignore later parts of the conversation which point to a different conclusion.

Interrupting / Dominating A person who is interrupted will not be able to express his attitudes and feelings fully, and may eventually be discouraged from speaking at all. As well as verbal interruptions, our body language can make it difficult for the other person to continue speaking. Signs of restlessness and impatience in the listener are likely to cause the speaker to stop talking. On the other hand, speaking excessively and not giving the other party a chance to contribute also inhibits effective communication. A person who finds it impossible to get a word in will eventually give up trying.

Changing the subject A conversation 'meshes' if the participants are on the same wavelength and there is a clear and logical connection between their respective contributions. Changing the subject when it is inappropriate to do so prevents this meshing taking place. It creates confusion, can cut off discussion of an important topic prematurely and may discourage a client from speaking further.

Manipulation This occurs when a person dominates a conversation not by speaking too much but by leading and controlling the responses of the other participant. In a health and social care context it may involve manoeuvring the client into saying something that serves the care worker's needs and interests rather than the client's. The manipulation might for example take the form of a leading question:

'You feel better now, don't you?'

Or a threat:

'If you don't co-operate more we'll have to move you to a different ward.'

In each of these cases there is unfair pressure on the client to comply. When people are in unfamiliar surroundings or are anxious or confused, they are more easily influenced and controlled. Care workers must be sensitive to the vulnerability of their clients and avoid this kind of manipulation.

Specific difficulties/disabilities One or both of the participants may experience particular communication difficulties – impaired speech or hearing, for example. Ways of approaching the communication problems caused by such difficulties are discussed in the next section.

Communication with particular groups of individuals

Special considerations arise when the communication process involves *particular groups* such as the elderly or those whose speech or vision is impaired. The needs of some of these groups will be outlined in this section.

Children

Children need to be respected as individuals as much as older clients do. You should not assume that because a child is a certain age he or she will inevitably exhibit certain kinds of behaviour. Neither should you give children the impression that their feelings and opinions are of little importance. Rather, as with older clients, there should be *empathy* between child and care worker. This means trying to understand the child's point of view, and showing the child that you have this understanding. Empathy is a particular challenge with children because a child's view of the world is obviously very different from an adult's, and because very young children have little or no ability to express themselves through speech. Attention to the child's behaviour and non-verbal communication is therefore especially important. Correspondingly, we need to communicate ourselves in ways that the child is likely to understand. Body language and paralanguage (tone of voice and so on) assume greater importance in communication with a child.

The elderly

Empathy between a care worker and an **elderly** client can again be difficult to achieve, especially if the care worker is from a much younger generation. The care worker must show sensitivity to the feelings of loneliness, confusion and frustration that elderly people sometimes have. Elderly clients may have particular need of friendliness, warmth and reassurance. However, the individual needs and preferences of the client must always be respected. One elderly person may welcome behaviour (a friendly hug, for example) that another finds patronising or intrusive.

Foreign language speakers

If a person has **limited knowledge of English** it is essential that you check to ensure he or she understands what you are saying. This may involve repeating important points or explaining them in a simpler way. Do not show impatience – this will discourage the other person from continuing the conversation. It may be appropriate to ask the help of a friend or relative of the client who has a better command of English – but not if the subject of the conversation is sensitive or confidential. It may be possible to use an interpreter; lists of interpreters are often kept by health authorities and social services departments.

Hearing difficulties

The following measures can help to facilitate communication with those suffering from **partial or complete hearing loss**:

- Face the client and talk directly to him, so that lip movements and facial expressions are clearly visible. Avoid covering any part of the face with your hand.

- Reduce or eliminate background noise (televisions, radios etc.).

- Do not shout but speak slowly and clearly, with deliberate and well defined lip movements.

- Be prepared to repeat or rephrase words and statements that are not immediately understood.

- The spoken message can be supported by other kinds of communication (use of pen and paper, gestures, facial expressions etc.).

- Avoid turning away to speak to others during the conversation. This may cause the client to feel excluded.

Visual impairment

Because they are unable to perceive most elements of non-verbal communication, speech and those aspects of non-verbal communication that they are able to respond to (paralanguage, touch), are especially important to blind people. The following measures may help communication with those suffering from **visual impairment**:

- Do not raise your voice but remember that blind people are especially sensitive to paralanguage (tone, expression and so on).
- If the client is partially sighted, stand or sit directly in front of him and give facial expressions and gestures additional emphasis.
- Introduce yourself clearly to the client.
- Let the client know when you are leaving the room.
- Remember how important conversation is to the blind. Be prepared to spend time sitting and talking to a blind client, encourage others to do the same, and be prepared to listen.

Speech difficulties

Speech difficulties can have a variety of causes, including for example impaired hearing and partial or complete loss of speech due to a stroke. The inability to communicate effectively through speech can cause intense frustration, confusion and anxiety. The loss of a faculty that had previously been taken for granted often creates acute embarrassment and a feeling of diminished self-esteem. It is the task of the care worker to understand these feelings and to offer the client reassurance and support. Steps that can be taken to improve communication with someone experiencing speech difficulties include:

- Listen closely and observe the speaker's non-verbal communication (gestures, facial expressions) carefully.
- Use adult speech (do not address the client as if he or she were a child), but at the same time try to use direct, straightforward questions which can be answered with one or two words or with a movement of the head.
- If in doubt repeat words used by the speaker to check that you have understood. If necessary, politely ask the speaker to repeat what he has said (or to speak more loudly or more slowly).
- Be patient and do not give the impression that you are in a hurry.
- Make use of other methods of communication as appropriate (signs, gestures, pen and paper and so on).
- Speak to relevant therapists for more advice on how to communicate with the client.

Learning disabilities/The mentally handicapped

People with **learning disabilities** often find it difficult to articulate their thoughts and feelings. Instead, attitudes and emotions may be expressed by means other than speech – by behaviour or body movement, for example. The care worker needs through careful observation to develop an understanding of the individual client and of his particular way of communicating. Often there is also difficulty in understanding the speech of others – the care worker's non-verbal communication, and use of this to show support and reassurance, therefore become especially important. Above all, the client must be viewed as a whole person and not only in terms of his disability. Inability to express feelings as clearly as others does not mean that these feelings do not exist. The client's individuality should always be recognised, and his particular needs and preferences respected.

Respect for others and awareness of individual needs

As was emphasised in the previous section, none of the difficulties or disabilities that a client may have should prevent us from viewing the client as an individual. Respect for this individuality is one of the principal values underpinning health and social care. Communication with a client should encourage him to see himself not as a passive recipient of care but as someone actively involved in the caring process. This means respecting his opinions, giving him the opportunity to make decisions wherever possible and encouraging him to be independent. Other ways of showing respect include such simple points as addressing the client by name, arriving on time for appointments and not appearing preoccupied or in a hurry.

The client's social and cultural background also needs to be respected. We have all been influenced by the values, beliefs and customs of family, friends and community. The care worker's culture may well be different from the client's (for example, if the client is from an ethnic minority). The care worker should be aware of these differences, which might for example involve learning a little about the religious practices and dietary customs of the cultural group to which the client belongs. At the same time, you should always have regard for the client as an individual and should not make assumptions based on race, colour, sex or social class (that is, you should not *stereotype* the client).

Demonstrating respect for a client in the ways outlined above enhances the client's *self-esteem* (the worth or value which an individual considers he or she has). Receiving help from others sometimes threatens this self-esteem, because it may reduce the client's sense of independence and self-reliance. The situation is made worse if clients are made to feel that their individual needs and preferences count for little. Sensitivity to the client's wishes and a sympathetic response to the client's needs help to ensure that self-esteem is encouraged rather than undermined.

Self-check ✓ Element 1

1. Which ONE of the following statements is correct?
    (a) A care worker should try not to be conscious of her own non-verbal communication but should pay close attention to the client's non-verbal communication.
    (b) A care worker should note the client's non-verbal communication and also be aware of her own.
    (c) A care worker should listen to what the client says rather than paying attention to the client's non-verbal communication.
    (d) A care worker should not observe the client's non-verbal communication as this will make the client nervous and uneasy.

2. How many of the following could be described as non-verbal communication?
    (a) The movements of a person's head
    (b) How loudly a person speaks
    (c) The words a person speaks.

3. Which ONE of the following should a care worker's speech to a client NOT be?
    (a) Warm
    (b) Free of jargon
    (c) Ambiguous
    (d) Expressing empathy.

4. Comment on the following, spoken by a care worker to a client, as examples of self-disclosure:
    (a) 'You think you've got problems – wait till you hear what happened to me yesterday!'
    (b) 'So as you can see I'm a bit of a mess as well. What do you think I should do?'
    (c) 'You'd be surprised how many people have days when they feel just like you do. Sometimes I wake up feeling I'd like just to stay in bed and not have to speak to anybody.'

5. Identify the type of question being used in each of these examples, using the categories listed earlier (i.e. closed question, open question, probing question, leading question):
    (a) 'You're feeling better today, aren't you?'
    (b) 'When is your baby due?'
    (c) 'How are you getting along with your new neighbours?'

6. How many of the following could be considered forms of reflection?
    (a) Paraphrasing what the client has said.
    (b) Repeating what the client has said.
    (c) Introducing a new subject into the conversation.
    (d) Repeating only the main points the client has made.

7. Comment on the following as ways that a care worker might end a conversation with an elderly, housebound client:
    (a) 'I might call in tomorrow if I get the chance.'
    (b) 'Remember to ask someone to get you those tablets. Bye!'
    (c) 'I'll see you on Tuesday at three. And don't forget – keep yourself warm!'

8. How many of the following kinds of behaviour are associated with active listening?
    (a) Concentrating fully on what the other person is saying.
    (b) Remaining silent even when the person speaking pauses.
    (c) Interrupting the other person when you feel it is time for you to respond.

9. What is meant by approaching a conversation with a client with preconceived ideas?
    (a) Beginning a conversation with a definite aim in mind.
    (b) Beginning a conversation with an open mind.
    (c) Beginning a conversation with ideas that are only half-formed.
    (d) Beginning a conversation having already made assumptions about the client.

10. Which ONE of the following statements is correct?

(a) If a child is not yet able to understand spoken language fully, paralanguage assumes greater importance when speaking to the child.

(b) If a child is not yet able to understand spoken language fully, we should not attempt to speak to the child.

(c) If a child is not yet able to understand spoken language fully, paralanguage becomes irrelevant.

11. Which ONE of the following statements is correct?

(a) When speaking to a visually impaired client it is important to raise one's voice.

(b) When speaking to a visually impaired client all aspects of non-verbal communication are irrelevant.

(c) When speaking to a visually impaired client paralanguage is especially important.

12. A good care worker encourages a client to believe which of the following?

(a) The client's needs are more important than anybody else's.

(b) The client's wishes are important and will be taken into consideration by the care worker.

(c) The client must co-operate or care may have to withdrawn.

2.2 Communication within groups

A great many of the points made in the preceding part of this Unit regarding communication between individuals have equal relevance to situations where more than two people are involved in the communication process. The essential principles of such skills as non-verbal communication, questioning and listening do not change because the interaction is of a group nature rather than one-to-one. However, **group communication** does have certain distinct characteristics and they will be considered in this second element.

What is a group?

Although in its loose everyday use the word 'group' can mean any collection of individuals, writers on human behaviour give the term a more precise meaning. Usually, a group is defined as three or more people sharing a common purpose or goal. Communication among members in order to achieve this purpose is another feature of groups. Thus a line of people queuing at a supermarket checkout may share a common goal but they cannot be considered a group.

In a health and social care context, groups sometimes consist exclusively of clients – the children in a playground, for example. Contrastingly, there are groups made up entirely of professionals – as when colleagues gather together for a case conference. The client and his family is another group commonly encountered by the care worker. The care worker may be readily accepted as a member of the group (as in the example of the case conference), or may need to win the trust of the other members before acceptance (the example of the client and his family). She may be on an equal footing with the other members of the group (the case conference) or she may be required to exercise leadership (the playgroup). In all these cases, some understanding of how group communication works would help the care worker to make a positive contribution to the business of the group.

Communication networks

The effectiveness of a group is heavily influenced by the way in which communication within the group is *organised* or *structured*. A **centralised network** of communication exists when communication is directed towards, and controlled by, a few members (or just one member) of the group. This occurs in the kind of network commonly known as the **wheel** as illustrated in Fig 2.2:

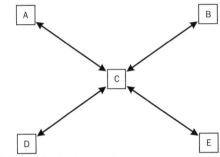

Figure 2.2   Centralised network

In this five-member group, communication is controlled by Member C. The other four members can communicate with Member C but not with each other.

In a **decentralised network** the communication channels are not centred upon a minority of the group in this way. An example of a decentralised network is the **circle** (Fig 2.3):

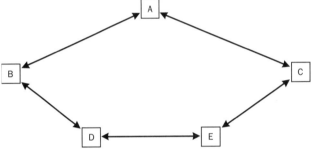

Figure 2.3   Decentralised network: the circle

Here each member communicates with two other members. Even more channels of communication are introduced if each member of the group is able to communicate with all the other members. This is known as the **all-channel** network (Fig 2.4):

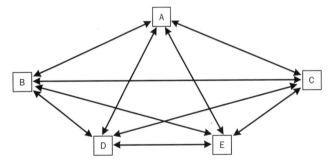

Figure 2.4   All-channel network

Of course many variations of these networks are possible, and many groups fall between the two extremes of the Wheel and the All-Channel network. For example, a group may have a central figure who controls most of the communication but the members of the group may still have some communication with each other. Here the degree of centralisation will depend on how far the leader exercises control and dominates communication within the group.

Research has been carried out into how *effective* these different kinds of groups are at performing tasks. It appears that centralised groups are efficient at performing simple tasks but that as tasks become more complex they become less efficient. This is possibly because more complex tasks place a greater burden upon the leader, and this burden eventually becomes excessive. It also seems that members of highly centralised groups tend to have low morale and to gain little satisfaction from group activities. This is understandable in view of the limited involvement each member has in the work of the group as a whole.

Research shows that a *decentralised group* in which the activities are not organised in any way is likely to be extremely inefficient. In such a group the members communicate with each other in an entirely random fashion and there is no coordination of group activity. You have probably at some time participated in a group discussion in which everyone tried to talk at once and which ended with you feeling that nothing had been achieved – this is an example of a decentralised group with no organisation! Research also suggests however that a decentralised group which is organised (with, for example, agreed procedures for decision-making) is capable of performing simple tasks and is actually more efficient than centralised groups at carrying out more complex tasks. The discussion group would have become organised if, for example, it had been agreed in advance that each member would be given an opportunity to express an opinion (and would be given a fair hearing), that the discussion would last a specific length of time and that a vote would be taken at the end. Such a discussion would be likely to have a more constructive outcome and would probably give the participants a greater feeling of satisfaction and achievement. Researchers have certainly found that members of decentralised groups tend to have higher morale, and are more likely to feel that they are making a worthwhile contribution to the work of the group.

Different situations give rise to different kinds of groups. Sometimes a leader who controls the communication that takes place is necessary, sometimes all members can participate as equals. For example, if a qualified instructor is demonstrating resuscitation procedures to a group of people with limited knowledge of first aid, the group is likely (initially at least) to be highly centralised, with most if not all communication channelled through the group leader. However, regardless of the structure or organisation of the group, two basic principles tend to be associated with successful group activity:

- A successful group is usually organised, and this organisation is directed towards achieving the purpose that the group has.
- The members of the group feel that their individual contributions are valued, and have a sense of involvement in the work of the group.

Participation

As indicated above, the effectiveness of a group is increased if all its members **participate** in the group's activities. This is partly because members who feel that they are making a positive contribution will gain satisfaction from this and will consequently work to make the group a success. The other reason is that participation by all ensures that the group benefits from the particular skills and expertise of each individual member. The individual member may well be able to offer the rest of the group specialist knowledge, relevant background information or simply a different point of view.

There are certain factors which frequently deter or prevent participation, and knowledge of these can help to ensure that they are avoided. They include:

- *Status* One or more members of the group may feel that others in the group have a higher status. As a result they may feel intimidated and reluctant to contribute. For example, if the family of a client is meeting a health or social care professional, they may regard the professional as very much the person in charge and may be unwilling to express their opinions or to ask questions. In such a situation the professional should try to put the family at ease and emphasize that contributions from them would be welcomed and valued. If a meeting consists entirely of professionals, some of the participants may defer to their more senior colleagues and feel that they have little or nothing to contribute. In fact, however, the more 'junior' members of the team are often closer to the client and therefore have a valuable contribution to make. For example, a nurse who is in regular daily contact with a patient may well have more insight into a patient's state of mind than a doctor who only visits the ward once a week. If a group has a leader, he or she may use this status to dominate the group and restrict the contributions made by other members. A good leader however will not do this – on the contrary, participation by all members of the group will be actively encouraged. (The qualities associated with good leadership will be discussed more fully later in the Unit.)

- *Personality*. Talkative, extrovert members of a group are likely to participate more than those who are quieter and more reserved. Here it is the responsibility of the group as a whole (and especially of the leader, if the group has one) to ensure that the group is not dominated by a few of its members, and that everybody is encouraged to contribute.

- *Physical position within the group*. This is related to the physical organisation of the group. For example, if people are seated in rows with the group leader seated at the front facing towards them, the greatest contribution is likely to come from the leader, while those at the back will be likely to contribute least. In contrast, sitting in a circle creates a feeling of equality and encourages freer communication between the members of the group. The **horseshoe** or **half-circle** arrangement is also common (Fig 2.5):

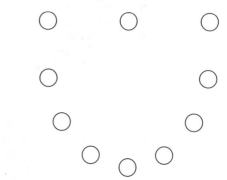

Figure 2.5   Horse-shoe arrangement

Here the leader is able to control or co-ordinate discussion when necessary, but the other members feel on an equal footing with each other and are able to communicate freely.

- *The size of the group.* Generally speaking, the larger the group, the more difficult it is for each individual member to make his or her presence felt. This is often impossible to control, but there are situations where it is advantageous for a large group to break up into several smaller groups, possibly coming together as a large group again later. This often happens in education: a teacher will divide a class into small groups, giving each group a different task; the groups then 'report back' to the class as a whole at the end of the lesson. This not only makes participation by every member of the class more likely; it also enables complex or time-consuming tasks to be sub-divided.

Roles within Groups

Another way in which the work of a group can be sub-divided is to assign a specific **role** to each member of the group. For example, if the staff of a day centre for the elderly are organising a trip to the seaside, one person might deal with the administrative arrangements (such as booking the coach), another might draw up a list of activities for the day, someone else might be asked to advertise the trip, and so on. This again ensures that all members of the group participate and is also a way of making sure that the particular skills of each member are utilised. If a group of professionals is dealing with a single client it is especially helpful for each professional to have a clearly defined role and for these roles to be explained to the client. This avoids creating confusion not only for the client but for the professionals also.

Experts on group interaction also use the word 'role' in another sense, to refer to the social behaviour of particular members. They have identified certain roles (or kinds of behaviour) as typical of small groups. For example, a group often has a critic, someone who frequently disagrees with the rest of the group and who seems always to look for the disadvantages of any proposed course of action. Other roles include the joker (whose contributions are usually lighthearted) and the harmoniser (who usually looks for compromise solutions and ways to bring the group together). The contributions of such group members can be positive: the critic can help to ensure the proposals are not accepted too readily and can point out difficulties that have been overlooked by other group members; the joker can release tension and help to create a relaxed atmosphere; the harmoniser can help to overcome conflict within the group. However, the behaviour of these same members can also be less beneficial: the critic may in some situations appear negative and obstructive; the joker's lightheartedness may sometimes seem inappropriate and a distraction; the harmoniser may seek to smother differences of opinion that ought to be aired more fully.

Do any of these roles match your own behaviour in group activity? (Or that of any other members of your course group?)

If you are a member of a group, you need to consider whether your behaviour tends to follow a certain pattern (always cracking jokes, for example!) and, if so, whether this behaviour is always helpful to the group as a whole. And while some acceptance of our own and others' failings is necessary in any group activity, the rest of the group (or the leader) should point out to a member when his or her behaviour is seriously impeding or disrupting the work of the group.

Group Conformity

Research has indicated that the decisions made by individuals when they are members of groups often differ significantly from the decisions they make when they are alone. In many groups there is a tendency towards **conformity** – that is, individuals will abandon (or modify) their own opinions and instead follow the views of the majority, or the views of the most influential members of the group. Conformity is especially likely in a group when some members have a higher status than the rest. Here the 'junior' members of the group may be reluctant to disagree with the senior members, or may assume that the senior members' judgement is better than their own. Conformity is also caused by social pressure – when everybody else in the group seems to be in agreement, it takes courage to be the odd one out and express an opposing view.

An *advantage* of conformity is that it creates a strong sense of group unity. As a result, members have a feeling of stability and security and the group presents a united front to the outside world. The business of the group is conducted smoothly and efficiently, unimpeded by conflict and disagreement.

However, group conformity can also have several *disadvantages*. It can lead to bad decisions, because the members of the group are too anxious to avoid criticising each other and become complacent, resistant to change and reluctant to look at alternatives. I. Janis coined the word '*groupthink*' to describe what happens when group conformity obstructs sensible and effective decision-making. Healthy, constructive discussion is prevented because the open expression of individual opinion is discouraged. The pressure to conform causes individuals to suppress their doubts and reservations. (A comparison can be made here with crowd behaviour: individuals caught up in a riot may behave very differently from when they are alone, and in ways which they later regret.)

It is important to try to avoid these negative consequences of group conformity. The atmosphere within the group should be such that the honest expression of opinion is encouraged, and there is a willingness to consider fresh ideas and alternative approaches. Disagreement with another's point of view should not be seen as personal animosity and criticism should not be regarded as disloyalty to the rest of the group. If you are a member of a group and have doubts about the position being taken by others, it is best to express these doubts at an early stage, before opinions among the group have become fixed. Group leaders, or high status members, should not seek to impose their own views on the rest of the group; they might help to ensure open discussion by asking the views of other members before expressing their own.

Leadership

Groups often have **leaders**, and leadership is often necessary to ensure that the group operates efficiently. The leader may be democratically elected by the rest of the group or appointed by an outside agency (as when the government sets up a committee to investigate an aspect of policy and appoints a particular individual as its chairperson). If the group is more informal, the personality of an individual member may cause him or her to emerge as leader, and to be accepted as such by the rest of the group. Leadership sometimes moves around a group, according to the activity the group is engaged in and the expertise of individual members.

If you work in the field of health and social care you may find yourself leading a group of clients, or leading a group of fellow professionals. In either case, it will help to know the qualities associated with good leadership, and the pitfalls to avoid.

Qualities of a good leader

Effective leadership often requires *preparation*. If you are chairing a meeting you may well need to prepare an agenda (a list of the items to be dealt with at the meeting) and to distribute these in advance to those who will be attending. You will need to think about the best order for the agenda items, and the approximate amount of time that is to be devoted to each. For any kind of group activity, you should ensure that you have all the information you are likely to need, as well as any other materials or resources that might be required (copies of charts or graphs for distribution to the group, for example). Preparation also involves anticipating any problems that might occur and planning how you will tackle them (for example, if there is disagreement over a particular proposal, will you be able to suggest a compromise?).

A good leader helps a group to *accomplish its objectives*. This means the leader must have a clear understanding of what the group's objectives are, and must ensure that the group understands them also. At a meeting, it is often appropriate to begin, after welcoming those in attendance, by clarifying the meeting's purpose ('We are here to consider...'; 'We need to decide today...').

As was established earlier in the Unit, a group functions more effectively if there is a high level of *participation* by its members. Encouraging and facilitating this participation is an important responsibility of the group leader. The leader should seek to create a relaxed, friendly atmosphere in which group members interact freely. He needs to ensure that the particular knowledge and expertise of each individual member are utilised by the group and he can help to achieve this by showing that each member's contribution is valued. Members will be less likely to contribute fully if the leader has a domineering, dictatorial attitude. Research indicates that, on the whole, democratic leadership of a group is more effective than autocratic leadership (see 'The Lewin, Lippit and White Experiment' below). A member who is contributing little needs to be encouraged to participate; correspondingly, a member who is dominating the proceedings needs to be quietened down. In both these situations tact is required: 'How do you feel about this, Susan?' is a better way of encouraging participation than a blunt 'Haven't you got anything to say?'. Similarly, the contributions of a dominant member need to be curtailed in such a way that he or she is not discouraged from participating altogether.

The Lewin, Lippit and White Experiment

This influential and widely-quoted experiment to discover the effectiveness of different leadership styles was carried out in the United States in 1939. The researchers focused upon three types of leadership:

- *Autocratic* – where the leader was authoritarian, making all important decisions and giving orders to the rest of the group.
- *Democratic* – where the leader was friendly, encouraged group involvement in the decision-making process and gave help and guidance when requested to do so.
- *Laissez-faire* – where the leader was passive, leaving decisions entirely to the group and making no attempt to direct or co-ordinate group activity.

Three groups of ten and eleven year old boys were formed at a recreational youth club, each led by an adult adopting one of the above leadership styles. The three groups undertook similar tasks – carving models from soap. The study revealed that the different kinds of leadership produced dramatically different results. The *autocratic group* produced the most models but were very dependent on the leader, losing concentration and misbehaving when he was out of the room. They also gained little enjoyment or satisfaction from the activity, often destroying their models after making them. The boys in the *democratic group* showed more initiative, were more cooperative towards each other and continued working when the leader left the room. They produced fewer models, but the work was of higher quality and the boys were proud of what they had achieved. In the *laissez-faire* group the boys produced the smallest number of models and took little interest in their work, failing to complete successfully tasks that they were set.

The clear conclusion to be drawn from the study is that a democratic leadership style (that is, one which encourages initiative, independence and participation) has several advantages. Later research has painted a more complex picture, suggesting that different kinds of leadership are effective under different conditions. For example, individuals accustomed to autocratic leadership may, initially at least, respond less effectively to a democratic leadership style. It is also the case that autocratic leadership in some situations is not only more effective but essential – if a fire breaks out in a hospital ward, for example, the nursing staff must issue clear, unambiguous instructions to the patients. Nevertheless, it remains broadly true that in most group situations a democratic approach leads to the successful completion of tasks and results in a high level of motivation and commitment.

As well as encouraging participation by group members, the leader must of course participate himself. Because the leader has a unique position within the group, certain kinds of contributions are more likely to come from the leader than from anyone else. These include:

- *Giving information/guidance* Often at the beginning of a discussion a group will need some basic information on the topic to be discussed, and this will usually be supplied by the leader. For example, a group meeting to organise a Christmas party at a nursing home might initially be told by the leader how much money is available, how many people are expected to attend and so on. Some of this information might be provided at appropriate points during the course of the meeting rather than at the beginning. If a group is engaged in practical activity of some kind (a group of volunteers decorating a children's nursery, for example), they might look to the leader for some initial guidance on how to proceed.

- *Clarifying what has been said/what has taken place* In a discussion, the leader needs to ensure that each member of the group has a clear understanding of what is said. This means intervening to clear up possible sources of confusion by interpreting or repeating what members have said, and by asking members themselves to clarify their own statements and opinions. Here the skill of *summarising* (see below) is also relevant. If a group is engaged in a practical project, it is helpful to pause occasionally to 'take stock'. In this situation the leader will clarify what has been achieved and what needs still to be done.

- *Moving on to another topic or another activity* Although, as has been seen, a dictatorial approach is counter-productive, the leader does need to direct the group in a helpful and constructive way. If a topic has been exhausted or discussion has become repetitive, the leader should seek to move the discussion along by introducing a new topic, or a different perspective on the existing one. As stated earlier, the leader must have a clear sense of the group's objectives and sometimes it will be necessary to curtail, re-organise or re-direct the activities of a group in order to ensure that these objectives are met.

- *Summarising* It is helpful if the leader provides at appropriate points a clear summing-up of the group's position. Depending on the situation, this might for example involve summarising: points of view that have been expressed; what has been agreed; what has been proposed; activities that have taken place. Summarising is especially important at the conclusion of a group session or meeting, but summaries at earlier stages in the proceedings of the group help to give members a clear understanding of where the group has reached and the direction it is taking.

A leader's responsibilities do not necessarily end when the session is over and the group's members have dispersed. The leader may need to arrange for decisions that have been made to be implemented. He may also need to compile a written record of what has taken place (possibly in the form of minutes). If the group is to meet again, preparation for the next session will be needed. Finally, any leader can improve his own leadership skills, and the effectiveness of the group he is leading, by reviewing the activity that has taken place. He will ask himself such questions as:

- Did the session achieve its objectives?
- If not, why not?
- Did all members of the group participate?
- Does everybody have a clear understanding of the decisions that have been made and the actions that are to be taken?

Checklist: characteristics of good and bad groups

It might be useful to conclude our discussion of communication within groups with a brief **checklist** of the main charac-

teristics associated with successful and unsuccessful groups. This is given below.

A good group:	A bad group:
Has clear objectives	Lacks clear objectives
Is organised in a way that helps it to achieve these objectives	Is disorganised: group activity is muddled and chaotic
Has an atmosphere which is friendly and relaxed but also purposeful	Has a tense, argumentative atmosphere or one which is friendly and relaxed but non-productive
Has participation by all members	Is dominated by one or more members and has some members who contribute little or nothing
Encourages frank discussion and the open expression of opinion	Has members who are reluctant to question the views of others
Has a leader who encourages all members to contribute but who also directs and co-ordinates in a constructive way	Has a leader who is dominant and dictatorial or who offers no guidance or co-ordination
Has members who feel a high level of motivation, commitment and satisfaction	Has members who are discontented and uninterested and who feel they are achieving little
Completes tasks effectively and fulfils its objectives	Fails to carry out tasks efficiently and to fulfil its objectives

Can you think of any additions to this list?

Self-check ✓ **Element 2**

13. Which ONE of the following statements is correct?
    (a) A decentralised group is often more democratic than a centralised group.
    (b) A decentralised group is often less democratic than a centralised group.
    (c) Communication in a decentralised group is always tightly controlled.
    (d) In a decentralised group all communication flows outwards from the central member to the other members.
14. Which of the following communication networks are centralised, and which decentralised?
    (a) The Circle
    (b) The Wheel
    (c) The All-Channel Network.
15. Research indicated which of the following to be true?
    (a) Members of centralised groups are usually highly motivated.
    (b) Centralised groups are especially effective at performing complex tasks.
    (c) Members of decentralised groups usually have higher morale than members of centralised groups.
16. Participation by all members is helpful in group activity because:
    (a) It means the leader can hand all his responsibilities over to the group members themselves.

(b) It will soon become clear who isn't pulling their weight and these members can be asked to leave the group.

(c) The morale of the group is likely to be higher.

17 How many of the following are possible consequences of the leader of the group having a higher status than other members?

(a) Other members may be reluctant to express their own views.

(b) Members who have a valuable contribution to make may feel discouraged from doing so.

(c) If the leader has good leadership skills the disadvantages of his superior status will be overcome.

(d) The leader may use his status to become dictatorial, undermining the effective working of the group

18. Which ONE of the following statements is correct?

(a) It is better not to have a role within a group because our behaviour can become too predictable.

(b) In all groups it is essential for each member to have a separate, clearly defined role.

(c) In a caring situation it can be helpful for a client to know the role of each professional she has contact with.

19. You are due to attend a meeting and know that your views on an issue that is to be discussed are different from those of several other group members. You need to decide how you will approach the meeting. Comment on the following as possible courses of action:

(a) Make a clear statement of your position at the beginning of the meeting and continue to argue your case strongly whenever you get the chance.

(b) Express your views early on but accept that what is said by others might cause you to change them.

(c) Wait until the rest of the members have made up their minds and see if your views have been changed by what you have heard.

20. You are leading a group discussion and John, one of the group members, is dominating the conversation. Of the three verbal responses to John's behaviour given below, which would you choose? Give reasons for your answer.

(a) 'You've given us plenty to think about John, but I think we need to hear other people's views.'

(b) 'John's made his position clear. Perhaps we can hear someone else's view then John can respond.'

(c) 'OK John, you've more than had your say. The best thing you can do now is to shut up.'

21. Research indicates which of the following to be true?

(a) Autocratic leadership fails to motivate group members and leads to inefficiency.

(b) Democratic leadership is usually preferred by group members but is inappropriate in some situations.

(c) Laissez-faire leadership is the most effective at motivating group members because it does not force them to do anything against their will.

22. How many of the following are characteristic of good group leaders?

(a) Inviting the views of others but ensuring that his view always prevails.

(b) Leaving the direction that a meeting takes entirely to members.

(c) Encouraging all members to participate.

(d) Never openly disagreeing with the views of other members.

2.3 Analyse clients' rights in interpersonal situations

This third Element extends our discussion of interpersonal interaction in the previous two Elements to a consideration of **clients' rights** in interpersonal situations. We shall be looking at ways in which the values which underpin health and social care work can be applied in practice, and at problems and difficulties which may arise when doing this. The four values which are central to all health and social care work are:

(i) Supporting individuals through effective communication;

(ii) promoting and supporting individual rights and choice;

(iii) maintaining confidentiality of information;

(iv) freedom from any type of discrimination.

Did You Know ?

The Canadian nurse-philosopher M.Simone Roach argues that the essential principles of caring all begin with the letter c. The 'Five Cs' of caring are:

Compassion
Competence
Confidence
Conscience
Commitment

(M.S. Roach: The Human Act of Caring. Canadian Hospital Association, 1987)

Supporting individuals through effective communication

This has already been discussed in the first Element of the Unit. In interpersonal situations the care worker should always be sensitive to a client's feelings and opinions, and should encourage the client to express these. Communication with a client should be understanding and supportive, and should take account of the client's particular needs and abilities.

Promoting and supporting individual rights and choice

Client independence

A client has the right to *self-determination* and to involvement in the making of decisions which affect his or her care. In recent years there has been a strong movement away from the old **paternalistic** approach to caring, which assumed that those responsible for the delivery of care always knew more than those receiving it. In nursing and other areas of health work this has been increasingly replaced by the concept of **individualised care**. This means that each patient is respected as an individual and that care is carefully planned to meet the patient's particular physical, psychological and emotional needs.

Receiving help from others inevitably reduces our sense of independence. In a care situation, if a client is in ill health or feels anxious, distressed or confused, the loss of independence will feel that much greater. Being in unfamiliar surroundings (such as a hospital, nursing home or clinic) can increase the sense of helplessness and loss of self-control. In a hospital, such factors as lying down while having a conversation with a doctor who is standing, and wearing nightclothes while the hospital staff are in uniform, increase the client's vulnerability.

It is the duty of the care worker to ensure that the client retains as much independence as possible. This involves allowing clients to do as much for themselves as they can and avoiding situations which might threaten clients' dignity or put clients at a disadvantage (patients in hospital, for example, are increasingly encouraged to wear their usual clothes during the day).

Giving information to clients is important

An important means of reducing the feeling of dependence upon others that clients might have is to give them *information* about the care they are receiving. Clients have the right to be kept informed about the nature and purposes of the care that is planned for them. This might involve for example explaining how a particular medicine will help in the treatment of an illness, or describing the routines and procedures of a nursing home to someone who has newly arrived. Information about health and social care services can also be presented in the form of posters and leaflets, and in areas with a significant ethnic minority population these should be available in the relevant languages.

Involve clients in decision-making

Sharing information with clients helps to involve them in the *decisions* that are made about their own care. The client's opinions should be sought, and wherever possible the caring that takes place should be shaped and modified in the light of these. Where the physical or psychological state of the client limits his or her ability to participate in decision-making, it might be appropriate to consult the client's family.

There is much evidence to indicate that the provision of information is welcomed by clients. Surveys have repeatedly shown that lack of information is one of the main causes of dissatisfaction among users of the health and social care services. Research also suggests that lack of information can cause anxiety, while giving information to clients can have a therapeutic effect. A study carried out in the Psychology Unit of the Royal Free Hospital in London, for example, suggested that patients who feel in control of their own treatment tend to recover more quickly from illness.

Special considerations apply to children and the elderly

Special considerations arise where children and the elderly are concerned. It is sometimes necessary to be less frank with children and there are of course decisions which very young children cannot be expected to make. Nevertheless it should always be remembered that every child is an individual, with his or her own preferences, anxieties and needs. As much as adults, children are likely to respond positively if the care or treatment they are to receive is explained to them in ways they are able to understand. Where it is appropriate to allow the child some freedom of choice, this should be given. (For a fuller discussion of the rights of children see the section on Children's Rights on page 35).

Old age is often accompanied by an increased dependence upon the assistance of others, whether in the form of greater health care or help with everyday tasks such as dressing and shopping. This process can be accelerated by care workers who are over-protective and who do too much for their clients. Such care workers may believe they are acting in their client's best interests, but they should instead be seeking to preserve and, where possible, increase the client's independence. For a client recovering from an illness, this might involve setting realistic goals for the client to achieve (an example might be being able to put her shoes on unaided by a certain date). Patience and flexibility are needed here: clients should not be pushed into doing more than they can comfortably manage and they will need more help on some days than on others. Where help is necessary, clients should be given as much choice as possible: if a client is not able to dress herself, for example, she should at least be able to choose the clothes that she wears.

Consent

An important principle of health and social care is that a client should not receive care or treatment unless he or she **consents** to it. This is a right that is protected by law. In a hospital, for example, an operation under local or general anaesthetic may only be performed if the patient signs a CONSENT FORM. These vary slightly from hospital to hospital, but follow a fairly standard format. A form from the Royal Liverpool University Hospital is reproduced in Figure 2.6.

For consent to be meaningful it must be INFORMED. The treatment proposed must be explained to the client so that he is aware of the implications of his decision. In signing a consent form the patient declares that he has been given such an explanation.

Difficulties arise when a client is not in a position to make a decision regarding his care. A patient in a hospital, for example, may be unconscious. In a case such as this, responsibility for consent falls upon the next of kin. Legally, a patient can also be treated without consent in the following instances:

(i) If the patient has a notifiable disease or is carrying an organism capable of causing one.

(ii) If the patient has been detained under the Mental Health Act (1983).

Where a client lacks the mental capacity to make an informed decision about care or treatment, the care worker should always act in the client's best interests.

Adult patients also have the right to discharge themselves from hospital, unless they fall into one of the two categories mentioned above. If they do so against the advice of hospital staff, they will usually be asked to sign a form declaring this to be the case and accepting responsibility for the consequences of their action.

Did You Know ?

Despite being asked to sign consent forms, many patients do not receive a clear explanation of the operation that is about to be performed. A group of investigators interviewed 100 consecutive patients having operations in a Scottish surgical unit, two to five days after the operations had been performed. 27 did not know which organ had been operated on, and 44 did not know what procedure had been performed. (D.J. Bryne, A. Napier and A. Cuschieri – How Informed is Signed Consent? Institute of Medical Ethics Bulletin 37)

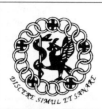

Royal Liverpool University Hospital

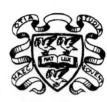

PRESCOT STREET LIVERPOOL L7 8XP TEL: 051-706 2000 FAX: 051-706 5806

CONSENT FORM

For medical or dental investigation, treatment or operation

Patient's Surname.. Date of Birth...

Other Names.. Unit Number...

Sex: *(please tick)* Male ☐ Female ☐

DOCTORS OR DENTISTS *(This part to be completed by doctor or dentist. See notes on the reverse)*

TYPE OF OPERATION, INVESTIGATION OR TREATMENT

I confirm that I have explained to the patient the operation, investigation or treatment, and such appropriate options as are available and that an anaesthetic may be required, in terms which in my judgement are suited to the understanding of the patient (and/or to one of the parents or guardians of an under-age patient).

Signature .... Date ....

Name of doctor/dentist ....

I confirm that I have explained the type of anaesthetic to the patient in terms which in my judgement are suited to the understanding of the patient (and/or to one of the parents or guardians of an under-age patient)

Signature .... Date ....

Name of anaesthetist ....

PATIENT/PARENT/GUARDIAN

Please read this form and the notes overleaf very carefully.

If there is anything you don't understand about the explanation, or if you want more information, you should ask the doctor or dentist.

Please check that all the information on the form is correct. If it is, and you understand the explanation, then sign the form.

I am the patient/parent/guardian *(delete as necessary)*

I agree ■ to what is proposed which has been explained to me by the doctor/dentist named on this form.

■ to the use of the type of anaesthetic that I have been told about.

I understand ■ that the procedure may not be done by the doctor/dentist who has been treating me so far.

■ that any procedure in addition to the investigation or treatment described on this form will only be carried out if it is necessary and in my best interests and can be justified for medical reasons.

I have told ■ the doctor or dentist about any additional procedures I would **not** wish to be carried out straightaway without my having the opportunity to consider them first.

Name .... Signature ....

Address ....

(if not the patient) ....

.... Telephone Number ....

WNN002 MED/01.562 (3/92)

Figure 2.6   Example of a consent form

Children's rights

Special guidelines and considerations apply when the client is a **child**. Sixteen and seventeen year old minors have a statutory right to give consent to treatment and this includes diagnostic procedures as well as medical treatment requiring the use of anaesthetics. For children under the age of sixteen the right of consent rests with the parents.

Nevertheless, a child below the age of sixteen who is capable of understanding the care or treatment he is receiving has a moral right to have that care or treatment explained to him. As in so many care situations, a combination of tact, sensitivity and simple common sense is needed. Obviously a nine month old baby is incapable of expressing an informed opinion. A twelve year old girl, however, can understand a great deal and should be helped to reach this understanding by having her treatment clearly and patiently explained to her. While parents have the legal right of consent, they should be encouraged to explain decisions to children, and to take their views and opinions into account. The principle of involving children actively in their own care is reflected in the **Children Act** (1989).

The Children Act 1989

This Act of Parliament replaced almost all of the previous legislation relating to children and created a single coherent framework for the welfare of children. The Act asserts that 'the child's welfare is paramount', and emphasises that when decisions are made that affect the welfare of a child the interests of the child must always come first. It stresses the importance of consulting children and taking account of their views. The idea that parents have rights over children is replaced in the Act by an emphasis on the *responsibilities* of parents towards children. Parents have a duty to care for their children and the role of the health and social care services is to help them in this task. Health and social care professionals should therefore work in partnership with parents and seek to involve them in the care of their children as much as possible.

Access to information

Clients have certain legal **rights of access** to records that are kept about them. These rights have been granted relatively recently. The idea that more information about their own care should be made available to clients reflects the growing belief that health and social care professionals should be more open with clients.

The Data Protection Act 1984 gives access to any information which is contained on computer. The Access To Health Records Act 1990 extends the right of access to handwritten records completed after November 1991. The Act applies to records compiled by or on behalf of a health professional. The term 'health professional' is broadly defined and includes for example doctors, nurses, midwives, health visitors and physiotherapists. It does not include social workers, though access to social work and housing records is granted under the Access To Personal Files Act 1987.

Access rights are however subject to important exceptions. In particular, records cannot be disclosed if disclosure is likely to cause serious mental or physical harm to the client. Another exception is where disclosure would lead to the identification of a third party who has not consented to the disclosure – someone who has given information in confidence, for example.

The right to choice

Closely linked to the right to independence is the client's **right to choice**. Wherever possible, clients should be made aware of the care options available to them and encouraged to make an informed choice between them. In recent years government legislation has deliberately sought to increase clients' freedom of choice. It has become easier to change one's GP, for example, and GPs are required to list the services they offer to help people decide which practice to join. Opticians are allowed to advertise and now compete for custom like other high street shops.

In practice, however, there are several limitations to client choice. GPs, for instance, are usually only willing to cover a defined geographical area and applicants from outside the district will be rejected. Financial considerations and the need for care to be delivered efficiently also restrict choice. A hospital patient may wish for a private room but in most cases such a room will not be available. If a nursing home has forty residents, it would be impractical to allow them all to choose their own meal-times. The needs of other clients are another constraint. One hospital patient may wish to watch a late night film on television, while another may complain that the noise of the television will make it difficult for her to sleep.

Complete freedom of choice is therefore impossible. The care worker should nevertheless seek to give the maximum freedom possible, while recognising that some constraints are inevitable. The scheduling of meal-times in the nursing home might allow for some flexibility for example, and it should be possible to offer some choice of food. The television in the hospital ward might be temporarily moved to another room, so that it will not disturb other patients.

Where alternative care options are available to a client, the care worker should explain clearly what these options are, providing the information necessary for the client to make an informed choice. If the care worker's own knowledge of a topic is limited, she might suggest to the client where the relevant information could be found. A number of bodies exist to advise and support clients, making it easier for them to exercise their right of choice. The Community Health Councils, for example, advise patients on health provision in their area and on complaints procedures.

The Patient's Charter

Many of the rights that we have been examining are contained within the **Patient's Charter**, issued by the Department of Health in 1991. This explains the rights of patients who use the National Health Service, and also sets national and local standards on such subjects as waiting for an ambulance and for outpatient treatment. The charter does not give any additional legal rights but it provides a standard against which care can be measured and can be used as a basis for complaints. It sets out seven existing rights within the NHS and establishes three new rights. In addition to the national charter there are local charters, in which individual health authorities set and publicise their standards for patient care. The main elements of the Patient's Charter are summarised below.

THE PATIENT'S CHARTER

Citizens' existing rights within the National Health Service

- to receive health care on the basis of clinical need, regardless of ability to pay
- to be registered with a GP
- to receive emergency medical care at any time, through your GP or the emergency ambulance service and hospital accident and emergency departments
- to be referred to a consultant, acceptable to you, when your GP thinks it necessary and to be referred for a second opinion if you and your GP agree this is desirable.
- to be given a clear explanation of any treatment proposed, including any risks and any alternatives, before you decide whether you will agree to the treatment
- to have access to your health records, and to know that those working for the NHS will, by law, keep their records confidential
- to choose whether or not you wish to take part in medical research or medical student training.

Three new rights

- to be given detailed information on local health services, including quality standards and maximum waiting times. You will be able to get this information from your health authority, GP or Community Health Council
- to be guaranteed admission for virtually all treatments by a specific date no later than two years from the day when your consultant places you on a waiting list
- to have any complaint about NHS services – whoever provides them – investigated by your health authority or general manager of your hospital

Nine standards of service which the NHS will aim to provide

- respect for privacy, dignity and religious and cultural beliefs
- arrangements to ensure everyone, including people with special needs, can use the services
- information to relatives and friends about the progress of your treatment, subject to your wishes
- an emergency ambulance should arrive within fourteen minutes in an urban area, or nineteen minutes in a rural area
- when attending an accident and emergency department, you will be seen immediately and your need for treatment assessed
- when you go to an outpatient clinic, you will be given a specific appointment time and will be seen within thirty minutes of it
- your operation should not be cancelled on the day you are due to arrive in hospital. If your operation has to be postponed twice you will be admitted to hospital within one month of the second cancelled operation
- a named qualified nurse, midwife or health visitor responsible for your nursing or midwifery care
- a decision should be made about any continuing health or social care needs you may have, before you are discharged from hospital

THE NAWCH CHARTER

- children shall be admitted to hospital only if the care they require cannot be equally well provided at home or on a day basis
- children in hospital shall have the right to have their parents with them at all times provided this is in the best interests of the child. Accommodation should therefore be offered to all parents, and they should be helped and encouraged to stay. In order to share in the care of their child, parents should be fully informed about ward routine and their active participation encouraged
- children and their parents shall have the right to information appropriate to their age and understanding
- children and their parents shall have the right to informed participation in all decisions involving their health care. Every child shall be protected from unnecessary medical treatment, and steps taken to mitigate physical and emotional distress
- children shall be treated with tact and understanding and at all times their privacy shall be respected
- children shall enjoy the care of appropriately trained staff, fully aware of the physical and emotional needs of each age group
- children shall be able to wear their own clothes and have their own personal possessions
- children shall be cared for with other children of the same age group
- children shall be in an environment furnished and equipped to meet their requirements, and which conforms to recognised standards of safety and supervision
- children shall have full opportunity for play, recreation and education suited to their age and condition

Maintaining confidentiality of information

Clients also have a right to **confidentiality**. The special circumstances of the client–care worker relationship mean that the care worker may well be given information which the client would not normally reveal to others. Further personal information about the client may be divulged by the client's family, or contained within medical or social work records to which the care worker has access.

There is a duty to regard such information as confidential. Only if the right to confidentiality is maintained can clients be expected to trust care workers and speak freely about their feelings and their needs.

Boundaries to confidentiality: sharing information with other professionals

There are however situations in which it may be necessary to share information about a client with others. The most common of these is when it is in the client's own interests for information to be passed on to other health and social care professionals. The care offered to a client who is in ill health, for example, may be improved by seeking the assistance of a doctor who specialises in a particular type of illness. Here the client should be told that the information is to be passed on, and the reasons for doing so should be explained.

The NAWCH Charter

A separate charter relating specifically to the care of children in hospital has been produced by the **National Association for the Welfare of Children in Hospital** (NAWCH):

Boundaries to confidentiality: legal requirements

There are also situations where the law may require information to be revealed. This is usually where the concealment of information is considered to be against the public interest. Public health legislation, for example, requires information relating to infectious diseases to be passed to the Community Medical Officer. AIDS and HIV–positive cases are covered by specific legislation. The Prevention of Terrorism and Misuse of Drugs Acts also require disclosure of information in certain circumstances. The legal limits to the confidentiality of social work files includes the requirement of disclosure if requested in the interests of national security, law enforcement or revenue purposes, or if ordered by a court.

Boundaries to confidentiality: safety of clients

Situations can arise where the client's own safety is at risk if information is not passed on to others. In cases of self-inflicted injury, for example, or where a child appears to be the victim of abuse, there is a moral as well as a legal obligation to take action to protect the client.

Boundaries to confidentiality: threats to the rights and safety of others

Information disclosed by a client may indicate that others are at risk, and here again the client's right to confidentiality will be overridden by the duty to protect the well-being of others as well as the client. If a client intends causing harm – to a member of his family, for example – action must clearly be taken to prevent this happening.

Freedom from any type of discrimination

In Unit 1 Element 2 **discrimination** was defined and various types and bases of discrimination were outlined. Discrimination usually occurs when we act on the basis of a prejudice, to the advantage of some groups and individuals and to the disadvantage of others. Discrimination can be *overt* (open and direct) or *covert* (hidden and subtle). Bases for discrimination (that is, the grounds on which people might be discriminated against) include:

- race
- gender
- age
- physical ability
- cognitive ability

A central value of health and social care work is that clients should not suffer any form of discrimination. Treatment of clients should be *non-judgmental*: that is, care workers should not make judgements about a client's lifestyle, culture, religion and so on. Britain is a multicultural society, and clients and care workers often come from different cultural backgrounds. It is important for care workers not to believe that their own beliefs and values are superior to those of their clients. Neither should they make assumptions about clients on the grounds of age, gender or any of the other bases for discrimination listed above. They should not assume, for example, that because a client is elderly his opinions are of less importance, or that a client with learning difficulties is entitled to less privacy than other clients.

Some forms of discrimination are obvious (verbal abuse, for example), but discrimination is frequently more subtle and often it is unintentional. Body language, for example, can indicate that a care worker has less respect for certain clients than others. The way that services and facilities are organised may mean in effect that certain groups have less access than others. A day centre may offer a restricted lunch time menu, excluding items required by the religion and culture of some members of the community. Posters and leaflets advertising local services may not be available in languages used by ethnic minority groups.

All forms of discrimination undermine the respect that should always be shown for the beliefs, values and opinions of the individual client.

 Self-check ✓ **Element 3**

23. Individualised care means:
    (a) In a group the needs of the group are more important than the needs of any one individual.
    (b) Care is designed to meet the particular needs of the individual client.
    (c) Care is the responsibility of the individual care worker.
    (d) Giving a hospital patient his or her own room.

24. How many of the following might help a hospital patient to retain a sense of independence?
    (a) Giving the patient a choice of menu at meal times.
    (b) Allowing the patient to wear his or her own clothes.
    (c) Involving the patient in the decisions that are made concerning his or her care.
    (d) Aiding the restoration of mobility after an operation.

25. Comment on the following statements about the care of children:
    (a) Children cannot exercise freedom of choice until they are sixteen.
    (b) Parents should leave all decisions regarding the care of their children to health and social care professionals.
    (c) Children are entitled to have their opinions taken into consideration.
    (d) Children are too young to be consulted about their care.

26. A Consent Form is used in a hospital:
    (a) When an operation under local or general anaesthetic is to be performed.
    (b) When a patient is about to be discharged.
    (c) When a patient is given tablets for the first time.
    (d) When a patient is moved to another ward.

27. The Children Act 1989:
    (a) Emphasises the rights that parents have over children.
    (b) Recommends stiffer punishment for children who play truant.
    (c) Emphasises the responsibilities that parents have towards children.
    (d) Emphasises that the rights and wishes of parents are paramount.

28. Comment on the following as ways of promoting clients' right to choice:
    (a) Insisting that one occupant of a shared room in a nursing home allows the other occupant to listen to the radio until midnight every night.
    (b) Explaining the care options available to a client so that he or she can make an informed choice.
    (c) When dealing with a group of clients, only taking decisions for which there is unanimous agreement.
    (d) Negotiating with a client convenient times for a health visitor to call.

29. Community Health Councils
    (a) Advise clients on health provision in a particular area.
    (b) Are run by locally elected councillors.
    (c) Are financed by voluntary contributions.
    (d) Control the budgets of local hospitals.

30. The Patient's Charter:
    (a) Replaces all local charters.
    (b) Lists patients' demands for a better Health Service.
    (c) Explains the rights of patients who use the National Health Service.
    (d) Is a guide to all services offered by the National Health Service.

31. The Patient's Charter asserts that within an urban area an emergency ambulance ought to arrive:
    (a) Within five minutes.
    (b) Within eight minutes.
    (c) Within fourteen minutes.
    (d) Within twenty minutes.

32. In how many of the following situations should confidential information about a client be disclosed?
    (a) When disclosure is necessary to protect the safety of the client.
    (b) When disclosure is necessary to protect the safety of others.
    (c) When information is requested by the client's family.
    (d) When information is requested by close friends of the client.

33. Non-judgmental behaviour in the care of clients means:
    (a) Assumptions based on prejudice are not made about clients.
    (b) Decisions made about care are not arrived at too hastily.
    (c) Clients are consulted before important decisions are taken.
    (d) An open mind is kept about the care that a client might need.

Answers to Self-check questions

1. (b)

2. (a) YES
   (b) YES This is an aspect of paralanguage, a component of non-verbal communication.
   (c) NO This is verbal communication.

3. (c)

4. (a) This is not the kind of self-disclosure a care worker should make. The client's problems are dismissed, when they should be the care worker's central concern. The care worker suggests that his/her own problems are more important, which a care worker should never do.
   (b) Again unsatisfactory. The care worker is burdening the client with his/her own problems and suggesting that the purpose of their conversation is to sort out the care worker's difficulties rather than to help the client.
   (c) A good example of helpful self-disclosure. The care worker is sympathetic and shows empathy. The care worker might go on to discuss ways of dealing with the kind of feeling that both care worker and client have experienced.

5. (a) Leading question
   (b) Closed question
   (c) Open question

6. (a), (b) and (d)

7. (a) This is unsatisfactory because the care worker is not definite enough. The client is left not knowing whether the care worker will call or not. 'If I get the chance' might also suggest that the client is low on the care worker's list of priorities.
   (b) A positive aspect of this conversation ending is that the care worker reminds the client of the need to obtain some tablets. However, 'ask someone' is much too vague – the care worker should have clarified with the client exactly who could be depended upon to get the tablets, and if necessary might have made the arrangements herself.
   (c) This is the best of the three. The client knows exactly when the care workers will next call. The final 'keep

yourself warm!' reminds the client of the importance of doing this and shows that the care worker is concerned about the client.

8. (a) YES
   (b) NO A pause is often an appropriate moment to offer the speaker encouragement, by saying something like 'Yes, I see' or 'Please go on'.
   (c) NO Generally, you should allow the other person to finish speaking before responding.

9. (d)

10. (a)

11. (c)

12. (a) NO The client's needs are important, but do not necessarily override those of other people. A patient in a hospital ward, for example, should not be encouraged to believe that his needs are more important than those of the other patients.
    (b) YES
    (c) NO This kind of threat should not be used.

13. (a)
14. (a) Decentralised
    (b) Centralised
    (c) Decentralised

15. (a) FALSE
    (b) FALSE
    (c) TRUE

16. (a) NO Although a good leader encourages participation, he still has his own particular responsibilities to fulfil.
    (b) NO If members are not 'pulling their weight' attempts should be made to increase their involvement in the activity of the group.
    (c) YES Participation in group activity does increase members' morale.

17. (a), (b), (c) and (d)

18. (c)

19. (a) The first part of this proposed course of action ('Make a clear statement of your position at the beginning of the meeting') is sensible. However, the second part ('continue to argue your case strongly whenever you get the chance') would suggest that you approach the meeting with a closed mind. You ought to be prepared to change your mind if the arguments put forward by others are persuasive enough.
    (b) A sensible course of action. You make sure your views are known but do not adopt a rigid and inflexible approach. Listening to others may change your views or persuade you to agree to a compromise, and you accept this.
    (c) Not a wise approach. If you wait until others have made up their minds you are unlikely to be able to persuade them to change them!

20. (a) This is a good response. It acknowledges the contribution John has made but makes clear that it is now time for others to be heard.
    (b) This does invite someone else to contribute but asking John to respond to this contribution suggests that the focus of attention will soon return to him and he will continue to dominate the meeting. The leader is allowing the discussion to revolve around one person.
    (c) An unsatisfactory response because it is blunt and discourteous. It may well deter John from making any further contributions to the group.

21. (a) FALSE
    (b) TRUE
    (c) FALSE

22. (c) only.

23. (b)

24. (a), (b), (c) and (d)

25. (a) This is too sweeping. It is true of some situations (e.g. a child cannot choose to leave school until the age of sixteen) but not of others. In a caring context, there are many situations where a child below the age of sixteen could and should be given freedom of choice.
    (b) No. Parents should be involved in the care of their children and share in decision-making.
    (c) Yes. This is an important principle in health and social care.
    (d) Again this is too sweeping. It depends on the age of the child – a six month old baby clearly cannot be consulted, but a fourteen year old girl should be.

26. (a)

27. (c)

28. (a) This affords choice to the client who listens to the radio but not to the other occupant of the room! A compromise solution, respecting the wishes of both individuals, should be reached. The client who listens to the radio might for example obtain a set of headphones.
    (b) This is a good way of promoting the right to choice.
    (c) This is impractical. It would be better to take democratic decisions (based on the will of the majority) or, where there is disagreement, to seek compromise solutions.
    (d) Like (b), this is a good way of promoting the right of choice.

29. (a)

30. (c)

31. (c)

32. (a) and (b). Disclosure to a client's family or friends ((c) and (d)) should only take place with the consent of the client.

33. (a)

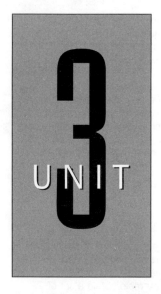

Physical aspects of health

Getting Started

Element 1   How body systems inter-relate.
Element 2   Human disease.
Element 3   Components of a healthy diet.

This unit will look at the functions of the **body systems,** in particular the heart and lungs. It will also look at the degenerative changes that are associated with the body systems during various life stages, and how the body can be affected by a person's choice of life-style.

Unit 3 will also examine the importance of taking responsibility for one's own health, by understanding the importance of a balanced diet, regular exercise, not smoking and the avoidance of stress. This unit will also look at the prevention and control of common diseases, and how nutrition and socio-economic factors can affect the pattern of disease.

Useful Cross-references

Unit 4 Element 3   Health maintenance, life event threats, stress related illnesses.
Unit 5 Element 2   Health and promotion advice.
Unit 5 Element 3   Substance abuse, risk from unsafe sexual practices.

Aerobic Involving the use of oxygen.

Anaerobic Taking place without the use of oxygen.

Arteries A type of blood vessel carrying blood away from the heart.

Assimilation Food absorbed and utilised by the body.

Balanced diet A diet which contains the correct types of food in the correct proportions for that individual's needs.

Capillaries A type of blood vessel carrying blood *away from* the heart.

Cardiac cycle Each complete beat of the heart.

Contagious disease A disease spread by direct contact.

Degenerative changes Changes associated with the ageing process.

Diastole When parts of the heart relax.

Disease A condition in which an organism is not functioning properly.

Exhalation Breathing out; sometimes called 'expiration'.

Health A state of complete physical, mental and social well-being, and not merely the absence of disease or infirmity.

Infectious disease A disease which can be transmitted from one person to another.

Ingestion The breaking down of food so that it can be absorbed.

Inhalation Breathing in; sometimes called 'inspiration'.

Respiration The release of energy from the breakdown of food molecules within living cells.

Systole When parts of the heart contract.

Vegan A diet which excludes any product which involves the 'exploitation' of animals.

Veins A type of blood vessel carrying blood towards the heart.

Essential Principles

3.1 How the body systems inter-relate

In this element we will look at the **body systems,** how they work together, and at the degenerative changes that occur. We will also look at lifestyle choices and how they effect one's health.

To be able to do this we must understand:

- the functions of the body's systems.
- the structure and the function of the heart, blood vessels, air passages and lungs.
- the degenerative changes during various life changes.
- the changes associated with body systems as a consequence of life-style choice.

Functions of the body systems

The functions of the body can be broken down into the following key systems.

- **Circulatory System** – This system transports substances around the body, in blood. For example it carries oxygen, glucose and amino acids to cells and carries waste away from the cells, such as urea and carbon dioxide.

- **Digestive System** – This system breaks down the food we eat and absorbs the digested food into the blood.

- **Excretory System** – This system removes unwanted and harmful waste products; e.g. urea produced by the liver is removed by the kidneys.

- **Reproductive System** – This system produces eggs or sperm that pass on genetic information to create future generations.

- **Skeletal System** – This system protects and supports the organs and muscles and enables the muscles to move the body.

- **Nervous System** – This system controls all the organs in the body and enables the body to respond to information received by sensory cells.

- **Respiratory System** – This system takes in oxygen and removes carbon dioxide.

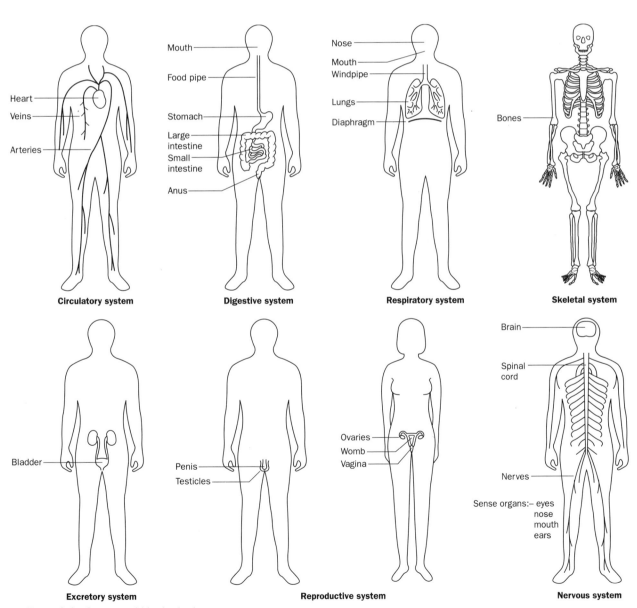

Figure 3.1   Systems within the body

The structure and function of the heart

We are now going to look at the **cardio-vascular** and **respiratory** systems in rather more detail.

The Heart

The **heart** lies in the *thoracic cavity* between the lungs. It is a muscular pump which keeps the blood moving around the body, through the circulatory system. The heart consists of 2 fused pumps which pump either *oxygenated* (oxygen containing) blood to the body (from the left side) or *deoxygenated* blood to the lungs (from the right side).

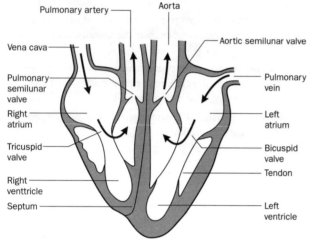

Figure 3.2   The heart

The heart (Fig 3.2) is further divided into 2 components, Right and Left *atrium* and Right and Left *ventricle* which allow the blood to be pumped in 2 stages (Fig 3.3). The atria pump blood into the ventricles. The ventricles then pump blood to the lungs (right ventricle) or round the rest of the body (left ventricle). The left ventricle has a thicker and more muscular wall than the right ventricle, because it has more work to do.

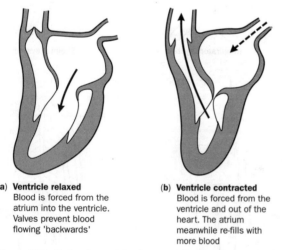

(a) Ventricle relaxed
Blood is forced from the atrium into the ventricle. Valves prevent blood flowing 'backwards'

(b) Ventricle contracted
Blood is forced from the ventricle and out of the heart. The atrium meanwhile re-fills with more blood

Figure 3.3   Role of ventricles in pumping blood

Valves

The **heart valves** keep the blood moving in the correct direction and prevent back-flow.

There are 4 main valves (see Fig 3.2 above)

(1) **Bicuspid (mitral)** – This is the valve between the left atrium and left ventricle.

(2) **Tricuspid** – This is the valve between the right atrium and right ventricle.

(3) **Aortic semilunar** – This is the valve between the left ventricle and the aorta.

(4) **Pulmonary semilunar** – This is the valve between the right ventricle and the pulmonary artery.

Blood travels towards the heart with the assistance of pressure from surrounding skeletal muscle (see Fig 3.4). Deoxygenated blood from all parts of the body enters the right side of the heart via the vena cava into the right atrium; the right atrium contracts and the blood then passes through the tricuspid valve into the right ventricle. Due to the contractions and gravity of the arterial wall in the right ventricle, blood is driven into the pulmonary artery. This divides into two branches, the right and left pulmonary arteries, which carry the blood to the lungs, and oxygen is taken in and carbon dioxide is given off. Blood is collected into the four pulmonary veins, which empty into the left atrium. The left atrium contracts and drives blood into the left ventricle. The left ventricle contracts and drives blood into the aorta. Blood is then distributed to all parts of the body to supply the tissues with oxygen, foods and water and to remove waste products.

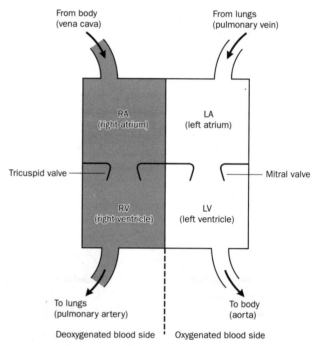

Figure 3.4   Blood flow

Cardiac cycle

The **heart beat** is controlled automatically in a continuous series of rhythmic muscular contractions, which is generated within the muscle itself and is not due to a nervous stimulus. Each repeating sequence is called a **cardiac cycle**. The frequency and power of each contraction depends on the body's need for blood and it is regulated by the brain. An adult heart beat is approximately 60 – 80 beats per minute. A normal pulse rate for an infant is 100 – 120 beats per minute and for a child aged 6 – 10 years old it is 80 – 100 beats per minute. The heart beat can also be increased by exercise. The heart can also regulate itself by a specialised cardiac fibre called the **Sino-Atrial Node** (see below) which acts as a pacemaker embedded in the right atrium. If a person's pacemaker fails to work, an artificial one can be implanted.

- **Cardiac muscle**
  The heart can continue to contract rhythmically for a very long time without tiring, possibly because of the nature of the **cardiac muscle**. This muscle consists of a network of interconnected fibres. The rhythmical contractions of the cardiac muscle are generated within the muscle itself and are not due to nervous stimulation.

- **Pacemaker**
  We have seen that in the wall of the right atrium there is a region of specialised cardiac fibres called the **sino-atrial node (SAN)** which acts as a **pacemaker** and initiates the heartbeat. A wave of electrical stimulation arises at this point and then spreads over the two atria. This causes the atria to contract. The stimulation reaches another specialised region of cardiac fibres, the **atrio-ventricular node (AVN)**, and causes that to pass on the stimulation to specialised tissue in the ventricles. From the AVN, the stimulation passes along the **bundle of His** and then spreads through the **Purkinje tissue** in the walls of the ventricles. As with the atria, stimulation is followed by contraction and the walls of the ventricle contract simultaneously.

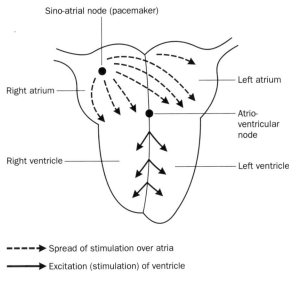

Figure 3.5 The heartbeat

- **Heart rate**
  The *rate* at which the heart beats can be modified by the nervous system; stimulation of the **vagus nerve** will slow down the heartbeat, but stimulation of the **sympathetic nerve** will accelerate it. The heartbeat can also be influenced by many non-nervous stimuli, such as temperature and hormones.

- **Systole and Diastole**
  A single cardiac cycle (single heartbeat) consists of **atrial systole**, when the atria contract, **ventricular systole**, when the ventricles contract, and **diastole**, when both pairs of

chambers relax. The whole process takes about 0.8 seconds, and as we have seen it is maintained by the heart's own pacemaker acting on the cardiac muscle.

> REMEMBER THE FOLLOWING: When parts of the heart CONTRACT it is in a state of SYSTOLE. When parts of the heart RELAX it is in a state of DIASTOLE.

Structure and function of the heart
The following chart outlines the main components of the heart and their various functions.

Heart	Function
Aorta	Carries oxygenated blood to all the organs except the lungs. It is the largest artery in the body.
Pulmonary artery	Carries deoxygenated blood to the lungs.
Pulmonary vein	Carries oxygenated blood from the lungs to the left atrium of the heart
Left atrium	Receives oxygenated blood from the lungs via the pulmonary veins.
Left ventricle	Pumps blood to all parts of the body except the lungs, via the aorta.
Bicuspid (mitral) valve	Prevents the back-flow of blood to the left atrium when the left ventricle contracts
Bicuspid (mitral) valve tendons	Prevents the bicuspid (mitral) valve from turning "inside out" when the left ventricle contracts.
Right ventricle	Pumps deoxygenated blood to the lungs via the pulmonary arteries.
Tricuspid valve	Prevents the back flow of blood to the right atrium when the right ventricle contracts
Semi-lunar valve	Prevents the back flow of blood from the pulmonary arteries when the right ventricle relaxes.
Right atrium	Collects deoxygenated blood from the organs of the body, but not the lungs, via the venae cavae.
Venae cavae	Returns deoxygenated blood to the right atrium.

The structure and function of blood vessels

Blood vessels are hollow tubes which carry many substances such as oxygen, carbon dioxide, glucose, salts, amino acids, vitamins, hormones and urea to and from the cells of the body.
There are 3 types of blood vessels.

- **Arteries**, which carry blood *away from the heart*
- **Veins**, which carry blood *towards the heart*
- **Capillaries**, which connect arteries with veins

Blood flows in one direction, with blood vessels either branching repeatedly (i.e. the arteries) or re-joining before returning to the **heart** (i.e. the veins). Capillaries form a network of fine tubes; these 'leak' the liquid part of blood into surrounding tissues. Exchange of materials occurs between the blood and these tissues. Much of the blood drains back into the blood system. The remainder drains into the **lymphatic system**, and eventually back into the heart.

The Table below (Table 3.1) compares these three types of blood vessel.

Comparison	Artery	Vein	Capillary
Cross-section	Muscle / Fibrous coat / Lumen		Single cell
Internal (lumen) diameter	Fairly narrow; can expand (= pulse)	Fairly wide	Very narrow; red blood cells squeeze through
Wall structure	The wall is relatively thick and also elastic, to withstand pressure	The wall is relatively thin; there are valves to keep blood moving in one direction	Wall is composed of a single cell layer; gaps between cells allow exchange of materials with surrounding tissues
Blood direction	Blood flows away from the heart	Blood flows towards the heart	Blood flows from arteries to veins
Blood pressure	High	Low	Very low
Blood flow rate	Rapid, irregular	Slow, regular	Very slow

Table 3.1 Comparison of the main types of blood vessel

The position and function of the various arteries and veins in the blood system is indicated in Fig 3.6.

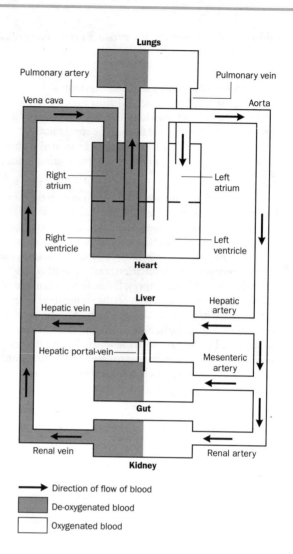

Figure 3.6 Position and function of various arteries and veins

Circulation and Blood Disorders

Humans (and other mammals) have a *double circulation*. This means that blood must pass through the *heart* twice on its way round the body (Fig 3.7). The blood circulates through the **pulmonary circulation** to the *lungs* to be oxygenated. It then returns to the left side of the heart, and is pumped to the body organs and tissues via the **systemic circulation**. Deoxygenated blood returns to the right side of the heart, and is pumped again to the lungs. The heart is the muscular pump which causes the blood to circulate.

A number of circulation and blood **disorders** are indicated in Fig 3.8 on page 45.

The respiratory pathway

The **respiratory system** (Fig 3.9) including the lungs is situated in the thorax. Air passes to the alveoli via the nostrils, nasal cavity, trachea and 2 bronchi which have many branches and millions of bronchides. Bacteria and dust can be filtered out by a mucus in the nasal cavity; also the trachea cilia (hairs) push sputum upwards. Respiration is the way in which cells can obtain energy for their activities.

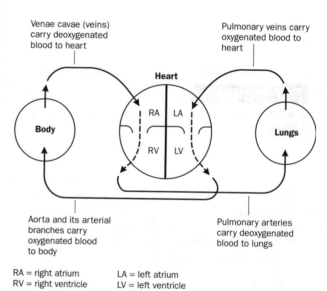

Figure 3.7 Pulmonary circulation

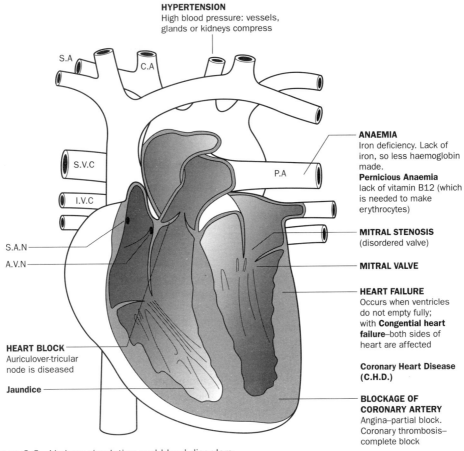

HYPERTENSION
High blood pressure: vessels, glands or kidneys compress

S.A
C.A
S.V.C
I.V.C
P.A
S.A.N
A.V.N

ANAEMIA
Iron deficiency. Lack of iron, so less haemoglobin made.
Pernicious Anaemia lack of vitamin B12 (which is needed to make erythrocytes)

MITRAL STENOSIS (disordered valve)

MITRAL VALVE

HEART FAILURE
Occurs when ventricles do not empty fully; with **Congential heart failure**–both sides of heart are affected

Coronary Heart Disease (C.H.D.)

BLOCKAGE OF CORONARY ARTERY
Angina–partial block. Coronary thrombosis–complete block

HEART BLOCK
Auriculover-tricular node is diseased

Jaundice

Figure 3.8   Various circulation and blood disorders

Components of the respiratory system

There are ten main components in a respiratory system as shown in the following chart.

Component	Description
Nasal Cavity	Hairs in the nose filter the air that is breathed; it is moistened by mucus and warmed by the blood capillaries that line the nasal cavity. We can breathe while chewing; this is interrupted by swallowing.
Epiglottis	Works like a trap door; it is a muscular flap which automatically closes off the trachea during swallowing.
Trachea	This is the windpipe which connects the mouth and nose cavity to the lungs. Bacteria, dust, etc can be filtered out by mucus and cilia (very fine hairs) which cover the lining of the trachea.
Lungs	Contain alveoli and bronchioles. The linings are elastic and are covered by a double pleural membrane which enclose the pleural fluid, which protects the lungs.
Bronchi	Connect the bronchial network with the trachea. These are non-collapsible because they are strengthened by cartilage.
Bronchioles	Bronchioles are a branching network of tubes which carry air to and from the alveoli. They are elastic tubes; the wider branch bronchioles are strengthened with cartilage.
Alveoli	These are collapsible air sacs involved in gaseous exchange. In the linings of the lung there are approximately 700 million alveoli with, a surface area of 80m^2.
Intercostal muscles	2 sets of antagonistic muscles between the ribs. *External* – raise ribs, causing inspiration. *Internal* – lowers ribs, causing expiration.
Diaphragm	Muscle sheet. When relaxed it is domed in shape; less so when contracted, causing inspiration and an increase in chest volume.
Ribs	Ribs protect the lungs and heart and are beneficial in breathing. They can move at the point of attachment to the vertebral column (backbone and sternum).

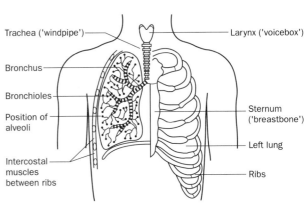

Trachea ('windpipe')
Bronchus
Bronchioles
Position of alveoli
Intercostal muscles between ribs
Larynx ('voicebox')
Sternum ('breastbone')
Left lung
Ribs

Figure 3.9   Respiratory pathway

Respiration cycle

Breathing involves the contraction and relaxation of muscles associated with the ribs and diaphragm (Fig 3.10).

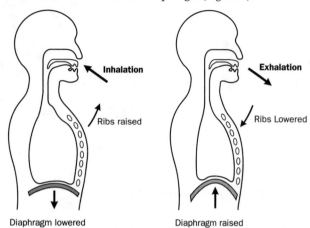

Figure 3.10   Breathing

Breathing is rhythmic, and is an alternating process involving **inhalation** (breathing in – *inspiration*) and **exhalation** (breathing out – *expiration*). The breathing rate in an adult is about 16 cycles per minute when resting. The depth and rate of breathing can vary according to an individuals needs for energy. The cycle is mostly co-ordinated by involuntary control.

The **depth** of breathing varies. The average capacity of an adult's lungs is about 5dm³. During normal (quiet) breathing about 0.5dm³ of air (**tidal volume**) is breathed in. This is increased to 4.5dm³ (the **vital capacity**) if more energy is needed. Some air (about 0.5dm³ during exercise) normally remains in the lungs at all time. This is called **residual capacity**.

The effect of the breathing movements shown in Fig 3.10 is to change the volume (and therefore the pressure) of the chest cavity (*thoracic cavity*). When the volume of the chest cavity is increased, the pressure is reduced and air enters from outside the body. The opposite happens when the volume is reduced. Table 3.2 summarises the main changes involved in breathing.

Change	Inhalation	Exhalation
intercostal muscles	**external** muscles contract, causing the ribs to move upwards and outwards	**internal** muscles contract, causing the ribs to move downwards and inwards; gravity may assist this
diaphragm	contracts and flattens, pushing down on the contents of the abdomen below	relaxes and becomes domed; displaced contents of abdomen push from below
lungs	become inflated against their elastic tendency	elasticity of lungs causes them to become deflated
volume of thorax	increases	decreases
pressure in thorax	decreases	increases

Table 3.2   Summary of breathing

Exchange of gases

Respiration occurs in all organisms and usually involves the gases *oxygen* and *carbon* dioxide. These respiratory gases enter or leave the organism at a *respiratory surface*. The gas exchange surfaces within the lungs of humans are the **alveoli** (Fig 3.11).

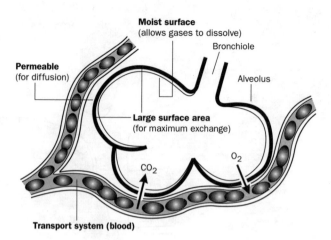

Figure 3.11   An alveolus

Alveoli have a good supply of blood capillaries which take *oxygen* into the body tissues and which bring *carbon dioxide* from the body tissues.

Approximately 70% of inhaled air reached the alveoli. The remaining 30% of inhaled air occupies the dead space of impermeable tubes which lead to the alveoli.

Composition of inhaled/exhaled air

Table 3.3 compares air inhaled and exhaled.

Component	Exhaled	Inhaled air
oxygen	16%	21%
carbon dioxide	4%	0.04%
water vapour	saturated = 6.2%	variable, depends on humidity; average = 1.3%
temperature	38°C	ambient

Table 3.3   Relative composition of inhaled and exhaled air in humans

Aerobic respiration

Aerobic respiration involves the use of oxygen to break down fats and carbohydrates to release energy. Aerobic respiration takes place in the cells of the body. The blood carries oxygen and food to the cells and takes away the waste water and carbon dioxide which are then removed by the lungs.

Aerobic respiration is characterised by the release of a relatively large amount of energy. Aerobic respiration is comparable with 'burning' a glucose in oxygen, producing the 'combustion products' of carbon dioxide and water and releasing energy.

$$\text{Glucose} + \text{Oxygen} \rightarrow \text{Carbon} + \text{Water} + \text{Energy}$$
$$C_6H_{12}O_6 \quad 6O_2 \qquad \text{dioxide} \quad 6H_2O$$
$$6CO_2$$

Anaerobic respiration

Anaerobic respiration (example via vigorous exercise) is a type of respiration involving the breakdown of fats and carbohydrates to release energy but *without using oxygen*. Less energy is released compared to aerobic respiration which uses oxygen.

During vigorous exercise not enough oxygen is supplied to the muscles to break down the food quickly enough and release the energy the body needs. This lack of the oxygen required is called the **oxygen debt**. If insufficient oxygen is available then glucose may be broken down to *lactic acid*.

$$\begin{array}{ccccc} \text{Glucose} & \rightarrow & \text{Lactic acid} & + & \text{Energy} \\ C_6H_{12}O_6 & & 2C_3H_6O_3 & & \end{array}$$

The accumulated lactic acid (which is toxic) in the tissues (e.g. the muscles) causes muscle ache or fatigue. After exercise, when demand for energy decreases, the lactic acid can be broken down (20%) or converted back to glucose (80%) in the liver. The time required for this is called the **recovery period**.

Healthy people tend to have lower pulse and heart rates than less healthy people, partly because exercise develops all muscles including the heart muscle. Non smokers and the healthy regain their resting pulse rate quicker than smokers and the unfit. A well balanced diet, exercise and avoiding smoking can all contribute to reducing the risk of heart problems.

Diseases of the respiratory system

Fig 3.12 outlines some of the main diseases of the respiratory system.

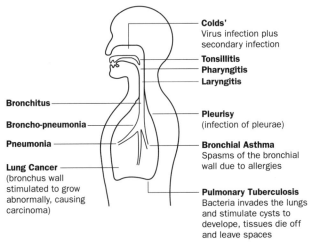

Figure 3.12   Some diseases of the respiratory system

Symptoms of these various diseases of the respiratory system could include:

- coughing due to irritation of the bronchi
- mucous congestion
- an increased respiratory rate
- breathlessness (dyspnoea)
- pain in the chest
- skin turning blue (cyanosis)
- coughing blood (severe cases)
- abnormal heart rate

Degenerative changes

Some **degenerative changes** that occur during the *ageing process* are as follows:

- The rate of skin replacement slows down. The epidermis becomes thinner.
- Some of the hair follicles stop producing hairs.
- The tissues lose elasticity, skin becomes wrinkled.
- Cells are not replaced by cell division.
- Reaction time and powers of concentration are less.
- A loss of short term memory may occur.
- Capacity of the bladder decreases.
- Hearing and vision become less acute.

- The eye lens loses some of its accommodation.
- The re-absorption of bone occurs quicker than replacement, hence bones become less dense and more easily broken.

Blood system and degenerative change

If the blood supply to the heart is reduced then the heart muscle cannot function correctly. Many of the following diseases affecting the blood system are related to degenerative change, ie the ageing process.

- **angina pectoris:** a severe pain or tightness in the centre of the chest. Angina occurs when the blood supply reaching the heart muscle through the coronary arteries is insufficient to meet the heart's demands for oxygen and nutrients

- **atherosclerosis:** the term used to describe the degeneration of the walls of the arteries

- **atheroma:** a fatty patch or plaque forms on the wall of an artery. As a result less oxygen gets to the tissues and they can be damaged or destroyed. The cause of deposits on artery walls is thought to be in part due to cholesterol present in blood, due to heavy smoking, stress, age and hereditary factors.

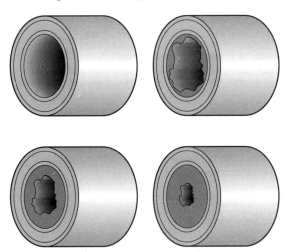

Figure 3.13   Progressive blockage of the arteries

Inner walls of the arteries are coated with a type of plaque. This increases the risk of total blockage of vital arteries (**thrombosis**). Alternatively such deposits weaken the artery walls causing them to bulge (**aneurysm**) and eventually rupture.

- **chronic heart disease:** a chronic or lingering heart disease is one that develops very gradually over a long time.

- **congenital heart disease:** a heart disease (or disorder) that is inborn, or present from birth.

- **coronary artery disease:** the narrowing of the arteries bringing the blood to the heart so that insufficient blood is supplied to the heart muscle.

- **coronary thrombosis:** the formation of a 'thrombus' or blood clot on the inner wall of the coronary artery.

- **myocardial infarction:** the death of an area of heart muscle as a result of an inadequate blood supply to that part of the heart. Myocardial infarction is more usually called a **heart attack**.

Body system and life style choice

This section focuses on the following areas:

- Exercise
- Diet
- Stress
- Smoking

Exercise

There are many reasons why people **exercise**:

- **Fun and enjoyment**   The feel good factor, mix with peers, to make new friends, and to belong to clubs.

- **General good health**   Exercise helps with digestion and reduces the risk of heart disease; it also encourages a supple, co-ordinated body, greater stamina, clear skin and glossy hair.

- **Mental health**   Exercise helps you relax and keeps you mentally healthy as well as physically healthy.

- **Heart and lungs**   Exercise on a regular basis increases the *efficiency* of the heart and lung muscles, as the more they are used the bigger they become. The respiratory muscles becomes more efficient; as a result the lungs are able to respond more quickly to any sudden change when required during exertion.

- **Muscles (power and endurance)**   Exercise helps the body to increase in size, strength and efficiency, in particular the arms and legs. Muscles are strengthened which help to keep the body in good working order.

- **Joints**   Exercise helps to keep the joints supple and prevent stiffness.

- **Motor skills**   These are enhanced by repeated practice of complex movement patterns.

The body during exercise

During exercise the body needs more food and oxygen to sustain the physical activity. Exercise helps the heart to work more efficiently and improves circulation, because it increases the rate at which blood flows round the body. The heart pumps blood faster (there is an increase in its stroke volume – volume of blood pumped per beat) through the body so that oxygen and food can get to the cells fast. The rate and depth of respiration also increase so that the lungs completely fill and almost completely empty themselves of air. More oxygen is breathed in and carbon dioxide is expelled. People who are fit, or become fit, generally have a lower heart rate and pulse rate than those who are less fit, because exercise develops the heart muscle as well as the bodily muscles. Non-smokers and fit people get back to their resting pulse quicker than smokers. Regular exercise, sensible eating, a well balanced diet which contains little fat, and not smoking can help to reduce the risk of heart disease. To keep fit, it is a good idea to exercise 20–30 minutes, 2–3 times a week.

Diet

A **diet** is made up of foods that are eaten. The body needs a variety of foods each day, that are essential for good health. A **balanced diet** should contain:

- Proteins
- Fats
- Starch
- Minerals
- Salts (iron and calcium)
- Vitamins
- Fibre
- Water

There are many reasons why we choose to eat foods that we do. It depend on a number of factors such as:

- Social economic groups
- Culture
- Advertising
- Peer pressure
- General health
- Availability
- Cost
- Climate
- Time factor – in preparation and consumption
- Life stage – youth, pregnancy (see section on life styles)

Diet is discussed in greater detail in Element 3 of this chapter.

Stress

Stress is similar to being excited and causes an imbalance in the internal environment. Stress can be the result of factors in the external environment, cold, heat, intense noise, a lack of oxygen or it may originate inside the body in the form of raised blood pressure, pain or even unpleasant thoughts. The body releases adrenaline under stress, resulting in an increased heart rate and blood being diverted away from the stomach and face to the brain, arm and leg muscles. The muscles tense and breathing increases and the skin becomes pale. The body gets ready for action. Homeostatic (self-regulating) devices oppose the forces of stress and bring the body's internal environment back into balance.

Stress can affect physical, mental and emotional health. The body's response to stress prepares us for "**FIGHT** or **FLIGHT**" but modern day living does not allow us to do either of these easily, so the body is left in a tense and alert state.

	Stress – fight or flight	
• BREATHING IS FASTER & GASPING		• HEART PUMPS FASTER
• NECK & SHOULDER MUSCLES TENSE	STRESS RESPONSES PREPARE A PERSON FOR BOTH **FIGHT** OR **FLIGHT**	• MUSCLES TENSE FOR ACTION
• PUPILS DILATE		• MOUTH IS DRY LIVER RELEASES GLUCOSE TO PROVIDE ENERGY FOR MUSCLES
• BLOOD PRESSURE RISES		
• SWEATING IS MORE PROFUSE		• SPHINCTERS CLOSE
• HORMONES ARE RELEASED		• DIGESTION SLOWS DOWN OR CEASES
• THE BRAIN MOBILISES THE BODY FOR VIGOROUS ACTION		

Table 3.3 gives some indication of the life-events most likely to create stress and bring about stress-related illness.

Table 3.3 Factors involved in stress

Some other causes of stress include:

- **Overcrowded conditions**; especially in cities via travel on the roads, underground, trains and buses.

- **Noise**; such as constant traffic or noise from neighbours.

- **Pollution**; (environmental) via industry and cars.

- **Competition**; keeping up with neighbours, etc.

Results of stress
People can adapt remarkably well, but *excessive* reactions can lead to various symptoms such as:

- Headaches – migraine
- Anxiety
- Diarrhoea
- Constipation
- Skin reactions: rashes, eczema,
- Asthma
- Lack of concentration
- Accidents
- Ulcers – in digestive tract
- High blood pressure: heart and respiratory disorders
- Withdraw into oneself
- Mental breakdown

Recognising the signs of negative stress
Do you have too many demands?
Can you cope?
The following chart considers a number of signs of negative stress.

Physical signs	Mental Signs	Behavioural Signs
Breathing & heart rate quickens	Anxious, nervous, worried	Short tempered Withdrawn
Poor circulation	Over excited	Accident prone
Cold hands, or feet		Achieving less
Dry throat	Irritable, depressed, bored	Forgetful
Biting finger nails	Apathetic, confused,	Lack of concentration
Feeling faint		
Upset stomach		May sleep less
Indigestion		(or more) often
Back Pain, muscle tension – shoulders and neck		May use alcohol or tobacco more
Headaches		(or less) often
Stammering		

Stress relievers

- **Relaxation techniques**; these will help to manage stress in the longer term

- **Physical activity**; this can relieve the symptoms of stress and encourage good health

- **Taking time out**; this may be for as little as a 10 minute walk in the fresh air.

- **Talk**; talking about the specific concern to someone prepared to listen. Talking is a great help especially between parents and children to get them into the habit of talking about their anxiety, fears, or aggressive behaviour.

- **Taking positive action to change the circumstances**; this can directly relieve stress

Stress can be either **positive** or **negative**. We need a certain amount for stimulation. Too much and we become overloaded. Under-stimulation can, however, be as stressful as over-stimulation. People who are prone to high blood pressure, should watch their smoking, drinking, eating habits, and avoid stress anxiety.

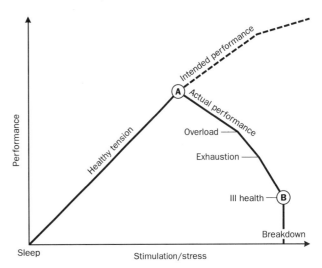

(A) a person must be aware of fatigue, going past this point increases one's inefficiency.

(B) even a minimal increase in stress may cause a breakdown

Figure 3.14 Achieving a stress balance

Smoking
Cigarettes can affect your health in many ways. Cigarettes are harmful – tobacco smoke consists of about 300 different chemicals; these substances enter the body through the mouth and lungs. Chemicals involved include nicotine, carbon monoxide, irritant substances and carcinogens. The lungs can be damaged by the constant irritation of tobacco smoke. Carbon monoxide and gas in cigarette smoke mixes with haemoglobin in the red blood cells and makes the blood less efficient for carrying oxygen. As a result blood vessels around the heart become weak and this may result in a heart attack. Smoking also lessens the resistance of the lungs to disease (by damaging the cells so that they can be attacked by pathogens). In particular, some lung diseases caused by bacteria and

viruses, like chronic bronchitis, can be linked with smoking, as can lung cancer.

There are 3 main diseases involving the *respiratory system* which occur more frequently in smokers than non-smokers. These are: bronchitis, emphysema, lung cancer.

- **Bronchitis.** This is an inflammation (swelling up) of the bronchi (tubes leading to the lungs), caused by irritants and infectious micro-organisms. This is accompanied by an accumulation of *mucus*. The result is a narrowing of the bronchi tubes which causes difficulty in breathing. *Cilia*, the fine hairs lining the respiratory tract, are gradually destroyed by smoke. The hairs remove dust and mucus, but become paralysed, so that sticky phlegm collects in the lungs, causing infection. Smokers try and cough it up, which damages the lungs even further and reduces the number of air sacs in the lungs. As a result there is less surface area for oxygen to diffuse into the blood stream, hence smokers become out of breath and may suffer from bronchitis. The larynx and trachea are also often affected, causing laryngitis and trachitis. Bronchitis can spread to the lungs, resulting in pneumonia.

- **Emphysema.** This is a condition which involves the breakdown of the alveoli walls. As a result the lungs are not properly emptied between breaths. It almost always occurs with severe bronchitis, resulting in the narrowing of the airways causing wheezing. Irritants in tobacco smoke induce coughing, which can damage the already weakened lung tissue.

- **Lung cancer.** This kills more people than any other cancer and 90% of all lung cancers occur amongst smokers. Smoking also increases the risk of cancer of the mouth, throat, oesophagus, bladder and possibly the pancreas, kidneys and cervix. The risk of lung cancer increases directly with the number of cigarettes smoked and the earlier that you start to smoke. In general: the more you smoke and the sooner you started smoking, the greater are the chances of contracting cancer. Smokers who give up, increase their life expectancy by reducing the chances of contracting lung cancer (Fig 3.15).

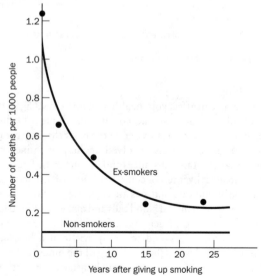

Figure 3.15   Benefits of avoiding smoking

- Smoking impairs athletic performance; gaseous exchange in the athlete becomes less efficient.
- Smoking during pregnancy reduces the amount of oxygen available to the developing foetus, which affects both physical and mental development.
- Pregnant women who have smoked can give birth to babies which are under sized and which are sometimes born prematurely.

Recent research has shown that mothers who smoke even affect the ovaries of their unborn daughters. When their daughters are pregnant, they have a higher chance of a miscarriage.

- **Passive smoking.** People who have worked with smokers for 20 years, but who were not exposed to cigarette smoke at home, have shown symptoms of lung damage similar to those of smokers who did not inhale. This damage to people who breathe smoke-laden air is called **passive smoking**.

- **ASH.** Action on Smoking and Health campaign (ASH) state that: "It is important that for non-smokers to avoid exposure to tobacco smoke, both at work and at leisure, segregation of smokers from non-smokers must become the norm."

Smokers who switch to lower tar cigarettes may offset the slight health advantage by smoking more, or by inhaling more deeply. There does not seem to be any evidence that switching to a lower tar brand of cigarettes reduces coronary heart disease, the main killer associated with smoking.

Certainly life expectancy is, on average, reduced by an increased rate of smoking (Fig 3.16).

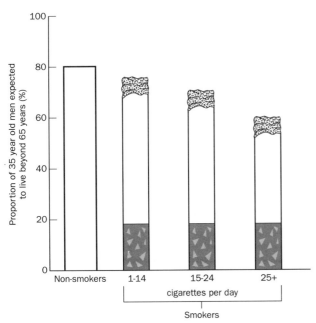

Figure 3.16   Life expectancy and rate of smoking

Useful information sources

Some organisations that you may find useful in your project work on topics in this Element include:

British Diabetic Association
10, Queen Street,
LONDON W1 0BD

British Heart Foundation
14 Fitzhardinge Street
LONDON W1 4DH

Coronary Preventation Group
60 Great Osmond Street,
LONDON W1H 3HR

Health Education Authority,
Hamilton House,
Mabeldon Place,
LONDON WC1H 9TX

ASH Action on Smoking and Health
5/11 Mortimer Street,
LONDON W1N 7RH

Pharmacy Healthcare
1 Lambeth High Street,
LONDON SE1 7JN

Sports Council
16 Upper Woborn Place
LONDON WC1 7JN

Self Check ✓ Element 1

1. What is the function of the valves of the heart?

   A   Decrease blood pressure
   B   Increase blood pressure
   C   Slow the blood flow down
   D   Stop the back flow of blood

2. Which artery has deoxygenated blood?
   A   Carotid artery
   B   Coronary artery

C   Pulmonary artery
D   Renal artery

3. Which two of the following are characteristic of arteries?
   A   Contain valves
   B   Carry blood away from the heart
   C   Contain deoxygenated blood
   D   Do not contain valves

4. Name the **blood vessels** in the following list:
   A   Arteries
   B   Red corpuscle
   C   White corpuscle
   D   Capillaries.

5. Repiration is the way in which cells can obtain energy for their activities. True or False.

6. Which of the following are components of the respiratory system:
   A   Epiglottis
   B   Trachea
   C   Alveoli
   D   Intercostal muscles

7. What is the function of the semilunar valves in the pulmonary artery and aorta?
   A   Increase arterial pressure
   B   Maintain the pulse in the arteries
   C   Prevent back flow of blood into the ventricles
   D   Separate atria (auricles) from ventricles

8. (a) Name the muscle of the heart wall.
   (b) What is its function?

9. Look at Fig 3.17

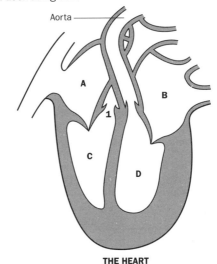

THE HEART

Figure 3.17   The heart

   (a) What is the function of the item labelled 1?
   (b) Which chambers contain the most oxygenated blood?
   (c) Which chamber produces the greatest pressure?

10 Look again at Fig 3.17 above. What route does blood take from the lungs to the aorta?

3.2 Investigation of human disease

In this Element we will look at the principles relevant to the prevention and control of disease, and how social and economic factors can affect the pattern of disease.

Classifying disease or ill health

The classes of disease or illness we shall review are:

- Physical illness
- Mental illness
- Infections
- Degenerative and inherited illness.

Health

Before we look at disease or illness we must first define what **health** is. The World Health Organisation (W.H.O) gave a definition of health as:

> *"Health is a state of complete physical, mental and social well-being, and not merely the absence of disease or infirmity"*

A quote from the former Health Education Council defined good health as occurring when you can:

> 'be all you can be'

Are you healthy because you do not feel ill, or because you never visit the doctor?

'Healthy' and 'Normal' are terms often used to mean the same thing, but:
What is healthy?   What is normal?

You must take into account cultural and social differences; also that peoples ideas of 'being healthy' vary dramatically. Self-perception of being healthy or ill may depend on the questions people ask.

"Are you mentally well because you have never had psychiatric help?"
"Do you see yourself as 'normal'?"

A general consensus seems to embrace the idea of *POSITIVE HEALTH* as involving social and mental well being, and being able to adapt constantly and continually to change. Fig. 3.18 presents a **holistic** (whole person) approach to health with all 4 'spokes' of the diagram closely associated with 'good' health.

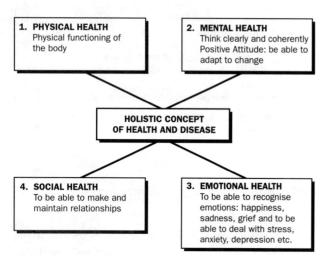

| 1. PHYSICAL HEALTH
Physical functioning of the body | 2. MENTAL HEALTH
Think clearly and coherently Positive Attitude: be able to adapt to change |

HOLISTIC CONCEPT OF HEALTH AND DISEASE

| 4. SOCIAL HEALTH
To be able to make and maintain relationships | 3. EMOTIONAL HEALTH
To be able to recognise emotions: happiness, sadness, grief and to be able to deal with stress, anxiety, depression etc. |

Figure 3.18   Holistic approach to health

Another spoke that could be added is:

> **Spiritual Health** Having a religious belief or a personal spiritual principle, i.e.: ways of thinking and behaving that bring peace of mind.

Another term that is often used to describe the holistic approach is PSYCHO-SOCIAL.

Physical illness

What is **physical ill health**? Is it a temporary condition such as not feeling well, having an illness, a disease or broken bones?

When we think in terms of physical ill health we often think of disease. A **disease** is a condition in which an organism is not functioning properly. The origin of the disease may be due to *internal* or *external* causes or a combination of the two.

Internal causes.   A person may inherit the disease itself, or the tendency to have the disease, from the parents. In some cases the likelihood of an individual having a particular disease is only slightly increased by inheritance. Examples: haemophilia, cancer, colour-blindness, some forms of mental illness.

External causes.   A person might be subjected to disease-causing agents in the environment: eg. radiation, mental stress, and disease-causing organisms or pathogens such as bacteria (eg Salmonella) and viruses (eg Herpes, HIV (aids)).

Disease is a major cause of death in natural populations. The body's natural defence against disease is the immune system.

Mental Illness

Mental illness is a condition that can affect more or less anyone at any age. It can range from mild anxiety or depression (*neuroses*) to being a violent psychopath (*psychoses*). In many cases it is self correcting, or curable.

Around half a million people are diagnosed as having a mental illness in England and Wales. Around 1 in 6 females and 1 in 9 males experience some mental illness or disabilities in their life time.

Neuroses. Can include depression, anxiety, claustrophobia, agoraphobia, compulsive cleanliness. Nevertheless, the person remains broadly in touch with reality.

Psychoses. A more serious form of lack of control, which can be more difficult to treat. For example with Schizophrenia the patient tends to lose contact with reality and suffers from hallucinations. Psychopathic personality behaviour is entirely governed by impulse and can lead to anti-social behaviour, and criminal behaviour without remorse.

Mental handicap. This is a result of retarded development of mental powers, which ranges from mild impairment to severe sub-normality and virtual helplessness.
Improvements in the condition is possible through special care and the use of tailored training programmes.

The following table (Table 3.4) compares mental handicap with mental illness, which is quite different.

Infections

Infections can be transmitted (infectious diseases) or not (non-transmissible infections), as the case may be.

An **infectious disease** can be transmitted from one person to another. The germs which cause infectious diseases are either bacteria, viruses or fungi. Germs enter your body through body openings or wounds (Fig 3.19).

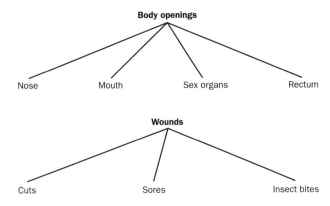

Figure 3.19   Transmission of infectious diseases

Infectious diseases are spread via contaminated air borne droplets, water, direct contact, food, animals, and insects. A time lapse may occur between the initial infection and the appearance of the symptoms of a particular disease. This is called the **incubation period**.

Diseases spread by direct contact are called **contagious**.

A **non-transmissible disease** can be caused by various factors. These may include nutritional deficiency (scurvy, kwashiorkor), hormone imbalance (diabetes), degeneration and senescence (arthritis), mental illness (depression), self afflicted disorders (alcoholism, drug abuse, obesity) and cell prohibition due to faulty gene control, as in cancers. *Genetic diseases* are caused by gene mutations and are not transmissible between individuals in the way that pathogens are, but can be transmitted from parent to offspring via the gametes.

Degenerative diseases (acquired disorders)

Some of the **degenerative diseases** are associated with old age and most people will experience them to some extent. Examples are atherosclerosis and osteoarthritis. A healthy diet and exercise may help to delay the onset of degenerative diseases.

Mentally Handicapped	*Mental Illness*
• Due to brain damage which affects development.	• Mental illness can often occur when a person cannot cope with the stresses and problems in everyday life.
• It is a permanent condition but the individual can be helped to overcome disabilities via various treatments, the use of specialist services, and education.	• It is often a temporary condition which in many cases can be treated successfully, though there is a possibility of a relapse.
• 1 in 100 people are born mentally handicapped.	• 1 in 6 people are affected by mental illness at some point in their life.
• Some women can run a slightly higher rate of giving birth to a handicapped baby, but it is difficult to predict which child will be mentally handicapped.	• Certain people are more likely to become mentally ill, however it is difficult to predict who will be affected.
• People are usually born mentally handicapped rather than develop the condition later in life. Problems can occur during pregnancy such as the mother contracting German measles, or a hormone deficiency which can result in a mentally handicapped child being born or a Downs Syndrome baby, caused by an extra chromosome.	• The reasons *why* people become mentally ill are vast. Family difficulties, pressures at school or work, poor housing conditions, isolation and loneliness, may result in stress that is difficult for some people to deal with. There are also biochemical causes (schizophrenia). Certain personality types are more likely to be affected; also people who have had an unstable family life are more at risk as they grow up. It is usually a *combination of factors* that affect people.
• Another way of becoming mentally handicapped is through injury, accidents, or disease such as meningitis and the side effects from vaccinations.	
• Being mentally handicapped is not an illness or a medical problem as such, hence no cures. Much can be done to improve everyday life, via social support, education in practical skills, etc, which help people lead as independent a life as is possible.	• The condition can be treated in many ways. Psychotropic (mood altering) drugs or electro-convulsive therapy (ECT) – a controversial form of treatment – are supposed to be effective in helping with severe depression. Talking therapy may be used – which helps people gain insight into the causes of their problems and to come to terms with them. Often a *combination* of the above treatments help people restore their way of life.
• Mentally handicapped people can become mentally ill, which can then be treated.	• Mentally ill people do not become mentally handicapped unless they suffer from brain damage via an accident or serious injury.

Table 3.4   A comparison of Mental Handicap and Mental Illness

Some of the acquired degenerative diseases have environmental causes, for example, bronchitis, emphysema, lung cancer and coronary heart disease.

Being exposed to certain chemicals or radioactive sources may increase the risk of cancer. There is evidence to suggest that diabetes and arthritis may be triggered by virus infections.

Inherited Diseases

Inherited diseases are passed on to the next generation by the offspring's parents; examples are blood conditions like sickle cell anaemia and haemophilia.

Sickle-cell anaemia is caused by gene mutation. The gene which is affected controls the production of haemoglobin in the red blood cells. The mutation causes the red cells to produce a defective form of haemoglobin which forms rod-like structures which damage red blood cells.

Genetic counselling can reduce the frequency of these diseases. Certain inherited disorders can be treated effectively such as haemophilia by injections of a blood-clotting factor.

Infectious diseases and the spread of disease

We now look at the following infectious diseases and at how to control and prevent them:

- Influenza
- Salmonella food poisoning
- Sexually transmitted diseases
- Diseases spread by airborne contamination and direct contact

Influenza (flu)

This is caused by a virus (which exists in 3 strains, A, B & C). The virus attacks the lining of the throat and the respiratory passages, which results in the inflammation of the trachea, bronchi and bronchioles.

- **Symptoms.** The symptoms of influenza can vary between a high temperature, headache, dry cough, a mild sore throat, and generally feeling unwell. Symptoms last 2–4 days, but damage to the respiratory lining may allow streptococci to invade, causing secondary bacterial infections.

No specific drugs are given, but aspirin helps to lower the temperature and antibiotics may be used against secondary infection. Having had the infection usually gives one immunity for several years. The 'A' strain undergoes mutation, and immunity to one form is not effective against other mutations. Sometimes there are epidemics of influenza; if the strain which is responsible can be identified, a vaccine can be given to those at risk.

Salmonella (food poisoning)

Food poisoning is caused by eating contaminated food. If food is not stored properly, cooked correctly or is prepared in a dirty kitchen, it can become contaminated.

- **Symptoms.** The symptoms can vary from mild headache to vomiting and diarrhoea which occurs between 12–24 hours after eating the contaminated food. Symptoms are unpleasant, but not often serious. Certain categories of people are more at risk from food poisoning than others,

such as babies, older people and pregnant women, due to their having less resistance.

Approximately 50 people per year die from food poisoning in the UK. Salmonella is one of the commonest forms of food poisoning. It is caused by the bacterium *Salmonella typhimurium*. The bacterium lives in the intestine of pigs, chicken, ducks and cattle. Humans contract food poisoning if they eat meat or eggs or drink milk which is contaminated with the salmonella bacteria from the alimentary canal of infected animals.

Salmonella bacteria is killed when meat is cooked thoroughly or milk is pasteurised (heated for 30 minutes at 62°C).

Infection occurs when milk is untreated, meat not properly cooked or cooked meat is contaminated with bacteria transferred from raw meat. Frozen poultry must be thoroughly defrosted before cooking.

To avoid disease all milk should be pasteurised, and meat thoroughly cooked. For example the inside of the chicken may not get hot enough during cooking to kill the salmonella. Do not handle cooked and raw meat at the same time and wash hands thoroughly between the two activities. The liquid which escapes when frozen chicken is defrosting may contain salmonella bacteria. Utensils used for defrosting chickens etc must not therefore come into contact with any other food, and care must be taken when the food is stored.

Sexually Transmitted Diseases (STD)

Sexually Transmitted Diseases (STD) include some which are called Venereal Diseases. STD are caught by having intimate sexual contact with an infected person. They include Gonorrhoea, Syphilis and Non Specific Urethritis (NSU). Also Thrush and Aids (AIDS is discussed further in Unit 5).

- **Gonorrhoea.** This is a disease caused by the bacterium *neisseria*. In men it appears within 2–10 days after being infected. The symptoms include pain when passing urine and a yellow discharge from the penis. The resulting complications are that the disease can lead to blockage of the urethra and sterility.

  In women there is no obvious symptom in the early stages. In the later stages the symptoms are an infection in the opening of the womb which is not usually painful and a discharge which may not be noticed. Sometimes the germ causes inflammation of the bladder and pain may be felt when passing urine. A woman can pass on the disease to her baby, during child birth. The disease invades the baby's eyes and causes blindness.

  If the disease is not treated, the germ will cause inflammation in other parts of the body in both women and men, resulting in general ill health, swollen joints and damage to the reproductive organs. It can stop both male and females from being able to reproduce. The disease can be cured with penicillin but some strains of neisseria have become resistant to this antibiotic and therefore other antibiotics are required. There is no immunity; having had the disease once does not prevent you contracting it again.

- **Syphilis.** This is caused by the bacterium *Treporema palladium*. In men it appears from 10 days, and with women from approximately one month after being infected. In men a painless sore (chancre) appears on or near the penis. In woman the sore appears around the vulva and therefore woman may not be aware of its presence. After a few days to 6 weeks the sore clears up. But this does not mean it is cured. Males and females affected must have treatment for the disease or it will spread to other parts of the body. A few weeks later the disease enters the 2nd stage. Here the symptoms are a skin rash, mouth sores, swollen lymph nodes, fever, sore throat and a feeling of ill health. These symptoms again disappear with time.

The 3rd stage is when the germ continues to attack the body with *no visual symptoms*. This stage can last for many years. It can then severely damage every part of the body and can cause paralysis, blindness, insanity and death.

In pregnant women, the bacteria can get across the placenta and infect the foetus. Antibiotics will cure syphilis if used in the early stages. Otherwise permanent damage can occur.

The only way of making sure you do not contract an STD. is to avoid having sex with an infected person. You can limit the risk to yourself by keeping to one sexual partner. Less risk also occurs if a man wears a condom.

Spread of disease by airborne contamination, and direct contact with people

- **Airborne contamination.** Airborne 'droplets' or aerosol infections are spread by coughing, sneezing, laughing, talking and even breathing out, which produces a fine spray of liquid drops into the air that remain there, floating around for a long time. The droplets can be breathed in by other people or fall onto exposed food. If these droplets contain viruses or bacteria, they can cause disease if inhaled or eaten.
- **Viruses** like the common cold, flu, chicken pox, measles are also spread in this way, as are **bacteria** such as streptococci which causes sore throats. As the water in the droplets evaporates, the bacteria often dies. Viruses however remain infectious, floating in the air. Places which are warm and moist are often full of floating droplets. In these places, such as buses, tubes, trains, discos and cinemas, one's chances of picking up an infection are increased.

Did You Know ?

AIDS is caused by a virus but cannot be spread by airborne transmission.

- **Fungi** Most fungi are harmless and can be useful to man, but some cause disease, eg ringworm and athletes foot. Fungi reproduce by putting tiny spores into the air. When the spores land they can be picked up by other people.

- **Direct contact contamination.** Here the source of disease is direct contact with the person involved, or with food, clothing, towels, used by the infected person.

The faeces of infected people contain bacteria that cause typhoid, salmonella, etc and these can be spread to food if hands are not washed. When infected food is eaten by healthy people the bacteria will multiply in their bodies and give them the disease. It is important that people working with food in shops, factories etc should have high standards when it comes to personal cleanliness.

Certain forms of food poisoning result from the *toxins* that are produced by bacteria that get into food. Cooking can kill the bacteria in food but may not destroy the toxins which cause the illness (e.g. botulism food poisoning can be highly dangerous).

Vectors are animals or insects which carry pathogens from one person to another and these may be involved in direct contact contamination. For example mosquitoes carry protozoa which cause malaria; houseflies pick up bacteria on their feet or mouth parts and transfer the bacteria to food; fleas on rats carry the bacteria causing bubonic plague; etc.

Control and prevention of infectious diseases

This section will explain the control and prevention of infectious diseases by looking at the following:

- Recognising, controlling and preventing disease
- Incubation periods
- Hygiene and Lifestyle
- Chemotherapy
- Immunisation
- Contact Tracing

Recognising, controlling and preventing disease

Recognising, controlling and preventing disease can be broken down into three separate categories, as shown in the following diagram (Fig 3.20). Namely primary, secondary and tertiary prevention.

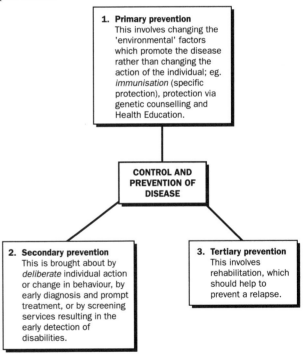

Figure 3.20 Stages in the control and prevention of disease

- **Preventing the spread of disease by using the body's own defences.** The body has its own **natural defences** in preventing the spread of disease (Fig 3.21). If germs which can cause an infectious disease enter the body, the white blood cells which produce **antibodies** try to make them harmless and destroy them. Once produced the antibodies stay in the blood to protect the body from getting that disease again; the antibodies have made the body *immune* to that disease.
- The **skin** acts as a barrier that stops the bacteria that live on the surface of the skin (epidermis) entering the body. If

the skin is damaged or cut, bacteria can enter the deeper tissue and can cause infection.

- **Sweat glands** and sebaceous glands produce substances which kill bacteria. Tears contain the enzyme *lysozyme* which protects the eyes from infection.
- The **stomach** produces acids which destroy bacteria in food. Nasal passages contain a moist lining that traps bacteria. The trachea and bronchi also contain musses, the ciliated cells which carry the trapped bacteria away from the lungs. If bacteria get through these barriers there are 2 more lines of defence, white cells and antibodies.

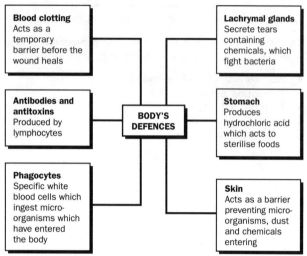

Figure 3.21 The body's defences to disease

Incubation Periods

An **incubation period** is the time delay between the *initial infection* by a disease-causing organism and the appearance of the *symptoms* of the disease.

Hygiene and Lifestyle

- **Personal Hygiene.** People who work with and handle food must be very careful with their personal hygiene. They must wash their hands often and always before touching food, especially if handling cooked and raw meat (particularly poultry). Some people carry intestinal pathogens but do not show symptoms; these people should not work with food. Hands must be washed after visiting the toilet. When you have a cold, it is a good idea to use a handkerchief and also to avoid crowded, humid, and poorly ventilated places.

  There is no way to prevent the spread of airborne pathogens, except by immunisation against individual diseases. People with infectious diseases often stay off school or work. It is often better to catch childhood diseases (chicken pox, rubella etc) when young, so as to develop immunity. Adults are more severely affected by such diseases.

- **Using chemicals.** A variety of chemicals can be used to prevent the spread of disease.

  Soaps: bacteria and dirt are trapped in the lather and wash off.
  Disinfectants: reduce the number of live micro-organisms
  Antiseptics: inhibit the growth of bacteria by preventing the production of micro-organisms.
  Germicides: strong chemical substances that kill bacteria.
  Detergents: substitutes for soaps (eg washing clothes).

- **Using specified methods and techniques**

  Dry heat: raising the temperature to 150°C will kill bacteria in discarded contaminated dressings as will incineration in a furnace.
  Drying: used in food industry. Bacteria cannot live without moisture.
  Light: ultraviolet light kills bacteria (a reason for sunlight in homes).
  Pasteurisation: milk is heated to 72°C for 15 seconds then cooled rapidly to 10°C, killing bacteria.

Chemotherapy

This is the use of chemical drugs to treat disease, by killing pathogenic micro-organisms or by selectively inhibiting the growth of specific cells, example carcinomas.

Immunisation and immunity

Vaccines can be given to protect the body from catching certain diseases. Some vaccines *contain* antibodies; other vaccines work by making *your body* produce the antibodies it needs. *Immunity* is a result of a particular immune response which the body 'remembers' and can use again if necessary, so preparing the body for prompt reaction to a disease.

Immunity can result from direct or indirect exposure to disease (*active immunity*), or can be 'borrowed' from another organism (*passive immunity*). Table 3.5 looks at different types of immunity.

Type of immunity	Description and examples
non-specific immunity	involves mechanisms which respond generally to non-self proteins. Examples: the action of phagocytes, also the action of chemicals such as interferon and lysosyme produced by the body
specific immunity	involves mechanisms which respond specifically to non-self proteins
active immunity	is based on antibody production and action *within one organism*; the immune response
active natural immunity	involves the immune response resulting from a naturally occurring infection by a pathogen (disease-causing) organism. Examples: immunity to German measles (rubella), whooping cough
active induced (acquired) immunity	involves the immune response resulting from an artificial introduction, e.g. by vaccination (inoculation) of a modified type of antigen. Example: cowpox, polio vaccine; much 'weaker' than the actual pathogen
passive immunity	is based on antibodies *produced by another organism* which then have their action within a particular individual. This provides immunity for a fairly limited period
passive natural immunity	involves the transfer of antibodies from a mother to a foetus across the placenta. Examples: measles and polio
passive induced (acquired) immunity	involves the transfer of antibodies by injection, e.g. of serum. Example: diptheria

Table 3.5 Summary of human immunity

Contact tracing

Contact Tracing is when a person who has contracted a disease such as one of the sexually transmitted diseases discussed in this section is encouraged to give the names and addresses of previous sexual partners. These partners would then be contacted on a confidential basis, advised of the situation and informed of help that is available, such as medical testing, treatment and counselling.

Social and economic factors which affect the patterns of disease

This section will review a variety of social and economic factors which affect the patterns of disease. Here we look at the following: Social Class, Housing, Expenditure, and Diet.

It can be argued that an individual's circumstances or 'environment' is largely out of their control, and that many such factors can influence their well being. Figure 3.22 shows a range of different influences on an individual.

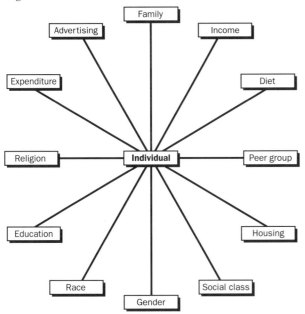

Figure 3.22 'Environmental' factors and the individual

The idea here is that it is the *setting* into which one is born or in which one is reared that can determine your life-chances and, in this context, your health prospects. Many reports (eg. Black Report, 1980) and statistics have shown that the health and welfare of an individual can be directly affected by the factors listed in Figure 3.22. Here we look at a selection of data linking individual health and welfare to a range of social and economic factors.

Social Class

Many bases have been suggested for placing individuals (or families) into *social class* groups. Although there is no agreed definition, the individual's *occupation* is widely used, as in the Registrar General's Classification below.

Social Class based on Occupation 1991	
Registrar General's classification	
I	PROFESSIONAL, ETC
II	MANAGERIAL AND TECHNICAL
III (N)	SKILLED NON-MANUAL
III (M)	SKILLED MANUAL
IV	PARTLY SKILLED
V	UNSKILLED

There is considerable evidence to link health to membership of one of these particular social class groups. For example the **Standardized Mortality Ratio** (SMR) can be calculated for each class group; The SMR is an index, with 100 indicating an *average* mortality for that class group. An SMR *below* 100 means that mortality is less than average for that group (even after taking into account age and sex differences). An SMR *above* 100 means that mortality is more than average for that group.

In Fig 3.23 we can see that the lower social class groups have the higher mortality rates, with the SMR for *unskilled men* (class V) over 2½ times that of *professional* (class I).

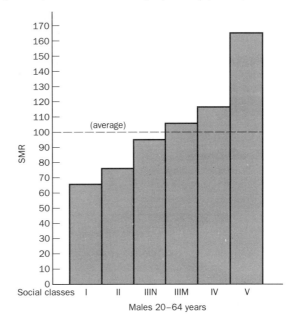

Figure 3.23 Mortality rates of social class groups

A similar picture can be seen with regard to the *rate* of serious illnesses (chronic, handicapping and acute) which is higher for the lower social class groups (Fig 3.24).

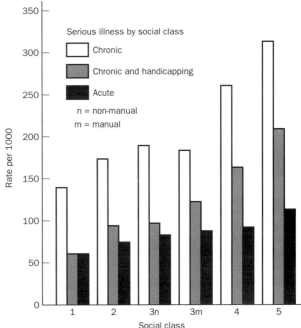

Figure 3.24 Serious illness by social class

Housing

As the following two extracts indicate, *housing* also varies considerably in quality between individuals/families and has a clear link to health.

The 1986 English House Condition Survey estimated that 2.9 million dwellings in England were in a poor condition. This was 15 per cent of all dwellings. Three measures of poor condition were used: unfit dwellings, lacking basic amenities, and in poor repair. Private rented dwellings were the most likely to be in a poor condition in 1986 (42 per cent) and housing association dwellings were the least likely (7 per cent)

(From *Social Trends*, 1991)

The death rate in Sheffield is still above the national average by about 10 per cent. Life expectancy is on average 68.4 years for men, 74.9 for women but is still unequally distributed. The central areas of the city have much higher death rates than other areas. Life is healthier generally in Sheffield today but still very unequal. Working-class people are most likely to live in the unhealthy districts.

(Adapted from *Survivors of Steel City*, Geoffrey Beattie, Chatto & Windus)

Expenditure/Income

Again the following extracts indicate a linkage between **poverty** and health, which is supported by a variety of other studies.

"Deprived kids are far more likely to die"
Britain is STILL a country where the rich live longer and the poor die sooner. And the gap has grown. Poverty is a killer, while the wealthy are able to buy health. The survey concludes:

"Social inequalities increased during the 1980's. And so has the health gap between rich and poor."
Today all the major and minor killers – notably lung cancer and coronary heart disease – hit the poor hardest.
(From an article on a survey by the Association of Community Health Councils for England and Wales, *Daily Mirror* 2/1/91)

PEOPLE living in deprived parts of the Edinburgh area are twice as likely to die prematurely as those who live in more affluent communities, a report revealed yesterday.
A strong link between poverty and early death has been established by the Lothian Regional Council.

(*The Scotsman*, 12/4/90)

The link between **diet** and health is considered further in the next Section.

Self Check ✓ Element 2

11. Which one of the following is False about the mentally handicapped?
    A   It is due to brain damage which affects development.
    B   It is a permanent condition but the individual can be helped to overcome disabilities via various treatments.
    C   1 in 100 people are born mentally handicapped.
    D   It is often a temporary condition which can often be treated successfully, though there is a possibility of a relapse.

12. Which statement is False about Mental illness?
    A   It can often occur when a person cannot cope with the stresses and problems in everyday life.
    B   1 in 6 people are effected by mental illness at some point in their life.
    C   People are usually born mentally ill rather than develop the condition later in life.
    D   Psychotropic drugs or electro-convulsive therapy (ECT) are supposed to be effective in helping with severe depression.

13. Schizophrenia is associated with a person who:
    1.   Loses contact with reality.
    2.   Suffers from hallucinations
    3.   Cannot sleep
    4.   Sleepwalks
    Answer
    A   2,3,4
    B   1,2,
    C   3,4
    D   1,2,3,4

14. Is the following statement true or false? A freezer preserves food for much longer than a refrigerator because:

    Bacteria do not reproduce at the temperature at which freezers operate, but they reproduce slowly at refrigerator temperatures.

15. Foods cannot be preserved by the addition of:
    A   Salt
    B   Monosodium glutamate
    C   Sulphur Dioxide
    D   Carbon Dioxide

16. Most microorganisms are NOT destroyed by:
    A   Adding acid
    B   Dehydrating
    C   Freezing
    D   Boiling

17. Individual circumstances which can influence a person's wellbeing are:
    1.   Poor nutrition
    2.   Poor housing
    3.   Unemployment
    4.   Lack of social support

    A   1,2,3
    B   1,2,3,4
    C   1,2,4
    D   1,3,4

18. Link the type of immunity (A–D) with the description (1–4)

    Type of immunity
    A   Non-specific immunity
    B   Specific immunity
    C   Active immunity
    D   Active natural immunity

    Description
    1.   Involve mechanisms which respond specifically to non-self proteins.
    2.   Is based on antibody production and action within one organism, the immune response.
    3.   Involves mechanisms which respond generally to non-self proteins
    4.   Involves the immune response resulting from a natural occurring infection by a pathogen

    A   A1   B2   C3   D4
    B   A1   B3   C2   D4
    C   A3   B1   C2   D4
    D   A3   B1   C4   D2

19. Link the type of immunity (A–D) with the description (1–4)

    Type of immunity
    A   Active induced
    B   Passive immunity
    C   Passive natural immunity
    D   Passive induced acquired immunity

    Description
    1.   Involves the transfer of antibodies by injection
    2.   Involves the transfer of antibodies from a mother to a foetus across the placenta
    3.   Involves the immune response resulting from an arti-

ficial immunity introduction
4. Is based on antibodies produced by another organism which then have their action within a particular individual.

A   A4   B2 C3 D1
B   A1   C2 D4
C   A3   B1 C2 D4
D   A3   B4 C2 D1

20. What is the *best* way to prevent the spread of air borne pathogens?

A   Use of a handkerchief when sneezing
B   Stay away from crowded and poorly ventilated areas: eg. underground trains.
C   Immunisation against individual disease.
D   There is NO known way.

21. Contact tracing is:
A   checking the immunity a person has to a specific disease.
B   when a person who has contacted a disease from a previous partner is traced.
C   when a person asks for additional information on a subject and passes it on to other people.
D   when a person has an overseas trip and comes into contact with unusual diseases.

22. Children who live in deprived areas, could suffer from various ailments.

(a) give an example of a disease that is often found in children that live in deprived areas.

(b) give at least three reasons why they may have a poor diet.

3.3 Components of a Healthy Diet

In this element we will look at the components that go together to make a **healthy diet**. We consider the nutrients that we eat, the various life stages that we go through, and the dietary choices we make.

To be able to do this we must understand the following six sections:

- Factors that contribute to a healthy diet.
- Macro-nutrients.
- Micro-nutrients.
- Nutritional needs during different life stages.
- The factors which affect our choice of diet.
- The nutritional effects of special diets and measures required to maintain a health diet.

Factors that contribute to a healthy diet

Humans are **heterotrophic**, that is we require a constant supply of ready-made complex organic substances called *food*. Food supplies the body with materials that are chemically oxidised to release energy. We acquire the food by **holozoic nutrition** in 4 stages:

Ingestion – Food is eaten
Digestion – Food is broken down by chewing and by enzymes so that it can be absorbed
Assimilation – Food is absorbed and utilised by the body
Egestion – Matter that is not absorbed is eliminated, e.g. defacation

The body needs food for:
1. **Growth** – The initial increase in cells in order to grow to adult size and repair damaged or worn out tissue.
2. **Energy** – To drive the chemical processes, for the mechanical work of muscles and for the maintenance of body temperature.
3. **Health** – Protection against disease and to provide raw materials for the manufacture of secretions such as hormones and enzymes.

A **balanced diet** contains appropriate proportions of all the necessary nutrients for growth, and for correct physiological functioning for general good health.

Types of food which make-up a balanced diet
The body requires a balanced diet which should include a quantity of each of the following 6 types of food, and water.

- **Proteins** – Required in large quantities for growth.
- **Carbohydrates** – Required in large quantities for energy production.
- **Fats** – Required in relatively large quantities for energy production.
- **Vitamins** – Required in small quantities to maintain health.
- **Minerals** – Required in traces for vital processes.
- **Roughage** – Required for bowel movement.
- **Water** – Required as a solvent for chemical reactions.

A balanced diet should consist of approximately the following:

(i)   20% fat
      20% protein
      60% carbohydrate.
(ii) Around 10500 – 14000 kilojoules a day is required to allow energy to be released for metabolism. Joule = unit of energy
(iii) The diet must also be palatable and easy to digest.

The table below indicates that the *daily* energy needs in kilojoules (KJ) of individuals vary by gender and type of activity

Women (metabolism needs)	8800	KJ
Man (metabolism needs)	10500	KJ
Man heavy work (total)	18900	KJ
Man sleeping (8 hrs)	2000	KJ
Man sitting	5	KJ (per minute)
Man walking (5km/p.h.)	18	KJ (per minute)
Man playing football	30	KJ (per minute)
Man cooking	8	KJ (per minute)
Man dancing	20	KJ (per minute)

Useful facts

Joule (J)	= unit of energy
1000 Joules	= 1 Kilojoule
Calorie	= amount of heat energy required to raise the temperature of 1g of water through 1°C.
Kilocalorie	= 1000 calories
1 kilocalorie	= 4.2 kilojoules

Kilocalories are units of energy measurement equal to 1000 calories or 4.186 kilojoules.

Unbalanced diet and the link with disease

The western diet is high in fats, red meat, sugars, processed and refined foods. These foods have been linked with many diseases:

> Cancer
> Heart Disease
> Diabetes
> Obesity

They have also been linked with various diseases of the gut, such as colitis, diverticulitis, and with ulcers.

The National Advisory Committee on Nutrition Education (NACNE) suggest that we should eat:

- less sugar
- less fat
- more fibre
- less salt

Elements in the typical unbalanced diet

- **Excess Sugar.** A person living in Britain eats around 38kg (84lbs) of **sugar** a year, plus more in the form of glucose and honey. A lot of the sugar is hidden in foods and it is not always obvious how much is being eaten.

Our bodies need energy to work properly, and sugar is a source of energy. But unlike most other foods it does not contain any other nutrients; as a result it has a limited use to the body.

Sugar can have a bad effect on health, for example tooth decay and if it is not all used up for energy, the left over is stored as fat.

The following table shows the percentage of sugar in various types of food.

Food	% of Sugar	Teaspoonful
2oz Milk choc	45%	6
1 choc biscuit	33%	2
1 can coke	10%	7
1 cup drinking choc	75%	$2\frac{1}{2}$
1 tablespoon of peanut butter	3%	1
1 small fruit yoghurt	15%	$4\frac{1}{2}$
1 small ice cream	15%	2
1 medium size choc cake	26%	2
Cornflakes average portion	8%	$\frac{1}{4}$
Dried tomato soup 1 pkt	40%	8
Dried chicken soup 1 pkt	10%	2

- **Excess Fat.** Many foods contain **fats**, either as solid or liquid (oil). Some foods are composed almost entirely of fat: such as butter, margarine, suet and lard. Some foods contain hidden fats: such as cakes, crisps, sausages, ice cream, chocolate.

Fats are important in our diet for several reasons:

- provides energy (excess is stored as fat)
- foods containing fat contain vitamins A,D,E and K
- fat makes food palatable and easy to swallow

There is a link between the amount and type of fat we eat in different foods, and heart disease. It is recommended that the amount of fat that is eaten is reduced and to change the types of fat we eat, to lessen the risks to health. An example is to turn to polyunsaturated fats – found in plants, e.g. sunflower. Soya, corn (maize) oils and margarine surrains are made from them.

- **Lack of Fibre.** **Fibre** (roughage) is an essential part of the diet; it is not digested or absorbed. Roughage mainly consists of cellulose derived from plant cell walls. The body is not able to break the substance down so it passes through the body without being significantly altered. Roughage provides bulk, which presses against the gut walls, mainly in the large intestine. Hence regular daily bowel movement becomes easier. A deficiency of fibre roughage causes constipation.

- **Excess salt.** **Salt** is essential to control the osmotic pressure of fluids and the blood. Certain types of salt activate some enzymes. Too much salt can, however, lead to raised blood pressure.

Nutrients can be divided into two broad groups: *macronutrients* and *micronutrients*. We now look at these in more detail.

Macronutrients

Macronutrients are nutrients needed in relatively large amounts, such as proteins, fats and carbohydrates.

Proteins

Proteins are essential to life, for body growth and the repair of tissue. The chemical elements of proteins are carbon, hydrogen, oxygen, nitrogen, and sometimes phosphorus and sulphur. Proteins are absorbed as amino acids and are then assembled according to genetic instructions within the organism.

Adults require eight essential amino-acids and children need ten.

The eight needed by adults are:

- isoleucine
- leucine
- lysine
- methionine
- phenylalanine
- threonine
- tryptophan
- saline

The two extra which children need are:

- arginine
- histidine

These amino acids cannot be made by the body. They must be obtained from food.

The proteins having all ten essential amino-acids are called HBV (high biological value proteins). These are found mostly in animal foods, e.g. meat, fish, cheese, eggs and milk. Soya beans, a plant food, are also HBV. They are used to manufacture textured vegetable protein (TVP), which has a lower proportion of methionine and tryptophan. These may be added during manufacture.

Proteins which have one or more amino-acids missing are called LBV (low biological value proteins) and are found in plants: pulses (peas, beans and lentils), nuts and cereals.

Gelatin is an animal protein made from collagen, which is extracted by boiling the bones, horns, skin, etc., of various animals. It is of low biological value, even though it is of animal origin, but it is mainly used for its setting quality and not as a nutritional source. The vegetarian equivalent is agar-agar, which is extracted from seaweed.

Proteins of low biological value can supplement each other or compensate for each other's deficiencies if eaten together.

It does not matter, from the point of view of protein, whether you eat only animal foods, or vegetables, or a mixture of both. If you are a vegetarian you will need to *vary* your foods so that your diet makes up the eight essential amino-acids for adults or the ten for children. For instance, wheat protein is low in one essential amino-acid – i.e. lysine, but milk has plenty of it. So a wheat cereal *with* milk for breakfast would be a good combination. What *does* matter is that *some* protein is eaten every day. You should remember that babies, growing children, adolescents, pregnant and nursing mothers all need more than usual, and that the body cannot make protein itself.

Fats (Lipids)

The chemical elements present in **fats** are carbon, hydrogen, oxygen. They are absorbed as glycerol and fatty acids.

Fats have 3 important functions

(i) *For Respiration*; the energy yield is 39 kj/g (which is twice as much as carbohydrates or proteins).

(ii) *As a Component of cell membranes.*

(iii) *Insulation and protection.* Fat is stored under the skin for insulation, to absorb toxins, and around organs for protection.

- **Saturated fats** Tend to be solid at room temperature. A high intake of such fats in the diet, could be a factor in causing atherosclerosis (fatty deposits in the artery walls which impede the blood flow).

> *Food sources*: animal fats, meat, lard, suet, dairy produce, e.g. butter, cheese

- **Unsaturated fats.** Tend to be liquid at room temperature, and called oils.

> *Food sources*: peanut oil, corn oil.

Carbohydrates

Carbohydrates contain carbon (C), hydrogen (H) and oxygen (O) as shown in the formula: CH_2O

There are 3 main groups of carbohydrates (saccharides):

- **Monosaccharides** (simple sugars): Fruit, Honey

- **Disaccharides** (complex sugars): Cane sugar, Milk (Lactose)

- **Polysaccharides** (consists of a great many monosaccharide molecules linked together): Starch, Flour, Potatoes, Cellulose (important as roughage).

The main function of carbohydrates is to provide energy for respiration. The average yield is 17 KJ/g. Carbohydrates are not essential in the diet, but they are a convenient source of energy because they are readily available. They are the main components of all plants.

- Carbohydrates are relatively easy to digest.
- Carbohydrates which are not required immediately are stored as glycogen in the liver and the muscles.

Micronutrients

Micronutrients are nutrients needed in relatively small amounts, such as many types of vitamins and minerals

Vitamins

Vitamins are complex organic chemicals found in small amounts in many foods. They are essential nutrients because:

1 they regulate the building and repair of body cells
2 they help with the release of energy through chemical reactions in the body
3 they protect the body by preventing disease.

In general, the body is unable to synthesise (produce) them so that they have to be supplied by the diet. The main vitamins can be basically divided into two groups:

1 Fat-soluble vitamins: A, D, E and K
2 Water-soluble vitamins: B group, C.

- **Fat-soluble vitamins**

  Vitamin A, retinol, is found in animal foods. Oily fish is a particularly good source of retinol. In vegetables and fruit it is called beta carotene. Beta carotene in solution is yellow in colour and is responsible for giving margarine its yellow colour. Beta carotene is only about one sixth as effective as retinol.

  Vitamin A is important because it protects the eyesight, particularly in relation to night vision, and it is valuable in preventing disorders of the skin and mucous membranes.

  Vitamin D, cholecalciferol, is found mainly in animal foods and the synthetic form is added to some breakfast cereals and margarine. It can be formed by the action of ultra-violet rays in sunlight on the skin. The rays convert the pro-vitamin, 7-dehydrocholesterol in the skin to vitamin D. A range of animal products, such as butter, therefore have a natural vitamin D content. Vitamin D is concerned with calcification and the absorption of calcium and phosphorus by the gut wall. Vitamin D is stored in the liver and an excess of it is poisonous. It is particularly important to be aware of this if children are given supplementary vitamins, as in fish-liver oils.

  Vitamin E, tocopherol, is widely distributed in eggs, cereal oils, liver and meat. It is thought to influence human fertility, but this research has not yet been completed. There is no known deficiency as yet.

  Vitamin K is essential for the normal clotting (or coagulation) of the blood. It is widely distributed in foods like fish, liver, oils and green vegetables. The gut bacteria can synthesise vitamin K in the large intestine, so there is no known deficiency.

- **Water-soluble vitamins**

  The B group of vitamins. This group has eight vitamins all having similar functions. In general they are all concerned with the release of energy from food. They are not able to be stored so a daily dose is required. Since they are water soluble, any excess is excreted in the urine.

  The main vitamins in this group are:

  - thiamin or B1
  - riboflavin or B2
  - nicotinic acid or niacin.

  Other less important vitamins in the B group are:

  - pyridoxine or B6
  - pantotheric acid
  - biotin
  - cobalamin or B12
  - folic acid

Table 3.6 summarises the vitamins required by the body.

	Vitamin	Why?	Where from?	Deficiency will cause

FAT-SOLUBLE	A
	
	As retinol
		• eyesight
		• mucous membranes of throat, etc.
		• health of skin
			• animal foods: milk
			                    cheese
			                    butter
			                    egg yolk
			                    liver
			                    kidney
				• eye problems
				• very dry skin
				• retarded growth in children

	As carotene		• oily fish
			• plants: carrots
			           spinach
			           watercress
			           tomatoes	

	D Cholecalciferol	• formation of bones and teeth • absorption of calcium and phosphorus	• liver • oily fish • margarine • milk • dairy foods	• rickets (in children) • osteomalacia (in the elderly), ie weakening of bones
	E Tocopherol	• present in all cells • function not clear	• peanuts • royal jelly • lettuce • wheatgerm	• problems with plasma membranes • anaemia in premature babies
	K	• coagulation of blood	• spinach • liver • oils • fish	• delayed blood clotting and excessive bleeding
WATER-SOLUBLE	B1 Thiamin	• helps to release energy from carbohydrates • for nerves • growth of children	• wholegrain cereals and products • yeast • meat • eggs • milk	• depression • weakness • beriberi
	B2 Riboflavin	• for release of energy	• wholegrain cereals and products • yeast • meat • eggs • milk	• dermatitis • conjunctivitis • poor growth in children
	Nicotinic acid	• for release of energy	• liver • meat • bread • milk • potatoes • cabbage • salmon	• pellagra • dermatitis • diarrhoea
	B12 Cobalamin	• for the metabolism of amino-acids in the body	• liver • kidney • oily fish • eggs • fresh milk	• anaemia
	C Ascorbic acid	• to make connective tissue • for absorption of iron • growth	• blackcurrants • citrus fruit • green vegetables	• gums bleed • haemorrhages under the skin • new potatoes • scurvy • anaemia

Table 3.6   The main vitamins needed in the diet

Minerals

The body needs a large number of **minerals** to keep it in good condition.

Mineral elements are used in varying ways in the body, but there are three main headings under which they may be considered:

1 As part of the rigid structure of the body: **calcium** (Ca), **phosphorus** (P) and **magnesium** (Mg) are used in the formation of the bone structure of the body.
2 As part of the soft body tissue: **potassium** (K) is used in soft tissue and stabilises cell fluid.
3 As part of the fluid of the body; **sodium** (Na) and **chlorine** (Cl) are stabilising influences in body fluid.

Table 3.7 summarises the basic minerals required by the body.

Mineral	Why?	Where from?
Calcium	• for bones and teeth • muscles • blood clotting	• milk • cheese • tinned fish • added to bread
Phosphorus	• with calcium for bones and teeth • helps to produce energy	• cheese • eggs • fish • meat
Iron	• for making haemoglobin	• liver • kidney • corned beef • egg yolk • cocoa
Sodium	• to stabilise the composition of body fluids	• salt
Potassium	• to stabilise the composition of body fluids	• fruit and vegetables
Iodine	• for metabolism and the thyroid	• all seafoods • milk • spinach
Fluoride	• for teeth	• seafoods • water supply

Table 3.7   Some basic minerals

Nutritional needs during different life stages

The 5 stages of life are defined and developed as follows:

- Infancy
- Childhood
- Adolescence
- Pregnancy
- Old age

They are all different stages in our lives when our daily requirements will vary. We will now look at each one in turn.

Infancy

Infants which are full-term have about a 6 month store of nutrients, e.g. iron (Fe) and copper (Cu) (which are not in breast milk). Often semi-solid foods are introduced into the diet to supply these needs; semi-solids are not given before 3 months because the infant may develop food allergies. Vitamin drops (A, C and D) are often given to babies over one month especially those who are not being breast fed. An infant needs a higher intake of all vitamins than do school children and adults.

Childhood

Children need more nutrients than adults do, due to the rapid rate of growth. Young people need sunlight (for the formation of vitamin D). Some young children (for example Asian children) in the UK may need extra vitamin D supplement. To avoid rickets in children two micro nutrients should be taken in, namely calcium and vitamin D.

Pregnancy

Pregnant women require an increased intake of vitamin B group, including vitamin 12, folic acid, vitamins D and C. Nursing mothers need to keep up the increased intake of vitamins, to provide the essential vitamin content of breast milk, which also helps the babies develop passive immunity.

Did You Know **?**

Fibre intake is important during pregnancy because the muscles are slacker and constipation can be a problem. Iron supplements can be given to women during pregnancy if they are anaemic.

Table 3.8 identifies some important nutrients required during pregnancy.

Nutrient	Where found	Needed for	Deficiency will cause
calcium	milk cheese yoghurt bread	developing baby and maintenance of mother-to-be's own teeth and bones	rickets in the limbs of children (not only caused by lack of calcium)
iron	red meat liver cocoa corned beef green vegetables	making haemoglobin in the blood	anaemia
Vitamin D cholecalciferol	liver oily fish margarine dairy foods sunlight	the absorption of calcium and phosphorus	rickets

Table 3.8   Important nutrients during pregnancy

Adolescence

This is also a time of rapid growth, so plenty of protein is required to support body growth and cell repair. High biological value proteins can be taken in by ensuring an adequate intake of some combination of meat, fish, cheese, eggs, milk and soya beans. The adolescent will also need plenty of calcium and vitamin D to stengthen bones and teeth. Iron (for making haemoglobin) will be another important element in a balanced diet for adolescents, especially for girls, to replace that lost in menstruation.

Old age

The elderly and many adults may be at risk of vitamin deficiency if they are living alone and neglect to eat a sufficient amount of fresh fruit, vegetables and protein. A deficiency of vitamin C, D, B12, and folic acid may occur, with the consequent development of scurvy and anaemia. If a lot of fibre is eaten, the elderly may have difficulty in absorbing calcium. They should therefore drink extra milk or eat extra yoghurt.

The factors that affect choice of diet

In this section we will discuss general attitudes to food and the specific attitudes and requirements of Jewish, Moslem, Hindu and Christian cultures.

Attitudes to food

What we eat, how much we eat, and when we eat, are linked with many of the following:

- Rewards
- Punishment
- Celebrations
- Social occasions
- Certain activities, including watching TV, driving a car.
- Feeling of pleasure, self indulgence
- Being concerned with one's image, how you look,
- Being concerned about having control over your life, via your body.

This can lead to becoming anorexic, bulimia, obesity, alternative bingeing and fasting.

In excess, such attitudes can become obsessions and lead to eating disorders such as:

- **anorexia nervosa**: an overwhelming fear and loathing of body fat that leads to extreme dieting

- **bulimia nervosa**: closely related to anorexia, this 'gorge-purge' syndrome involves vomiting after eating in an attempt to lose weight.

Cultural and religious beliefs and customs

These can play a very important part in people's lives and in some cases influence what they choose to eat. Some festive occasions are not based on religious laws, but have ritual importance and food has an important part to play, for example the New Year, Halloween, and Bonfire night. Certain religions have special laws or specific instructions about the way that food is prepared and about what should or should not be eaten, and also when it can be eaten. Religious ceremonies celebrate important days such as birth, marriages or funerals by either a feast or fast. Many religious beliefs are associated with food, such as Jewish, Moslem, Hindu and Christian beliefs.

- **Jewish culture.** Many Jewish festivals are celebrated with special meals (e.g. Passover involving unleavened bread). There is also a special weekly meal in which all the family attend on the Sabbath day, which covers sunset on Friday to sunset on Saturday.

  The Jewish customs and dietary laws are laid out in the Old Testament of the Bible (see Deuteronomy chapter 16 and Leviticus chapter 11). Foods fulfilling the requirements of Jewish dietary laws are called *Kosher* foods. Only meat from cud-chewing, clove-footed animals may be eaten e.g. lamb, venison and beef, and clean birds (birds of prey and scavenger birds are not to be eaten). Forbidden foods in the Jewish faith include: ham, pork, bacon (pig), eggs with blood spots, gelatine, shellfish, eels. Certain foods should not be prepared or eaten together, like milk and meat.

- **Muslim culture.** Ramadan is the main fast of Islam which lasts for one month each year. Strict Muslims do not eat or drink anything between sunrise and sunset (meals are eaten at night).
  Forbidden food
  Many Muslims follow similar food laws to those found in the Jewish culture, e.g. they do not eat pig meat.
  Food allowed to eat
  Halal is the ritual slaughter of animals; animals killed in this way can be eaten. A certain amount of fish is eaten by some Muslims.

- **Hindu culture.** Cows are considered sacred, also used as a working animal on the land. Hindus do not kill cows for food.
  Forbidden food
  Any meat from cows, and from pigs which are classed as unclean
  Food allowed to eat
  Non-meat products from cows, butter, milk and in some cases cheese. Many Hindus will not eat any meat from animals that have been killed by ritual slaughter.

- **Christian culture.** Christmas, Easter and Harvest festival are important festive seasons and traditional food is prepared and eaten at such times. Certain foods used to be restricted on certain days and fish replaced meat on Friday; some people still continue this practice. Many practising Christians also give up certain foods during Lent. Many non-practising Christians still take part in the above celebrations.

Special diets

In this section we will look at the following diets:

- weight reducing/controlling
- diabetic
- low salt
- vegetarian
- vegan

Weight reduction/controlling diets

When weight becomes excessive (**obese**) it can be dangerous to the health. This is a common nutritional disorder in affluent, developed countries due to an excessive amount of food intake and therefore of body fat.

Weight is gained because we eat more food, with its associated energy (calorific) content, than the body needs. This results in *fat* which is stored under the skin (adipose tissue). Foods such as carbohydrates, fats, protein, ethanol (alcohol) have high calorific content.

Overeating occurs when energy intake *exceeds* energy output; any excess is converted into fat. If the body weight exceeds 15% of the ideal weight, the individual is classed as clinically obese.

Did You Know ?

About 20 tons of food are eaten during an average lifetime. A small imbalance between energy intake and energy output can have an enormous impact. For example an *extra* 50 calories per day (from an extra knob of butter at breakfast) can result in a weight gain of 20kg over ten years.

Being obese and overweight causes an increased load on the skeleton system, which can lead to various disorders and complications. Such as:

- *Support problems* – joint arthritis, flat feet, ruptures of the abdomen wall.
- *Circulation problems* – high blood pressure, heart disease, piles/haemorrhoids and varicose veins.
- *Digestive problems* – sugar diabetes, gout, cancer of the womb or uterus, gallstones, and gall bladder problems.
- *Respiratory problems* – breathlessness on exertion.
- *Dental decay* – excess refined carbohydrate, can lead to tooth decay.
- *Surgical procedures* – made more difficult.
- *Accidents* – stumbling, tripping, falls, resulting in fractures.
- *Emotional problems* – can be unhappy about appearance; may have difficulty finding fashionable clothes; could be teased, etc. This can lead to a vicious circle, whereby the overweight person turns to food for comfort, which only increases the problem.
- *Life span* – is shortened.

Weight reduction diets. Obesity develops over a long time, therefore it will take some time to reduce one's weight.

- The only way to lose weight is to eat sensibly: eat a varied diet; eat only when hungry; do not eat between meals. One can eat as many as 5 or 6 small meals a day instead of 3 larger ones; do not eat snacks; do not eat when bored; never over eat. If you eat more than 350 calories per meal, the excess is laid down as fat.
- Eat lots of fruit, vegetables, wholemeal bread, pasta, brown rice, fish, chicken.
- Eat less fats, sweet foods, red meat.

Crash diets can damage one's health. Many lack vital nutrients which can cause mood swings, irritability and depression. On crash diets people often end up overeating/bingeing, resulting in a cycle of bingeing, guilt, starving, dieting. The diet then starts to take over one's life.

Task:
(a) Find out about local and national organisations that help people lose weight, like Weight Watchers.
(b) How do they do this and how many people come for help?
(c) Are the benefits long term?

Diabetes

People with diabetes have a deficiency of insulin. This may be because too little is made in the pancreas or because body cells are unable to use insulin properly, so need larger amounts than are normally made. A lack of insulin results in an increase in glucose concentration in the blood. The kidneys are unable to re-absorb all the glucose and some appears in the urine. Diabetics can control the condition through low carbohydrate low-sugar diets and by regular injections of insulin.

Low salt diet

It is important to restrict the amount of sodium (salt) in the diet to help those who already suffer from high blood pressure. It is important to cut back on foods with a high salt content.

- **Foods high in salt.** Bacon, sausages, salami, corned beef, ham, margarine, salted butter, hard cheese, savoury biscuits, yeast extract, tomato ketchup, canned vegetables, plus any food to which salt has been added.

- **Reducing salt intake.** Reduce (or stop completely) the amount of salt added to cooking. It only takes a short while for the body to adjust to the reduction in salt. It can be as short as three days. Remove the salt pot from the meal table. Using salt is an activity that can be habit forming.

Vegetarian

A vegetarian is someone who does not eat any products derived directly or indirectly from the slaughter of animals, fish or birds.

Being a vegetarian has no nutritional difficulties. It can be a very healthy diet, low in fat, high in fibre and low in sodium. Many vegetarians do *not* have low blood cholesterol levels due to the fact that they often rely heavily on dairy produce, which contains large quantities of saturated fats.

Vegan

Vegans go one stage further than vegetarians by not eating any product which involves the exploitation of animals. This diet excludes all dairy products and eggs, as well as flesh, fish and fowl and, in some cases, honey as well.

The Vegan Society was formed in 1945 to describe those who avoid animal products for food, clothing and other consumer goods. Cholesterol levels of vegans are lower than vegetarians or meat eaters, due to not eating dairy produce. As a result vegans are less prone to heart disease and other diseases that affect meat eaters.

It is recommended that vegans should take vitamin B12 supplements.

Self Check ✓ **Element 3**

23. Which one of the following vitamins is manufactured in the skin due to the presence of sunlight:
    A   Vitamin A
    B   Vitamin B
    C   Vitamin C
    D   Vitamin D

24. Why is calcium an important part of our diet?
    A   For stabilising of body tissue fluids
    B   To prevent rickets
    C   To prevent beri beri
    D   For making bones and teeth

25. Roughage (fibre) is essential in the diet because:
    A   prevents diarrhoea
    B   prevents constipation
    C   a good source of Vit A
    D   a good source of Vit C

26. Roughage (fibre) is made – up of:
    A   plant material consisting mainly of cellulose
    B   dead cells of the gut wall
    C   dead organisms in the gut cavity
    D   tough food taken into the gut

27. Which one of the following foods produces most energy:
    A   1g protein
    B   1g of fat
    C   1g glucose
    D   1g vitamins

28. Which one of the following closely describes vitamins:
    A   complex naturally occurring chemicals
    B   necessary substance that humans can make themselves
    C   man made substances required by humans
    D   necessary substances which humans cannot make themselves

29. Which one of the following is the main constituent of fish or meat:
    A   vitamins
    B   fat
    C   protein
    D   carbohydrate

30. Which one of the following has the greatest amount of energy per unit value:
    A   corn oil
    B   potato
    C   lean meat
    D   sugar

31. People who consume a well balanced diet make sure that:
    A   energy intake exceeds energy output
    B   energy intake slightly exceeds energy expenditure
    C   energy intake is slightly less than energy expenditure
    D   energy intake is less than energy expenditure

32. Food is acquired by holozoic nutrition in four stages. Put the stages into a logical order:
    1.   Assimilation
    2.   Digestion
    3.   Ingestion
    4.   Egestion

    A   1,2,4,3
    B   3,1,2,4
    C   3,2,1,4
    D   1,2,3,4

33. Pregnant women should have Vitamin D in their diet …
    A   To aid with the blood formation in the foetus
    B   To aid bone formation in the foetus
    C   To give the mother more strength
    D   To give the mother more energy

34. (a)   On a reducing diet, why is it better to eat fruit rather than cereal and full fat milk for breakfast?
    (b)   Why does breakfast cereal provide roughage?
    (c)   Why does a woman need more calcium when she is:
          (i)   pregnant?
          (ii)   breast feeding a baby?
    (d)   Give one good source of protein

35. Name 3 other classes of food, in addition to protein, fats, and carbohydrate, which are essential for a balanced diet

36. (a)   What is a vitamin?
    (b)   Why should pregnant women have vitamin D in their diet?
    (c)   What precautions should be taken during cooking vegetables so that Vitamin C is preserved?

Unit Test Answer all the questions

Question 1 and 2
Diagram A shows a simplistic view of blood circulation round the body.

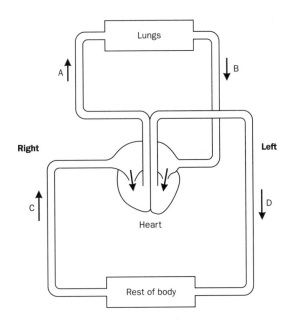

Question 1
Which of the lettered sections has blood vessels which carry deoxygenated blood? Is it:

A   A and B
B   C and D
C   A and C
D   B and D

Question 2
Which is the Pulmonary vein shown in diagram A. Is it:

A   A
B   B
C   C
D   D

Question 3
What are the functions of blood?

1. To prevent blockage in blood vessels.
2. To carry oxygen to the cells.
3. To carry oxygen from the cells.
4. To remove carbon dioxide

A   1,2,4
B   1,2,3
C   2,3,4
D   2,4,1

Question 4
What is the difference between arteries and veins?

A   Arteries do not have valves.
    Veins have valves.
B   Arteries have valves.
    Veins have valves.
C   Arteries have valves.
    Veins do not have valves.
D   Arteries do not have valves.
    Veins do not have valves.

Question 5
When air is breathed in, select (A) or (B) for what happens for each structure?

Structure	What happens	
1. Lungs	A. Expand	B. Contract
2. Rib	A. Raised	B. Lowered
3. Diaphragm Muscle	A. Contracts	B. Relaxes
4. Diaphragm	A. Raised	B. Lowered
5. Thorax – Volume	A. Increases	B. Decreases

Choice:
A   1.A   2.A   3.A   4.A   5.A
B   1.A   2.A   3.A   4.B   5.A
C   1.A   2.A   3.A   4.A   5.B
D   1.A   2.A   3.B   4.B   5.B

Question 6
An infectious disease can be transmitted from one person to another.

True or False?

Question 7
An incubation period is the time delay between the initial infection and the appearance of the symptoms of the disease.

True or False?

Question 8
The membranes surrounding the linings of the lung consist of:

A   The periosteum
B   The perichondrium
C   The pleura
D   The pericardium

Question 9
The process of anaerobic respiration

A   Occurs without using oxygen
B   Occurs using oxygen
C   Occurs inside & outside of cells
D   Occurs neither inside or outside of cells

Question 10
Aerobic Respiration can be shown by the following equation.

Glucose + ...→ Carbon dioxide + Water + Energy

From the list below complete the equation

A   Salt
B   Water
C   Protein
D   Oxygen

Question 11
Which one of the following contracts when you breathe in:

A   Ribs
B   Bronchus
C   Lungs
D   Diaphragm

Question 12
The origin of a disease may be due to the internal or external causes or a combination of both.

True or False?

Question 13
An example of an illness caused by a virus is:

A   Typhoid
B   Chickenpox
C   Ringworm
D   Whooping cough

Question 14
The incubation period of an infectious illness develops after:

A   The formation of antibodies in the blood
B   Entry of the infected organism into the body
C   Developing a high temperature
D   Developing a fever

Question 15
Food poisoning and dysentery may be spread by houseflies that land on food after they have:

A   Settled on human faeces
B   Sucked blood from an infected human or animal
C   Been sprayed with fly killer
D   Had sexual contact

Question 16
How are the following diseases spread?
(Match letters with numbers)

A   Influenza
B   Typhoid
C   Malaria

1.   Spread by female Anophles Mosquito and transmitted to humans when it bites them
2.   Caused by a virus which is spread by droplet infection during sneezing or other close contact between an infected person and a healthy person
3.   Spread by food or water which is contaminated by bacteria

Question 17
How is the spread of diseases controlled?
(Match letters with numbers)

A   Influenza
B   Typhoid
C   Malaria

1.   Vaccination and proper hygiene prevents the spread
2.   Controlled by killing the vector
3.   Prevention by vaccination which may last for 1–2 years. Also contact with people should be avoided for an isolation period of at least 7 days

Question 18
After having a disease like measles, a person is likely to have acquired:

A   Natural immunity
B   Artificial immunity
C   Active immunity
D   Passive immunity

Question 19
Passive immunity gives:

A   Long term protection
B   Short term protection
C   Gives no protection
D   Gives permanent protection

Question 20
How might a person become infected with the virus which causes AIDS?

A   By mixing body fluids during sexual intercourse
B   By blood to blood contact
C   By sharing public toilets
D   Sharing needles and syringes.

Is it
1.   A,B,C
2.   B,C
3.   A,B,C,D
4.   A,B,D

Question 21
The methods of preventing the spread of AIDS is by:

1.   Use of condoms during sexual intercourse
2.   Avoiding using public toilets
3.   Avoiding used needles and syringes
4.   Avoiding holding hands and/or cuddling
A   2 and 3
B   1,2 and 3
C   1 and 3
D   1,3 and 4

Question 22
During exercise which of the following factors is least likely to increase:

A   Breathing
B   Digestion of food
C   Pulse rate
D   Breakdown of glucose

Question 23
Why is fluoride in some areas added to drinking water?

A   To kill germs and bacteria
B   To make teeth white
C   To strengthen the enamel of teeth
D   To prevent mouth ulcers

Question 24
Roughage in our diet is important because

A   It is not digested and helps prevent constipation
B   It is not digested and provides extra carbohydrates
C   It is digested and helps prevent constipation
D   It is digested and provides extra carbohydrates

Question 25
Which of the following Nutrients provide the most energy per gram

A   Fats
B   Proteins
C   Carbohydrates
D   Vitamins

Question 26
From the list below, what combination is used for growth and repair of cells?

A   Fats
B   Starch
C   Proteins
D   Roughage
E   Minerals

1.   D, E, F,
2.   A, D, E,
3.   A, B, C,
4.   A, C, E,

Question 27
The following foods are unsuitable for slimmers.
Are the following statements True or False?

(i)   **Sugar** – Because it contains a lot of carbohydrate, which produces a lot of energy, which if it is not used up will be stored in the body.
(ii)   **Butter** – Because it contains a lot of fat, which if not used up will be stored in the body.

A   (i) True   (ii) False

B   (i) True   (ii) True
C   (i) False   (ii) True
D   (i) False   (ii) False

Question 28
Anaemia is caused by which particular substance missing from the diet?

A   Vitamin A
B   Vitamin D
C   Vitamin C
D   Iron

Question 29
A food which contains the substance required to avoid anaemia is:

A   Citrus fruit
B   Green vegetables
C   Dairy produce
D   Liver

Question 30
Scurvy is caused by a particular substance missing from the diet. What is it ?

A   Vitamin A
B   Vitamin D
C   Iron
D   Vitamin C

Question 31
A food that contains the above substance is:

A   Dairy produce

B   Fish
C   Citrus fruit
D   Liver

Question 32
Rickets is caused by a particular substance missing from the diet. What is it?

A   Vitamin A
B   Iron
C   Vitamin B
D   Vitamin D

Question 33
A food that contains much of this substance is:

A   Potatoes
B   Citrus fruit
C   Dairy produce
D   Meat

Question 34
Many forms of mental health are:

A   Treatable
B   Not treatable
C   Contagious
D   Fatal

Question 35
Mental illness can occur when a person cannot cope with the stress and problems of every day life. Mental handicap is, however, unlikely to be the result of an inability to cope.

Is this statement TRUE or FALSE?

Answers to Self-check questions

1. D

2. C

3. B and D

4. A and D

5. True

6. A, B, C and D (i.e. all)

7. C

8. (a) Cardiac
   (b) Helps continuous beat of heart (not subject to fatigue)

9. (a) To prevent back flow of blood on contraction of the ventricle (Chamber C)
   (b) B and D
   (c) B

10. See page 42

11. D. It is a permanent condition.

12. People are not normally born mentally ill. It can affect anyone at any time and varies in severity.

13. B

14. True

15. D it is a waste product.

16. C. The micro-organisms then stop reproducing.

17. B

18. C. See page 56

19. D. See page 56

20. C

21. B

22. Many possible answers here; e.g. (a) bronchitis (b) low income, lack of dietary awareness, unstable family routines (meal times) etc.

23. D. Due to a chemical process.

24. D. Also helps bones and teeth to overcome wear and tear.

25. B. Acts as the bulk stimulating bowel movement

26. A

27. B

28. D

29. C

30. A

31   B

32   C

33   B

34   (a) It would lessen the intake of carbohydrate and fat; fat is not present in fruit and carbohydrate only as a small amount of sugar (e.g. in grapefruit).
   (b) Because of the high fibre content
   (c) (i) To maintain calcium levels in her bones and for the foetal bones.
       (ii) To provide calcium for the growth of the babies bones.
   (d) Meat or Fish.

35   Vitamins, minerals and water.

36   (a) A vitamin is an organic chemical required in minute quantities by the body in order to perform essential chemical activities.
   (b) Vitamin D is important for bone formation. Although vitamin D will form in the skin of the women when exposed to sunlight, this will not be sufficient. The diet must be supplemented with vitamin D, e.g. to aid bone formation in the foetus.
   (c) Vegetables should be steamed or cooked in water: no additional substances should be added, such as salt/bicarbonate of soda which destroy vitamin C.
      – Vegetables not soaked before cooking
      – Minimal water necessary to cover vegetables
      – Boil before adding vegetables
      – Cooking should not be prolonged etc.

Answers to Unit Test

Question	Answer	Question	Answer	Question	Answer	Question	Answer	Question	Answer
1	C	9	A	16(B)	3	21	C	29	D
2	B	10	D	16(C)	1	22	B	30	D
3	C	11	D	17(A)	3	23	C	31	C
4	A	12	True	17(B)	1	24	A	32	D
5	B	13	B	17(C)	2	25	A	33	C
6	True	14	B	18	C	26	3	34	A
7	True	15	A	19	B	27	B	35	True
8	C	16(A)	2	20	4	28	D		

Unit Test Comments

Question 1
A and C carry deoxygenated blood to the heart and lungs.

Question 2
The pulmonary vein carries oxygenated blood from the lungs to the left atrium of the heart.

Question 3
The function of blood is to provide nourishment to the body's cells and to remove waste.

Question 4
Arteries do not have valves but veins do have valves to stop the backflow of blood.

Question 5
The lungs expand; the ribs are raised; the diaphragm muscle contracts; the diaphragm is lowered and the thorax volume increases.

Question 6
True. The germs which cause infectious diseases are either bacteria, viruses or fungi; germs enter the body through body openings or wounds, and can therefore be transmitted from one person to another.

Question 7
True. This is an accurate definition.

Question 8
See page 47.

Question 9
Unlike aerobic respiration, no oxygen is required.

Question 10
Oxygen is required for aerobic respiration.

Question 11
The diaphragm muscle contracts (flattens) when we breathe in, increasing the volume of the chest cavity and reducing the air pressure so that air enters from outside the body.

Question 12
True.

Question 13
Chickenpox is caused by a virus, as are measles and influenza.

Question 14
The incubation period begins with the entry of the infection into the body.

Question 15
Human faeces contain many disease carrying bacteria.

Question 16
A, 2 (as in answer 13 above)
B, 3 Typhoid is an infectious disease spread by contaminated food or water.
C, 1 Malaria is spread by a vector, in this case the mosquito.

Question 17
A, 3 Influenza can be controlled by vaccination and by avoiding contact with infected persons.
B, 1 Vaccination against typhoid will grant some immunity as will proper hygiene (e.g. avoiding bacteria in faeces etc. of infected persons).
C, 2 Spraying stagnant water in which mosquitoes breed and killing the vector helps control malaria.

Question 18
Antibody production in the infected person (i.e. active immunity) will protect against a recurrence of measles, etc.

Question 19
When antibodies have been produced by *another* organism, not the individual concerned, then immunity is likely to be relatively short-lived.

Question 20
Using public places, such as toilets, is not known to be a means of spreading the AIDS virus.

Question 21
Public toilets, hand holding and cuddling are not associated with the spreading of the AIDS virus.

Question 22
During exercise, breathing and pulse rate increase, as does the breakdown of glucose (anaerobic respiration). Digestion of food does *not* increase.

Question 23
Fluoride does not kill germs and bacteria, make teeth white or prevent mouth ulcers. It does strengthen the enamel of teeth.

Question 24
Roughage provides bulk which is not digested and does help bowel movement, preventing constipation.

Question 25
Fats are very high in calories (energy) per unit of mass.

Question 26
Roughage and minerals do not contribute in these respects.

Question 27
Both statements are reasons why the respective foods (sugar and butter) and unsuitable for slimmers.

Question 28
Lack of iron is a cause of anaemia.

Question 29
Liver is 'rich' in iron.

Question 30
A lack of vitamin C (e.g. citrus fruits) will cause scurvy.

Question 31
Citrus fruits contain much vitamin C.

Question 32
A lack of vitamin D will cause rickets.

Question 33
Dairy produce is 'rich' in vitamin D.

Question 34
Many mental disorders are treatable.

Question 35
True.

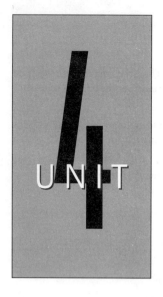

UNIT 4

Psychological and social aspects of health and social care

Getting Started

Element 1 Investigate the development of individual identity
Element 2 Investigate threats to maintaining individual identity
Element 3 Investigate the relationship of social and economic factors to health

This Unit examines a range of social and economic factors which are relevant to health and social care, together with some important aspects of human psychology. The study of this Unit should give you a greater insight into the ways clients might be influenced by their background, and consequently a greater awareness of client needs.

The first Element considers how the identity of the individual is formed, and looks at such topics as socialisation, cultural influences on the individual and the psychology of learning. The second Element is concerned with ways in which an individual might be threatened by stressful life events (such as bereavement or loss of health) and by various kinds of abuse. Ways of coping with such threats are also discussed. The third Element examines how the economic resources of clients can affect their ability to maintain good health and cope with stressful life events. The Unit ends with a consideration of stress-related illness.

Useful Cross-References
The following Elements from *previous Units* contain material relevant to this Unit:

Unit 1 Element 1 (Socialisation / Social role)
Unit 3 Element 2 (Influence of socio-economic factors on patterns of disease)
Unit 3 Element 3 (The components of healthy diet)

Coping mechanisms   Conscious and constructive ways of trying to deal with anxiety and stress.

Culture   A collection of beliefs, values and behaviours distinctive to a large group of people.

Defence mechanisms   Defences against anxiety that involve an individual deceiving himself about the reality of his situation.

Deviance   Behaviour which does not follow the norms and expectations of a particular society.

Identity   The physical, social and psychological make-up of an individual.

Labelling   When an individual is identified by another (or by others) as belonging to a particular group, and assumed to have the characteristics that other members of the group are believed to have.

Life events   Significant changes in a person's life which may occur through choice (such as marriage or moving house) or which may be unexpected (such as sudden bereavement or loss of employment).

Peer group   People occupying a similar position in society whom an individual associates with; usually the members of a peer group are also of a roughly similar age.

Role   The expected pattern of behaviour of someone occupying a particular position within a social group.

Self-concept   The image that an individual has of himself / herself.

Social network   The set of informal relationships that an individual has, including family, relatives, friends, neighbours and work colleagues.

Socialisation   The process by which an individual learns the norms and practices of the social groups to which he or she belongs.

Stereotyping   The act of assuming that all people who belong to a particular group have the same characteristics.

Stressor   An event or situation which threatens a person's well-being and gives rise to a stress reaction.

Essential Principles

4.1 The development of individual identity

What is identity?

The term **identity** refers to the physical, social and psychological 'make-up' of the individual. A person's identity is shaped by a multitude of factors, including for example their gender, temperament, social class and relationships with others. These factors interact in a unique way for each individual, a process which we shall examine in this Element.

Socialisation

Socialisation takes place when an individual learns the norms and practices of the social groups to which he or she belongs. The most important phase of socialisation occurs during infancy and childhood, and this is known as *primary socialisation*. During this period the child learns, usually from its parents, forms of behaviour that are considered acceptable and in this way is initiated into the customs of the wider society. The continued survival of any society is dependent upon socialisation, which ensures that one generation's patterns of behaviour will strongly resemble those of the next.

Any individual is a member not only of a society, but also of a diverse range of groups within that society. The first social group to which a child belongs is the family; later, it will become part of another group when it goes to school; later still, when it enters employment it will belong to an occupational group. The residents of a nursing home are a social group, as are the patients on a hospital ward. Each of these groups has patterns of behaviour which the individual must learn in order to integrate successfully with the group's other members. Further learning is necessary if an individual takes on an additional role within a group, of if the nature of the original role changes: within a family group, for example, a wife and mother may in later life become a widow and grandmother.

Socialisation is thus a lifelong process. The learning which takes place during childhood, however, has the most lasting significance. We shall now look at the main influences upon the developing child.

Influence of the family

The identity of the individual begins to be formed in childhood by the interaction that takes place with other **family members**, especially parents. The child's parents will encourage some kinds of behaviour and discourage others, and will serve as models for the child to imitate. They are likely to have a lasting influence on the child's attitudes and values: research comparing the attitudes of children and their parents has almost always shown a significant correlation, especially in political and religious attitudes. They are also likely to influence the child's perception of sexual role, so that the child will come to regard certain kinds of behaviour as appropriate for a boy, and other kinds as appropriate for a girl (for more on

this see the section on *Gender* later in this Element). During childhood three important types of learning occur:

> Classical conditioning
> Operant conditioning
> Imitation / Identification

Classical conditioning

The learning theory termed **Classical conditioning** was developed by the Russian physiologist Ivan Pavlov (1849–1936). His experiments with dogs showed the role of *conditioned reflexes* in animal and human behaviour. He began with the observation that dogs naturally salivate when presented with food. This natural behaviour could be described as an unconditioned response. He then sounded a bell immediately before giving food to the dogs. After repeating this procedure many times, he eventually found that the sound of the bell by itself was able to produce salivation in the dogs. He had thus *conditioned* the dogs to react in a certain way to the ringing of the bell – their behaviour could be termed a conditioned reflex, or conditioned response. The process is summarised in the box below.

Classical conditioning

STAGE ONE   Food (UCS) ⟶ Salivation (UCR)
STAGE TWO   Food (UCS) and Bell (CS) ⟶ Salivation
STAGE THREE   Bell (CS) ⟶ Salivation (CR)

UCS = Unconditioned stimulus   UCR = Unconditioned response
CS = Conditioned stimulus   CR = Conditioned response

The American psychologist J.B. Watson (1878–1958) demonstrated how children could acquire conditioned emotional responses in his famous 'Little Albert' experiment. Albert, who was nine months old, was observed reacting to the presence of a rat, a rabbit and a dog. He showed no fear, frequently reaching out to touch the animals. When a sudden loud noise was made, however, he naturally did appear frightened. By repeatedly pairing the loud noise with the rabbit, Watson eventually found that Albert responded with fear to the rabbit alone.

Classical conditioning helps to explain how *phobias* (a fear of spiders, for instance) can develop in childhood and persist into adult life. The same kind of conditioning can take place in later years: an especially painful visit to the dentist may give an adult a lasting aversion to dental treatment.

Such phobias and aversions need not be permanent however. In other experiments, children who have demonstrated fear in the presence of certain animals have been *desensitised* by associating the animal with a pleasant stimulus, such as sweets. Eventually the child is conditioned to react favourably to the animal. This desensitisation process is now frequently used in the treatment of phobias.

Operant conditioning

The theory of **operant conditioning** is especially associated with the American psychologist B.F. Skinner (1904–90). He stressed the importance of *reinforcement*: behaviour which is reinforced by something a person wants, needs or likes tends to be repeated, whereas behaviour which is not reinforced tends to die out.

In his early experiments Skinner placed a rat inside a box containing a food dispenser and a lever. This 'stimulus' produced a range of responses: scratching at the walls of the container, sniffing the floor and so on. After a time the rat accidentally pressed the lever and was rewarded with food. The rat soon learned that pressing the lever would cause food to appear and so it began pressing the lever more frequently – the behaviour was thus being repeated because it had been reinforced (by the reward of food). The process is summarised in the diagram below:

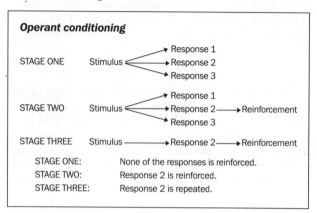

In human behaviour, reinforcement can take various forms. Examples of *material reinforcement* include giving sweets to a child who has been well behaved and paying a bonus to a salesman because his sales figures have improved. Another form of reinforcement is *social approval*: offering praise or congratulations, for instance. In all of these cases the behaviour which was reinforced is likely to be repeated.

Many lasting personality characteristics may be developed through operant conditioning. If a mother responds to a child's temper tantrums by giving the child sweets or by paying the child more attention, that behaviour is likely to be learned and repeated (because it has been rewarded). In later life the child may continue to use displays of temper as a means of trying to get what he or she wants.

Did You Know ?

A treatment technique known as the 'token economy' has become important in the practice of behaviour therapy in clinical institutions. A common feature of these tokens is that they can be earned for socially acceptable behaviour, and later exchanged for tangible rewards such as being allowed to watch a favourite television programme, home visits, sweets, cigarettes etc.

Imitation/identification

Another approach to child learning has been developed by Albert Bandura. He has studied the ways in which children imitate the behaviour of others. Everyday observation confirms that this kind of learning undoubtedly takes place: a child will copy adults when they wave goodbye, for example. Bandura calls this process **modelling**. A child's first models will be its parents; later, the influence of other members of the family will be felt; later still, friends, teachers and, in some cases, pop stars and sporting heroes will serve as models whose behaviour is imitated. What begins as simple imitation may become *identification*, which

occurs when the child or adolescent actually takes on one or more characteristics of another person so that the behaviour becomes a permanent feature of his identity. The behaviour has been *internalised* – the individual is no longer imitating others but expressing his own identity.

Bandura has particularly investigated whether children learn aggression from observing the behaviour of others. In one experiment children between three and six years old were divided into four groups. One group watched an adult behaving violently towards a rubber doll (punching it, hitting it with a hammer and so on). Another saw the adult behave in the same way, but on film. A third group saw similar behaviour towards the doll, but presented to them in the form of a cartoon. The final group were shown no aggressive behaviour at all. The children from all four groups were then given toys, including rubber dolls, to play with. The experimenters next deliberately frustrated the children by taking the toys away from them. When they were again allowed to play their behaviour was observed. The children from the first three groups behaved far more aggressively towards the dolls than the children in the fourth group.

In recent years there has been much debate about the effects of the explicit violence seen in 'video nasties' and on some television programmes. While some would argue that such violence is usually fictitious and therefore not taken seriously by the viewer, it is interesting to note that in Bandura's experiment the highest number of aggressive acts were performed by the children who had seen the cartoon, and the second highest by those who had watched the adult behaving aggressively on film.

Education

As a child grows older, the influence of parents and immediate family grows less, and with the onset of adolescence other social influences become increasingly important. One important influence in the development of the child's identity is **education**.

Much of the learning that takes place at school is formal and deliberate: the child is taught specific skills (such as reading and writing) and acquires knowledge about her own and other societies. As the child grows older, this kind of learning becomes increasingly specialised, so that education can be seen as preparing the individual for a specific role in society. In particular, a student who remains in education beyond the age of sixteen is likely to choose a course of study (such as GNVQ Health and Social Care!) suited to the career he or she wishes to follow.

The education system also helps to determine a child's attitudes and values. Again, this learning can be formal and deliberate, as when a school insists on certain standards of dress for its pupils, or emphasises to them the value of hard work. Often though this kind of learning is informal: observation of teachers, participation in school activities and the forging of positive relationships with teachers and other pupils can encourage the development of such values as co-operation and consideration for others.

Peer groups

As a child enters adolescence, he begins to spend less time at home with his family and more time with other members of his peer group – that is, with friends and acquaintances of roughly the same age.

> **Peer group** People occupying a similar position in society whom an individual associates with; usually the members of a peer group are also of a roughly similar age.

We belong to peer groups throughout our lives, though as our social circumstances change (as we move, for example, from school or college to work) so too will the groups to which we belong.

The influence of peer groups on the development of individual identity is at its greatest during adolescence. The kinds of influence a peer group can exert range from tastes in music and clothes to social and political attitudes. Closely-knit groups of friends (including gangs) are especially associated with the teenage years, as are style-conscious youth movements (past examples include mods and punks). The norms of behaviour of the peer group may conflict with those of the wider society, or with those of the adolescent's school or family. This means the adolescent must choose between these conflicting demands or, as is usually the case, attempt to strike a balance between them. This conflict may result in *deviant* behaviour.

> **Deviance** Behaviour which does not follow the norms and expectations of a particular society.

The adolescent may rebel against the rules and norms of family and society by playing truant from school for example, or by indulging in under-age drinking. Usually during this period the individual is attempting to find a stable identity, and may well experiment with a range of attitudes, roles and behaviours. As people enter their twenties, however, they tend to make firmer commitments – choosing a career, leaving the family home, marriage. As a result, the period of rebellion and experimentation ends, and the individual has a more secure identity and a greater acceptance of society's norms.

Social roles
Part of acquiring an identity is learning to identify with particular **social roles**.

> **Role** The expected pattern of behaviour of someone occupying a particular position within a social group.

Any one individual is likely to have many roles. A nurse, for example, will have this occupational role but she may also have other roles as a wife, mother, daughter, aunt, member of a union, neighbour and friend. In the course of an average day she is likely to fulfil yet more roles – as a customer in a shop, for instance, or a passenger on a bus. Society has expectations regarding how a person occupying each of these roles should behave. Thus a nurse is expected to be courteous and understanding towards patients, and to possess a certain amount of professional knowledge. As the individual's identity develops, she internalises these expectations and learns the correct patterns of behaviour for the roles she is to occupy.

Cultural Influences

Cultural influences: class, race, religion
Another set of norms and expectations comes from the **cultural groups** to which the individual belongs.

> **Culture** A collection of beliefs, values and behaviours distinctive to a large group of people.

As the above definition indicates, 'culture' is an extremely broad term. Cultural influences permeate all aspects of our lives: attitudes to diet, health, leisure and work are all expressions of a culture. Each nation or society has its own culture, its own set of beliefs, values and behaviours – British culture differs in many ways from Chinese culture, for example. Within the larger culture of a society, there also exist many smaller cultural groups (or 'subcultures'). Each of these groups will have its own distinctive attitudes, values and patterns of behaviour and the individuals belonging to these groups will inevitably be influenced by these.

One such cultural group is the **social class** to which the individual belongs. It is important not to assume that all members of a particular social class share the same beliefs and values, but there is an undoubted tendency for certain attitudes and patterns of behaviour to be associated with particular classes. Comparing middle and working class culture, for example, it seems that middle class families may attach more importance to educational achievement, while traditional, established working class neighbourhoods may have a stronger sense of community. Attitudes to health may also differ (for more on this see Element 3 in this Unit).

Ethnic groups are another cultural influence. Britain is a multicultural society, in the sense that people from many different ethnic backgrounds live here. Each ethnic group has its own values and customs (regarding marriage, dress and diet, for example). Difficulties can arise for the individual when these values and customs differ from those of the rest of society. A person who has grown up in Britain is likely to accept and adopt more aspects of British culture than a person who has spent only part of his life here. This in turn can lead to tensions between parents and children: young Asians, for instance, may come into conflict with their parents over the question of arranged marriages.

Religion is another important aspect of cultural background. Religious beliefs can have a wide-ranging influence, affecting for example a person's attitudes towards family planning, divorce and the upbringing of children. The beliefs of some religious groups affect attitudes towards health care, including the acceptability or unacceptability of certain kinds of treatment. Jehovah's Witnesses, for instance, may object to the use of blood transfusions. This sometimes leads to conflict with health professionals, especially when parents refuse treatment on behalf of their children.

Cultural influences: gender
Part of the socialisation process includes learning the different kinds of behaviour that society expects of **males and females**. This begins at an early age, when children are encouraged to rehearse their expected adult roles. Thus girls are given dolls and other toys which enable them to play at being mothers and housewives, while boys are given toys which encourage them to be more practical and aggressive, such as toy saws, hammers

and guns. Girls may also be taught to help their mother with cooking, cleaning and other domestic tasks.

Parents are now more aware of the influence of upbringing on attitudes towards gender, and sometimes make a deliberate effort to avoid pushing their children towards stereotyped forms of behaviour. There has also been a growing belief within society as a whole that men and women should break from their traditional social roles. Measures now exist which seek to ensure equal opportunities in employment, for example. Nevertheless, stereotypes of masculinity and femininity continue to be reinforced in a wide variety of ways (see the sections that follow on the media and language).

Cultural influences: the media

The **mass media** – advertising, television, radio, the cinema and newspapers – are another influence on the attitudes and behaviour of the individual. They help to create our view of society and often communicate beliefs and values. Sometimes this is done openly and explicitly, as when a newspaper during an election campaign carries a leading article on its front page urging readers to vote for a particular political party. Often, however, the values are hidden and implicit. A violent film, for example, may imply that violence is an acceptable (or even desirable) form of behaviour. Many people believe that media stereotypes of men and women encourage sexist attitudes. In advertising, for instance, women are often shown in domestic situations, while men are shown at work or driving fast cars.

A great deal of research has been carried out into the effects of the media on individual behaviour. However, a variety of problems make it difficult to arrive at definitive conclusions. One such problem is the impossibility of separating clearly the influence of the media and the influence of other factors, such as family and peer group. Nevertheless, that the media exert some influence is undeniable – television advertising unquestionably increases a product's sales, for example.

Cultural influences: language

The values of our society are reflected in the **language** that we use, and as children learn language they absorb also the values implicit in that language. Some of our language may serve to reinforce prejudices and stereotypes. It is often argued, for example, that much English usage stereotypes women, depicting them as the weaker and less important of the sexes. Evidence for this includes the use of 'man', 'men' and 'mankind' to refer to human beings in general (implying men are more important), and the use of patronising terms for women such as 'dear', 'love' and 'pet'. Another group to suffer in this way is the elderly, who could justifiably take exception to such expressions as 'silly old fool' and 'dirty old man' – even though users of these expressions are usually unaware that they might be offensive to old people.

Attempts have been made to change the language that we use in order to lessen the element of prejudice. Thus 'humankind' is now sometimes used instead of 'mankind', while the term 'senior citizens' accords more respect to the elderly than 'old age pensioners'.

Stereotypes/labels

Stereotyping occurs when we assume that all people who belong to a particular group have the same characteristics. As we have seen, stereotyping of men and women often takes place. Other common stereotypes are based upon age, racial group and sexual orientation.

Labelling is a closely related process. It occurs when an individual is identified as a member of a particular group, and assumed to have the characteristics that other members of the group are believed to have. A youth charged with theft, for example, might be labelled a 'delinquent' by his neighbours.

A danger of both labelling and stereotyping is that they can lead to false assumptions being made about an individual. People who are disabled, for example, are sometimes assumed to be helpless and completely dependent upon others, when in fact the degree of dependence varies considerably from one disabled individual to another.

Another danger is that the way victims of labelling and stereotyping see themselves can be affected. The youth labelled a 'delinquent' may come to share this view of himself and as a result go on to confirm the label by committing more crimes. A school pupil labelled 'slow' or 'of limited ability' by his teachers may lose confidence, lower his expectations and as a consequence perform poorly in his studies. Labels and stereotypes can thus contribute to the development of individual identity in that stereotyping or attaching a label to somebody may of itself cause the individual to conform to that label/stereotype.

Self-concept

All of the factors that have been discussed so far in this Element contribute to the development of the **self-concept** – that is, the idea that we have of ourselves. The social psychologist Michael Argyle has divided the influences upon an individual's perceptions of himself or herself into four main categories:

1. **The reaction of others** Initially, it is the reaction of parents that is important. A child repeatedly called 'stupid' by its parents will come to believe this is the truth and may well begin to act accordingly. Later, the attitudes of friends, teachers, workmates and so on become significant.

2. **Comparison with others** We can only see ourselves as fat, thin, attractive, ugly, clever, unintelligent and so on if we compare ourselves with others. Sometimes the comparisons are made for us: a girl who repeatedly hears others say that she is not as bright as her elder sister is likely to incorporate this into her self-concept.

3. **Social roles** As the individual grows older, he or she takes on an increasing number of roles. At first, when a role is new to us, the forms of behaviour associated with it are unfamiliar and we may be said to be 'acting out' the role. This occurs when a child first goes to school, for example, or when a woman becomes a mother for the first time. Eventually, however, we become used to the role, the behaviour associated with it is internalised and the role becomes an integral part of our personality – that is, it becomes incorporated into our self-concept.

4. **Identification** An individual tends to adopt the characteristics, attitudes and behaviour of others. The first models with whom we identify are our parents. Later models may include teachers, friends, figures in public life whom we admire and so on.

The time at which the adolescent's 'growth spurt' occurs may have an important effect on the adolescent's self-concept. The rate of physical development (especially in early or late maturers) can be a source of great anxiety and often becomes an important basis for adolescents making comparisons between themselves and other adolescents.

Self Check ✓ Element 1

1. Socialisation is a process by which the individual:
    (a) Acquires more friends and acquaintances as he or she grows older.
    (b) Learns how to form personal relationships.
    (c) Learns as a child to accept the authority of his or her parents.
    (d) Learns social norms and practices.

2. Identify each of the following as operant or classical conditioning:
    (a) A fear of heights that derives from a traumatic childhood experience.
    (b) Working harder in school because a teacher rewards effort with encouragement and praise.
    (c) Filling in a football pools coupon every week because you once won £500.
    (d) A love of long train journeys because as a child you always travelled by train to the seaside.

3. Which of the following statements is correct?
    (a) Imitation usually precedes identification.
    (b) Identification usually precedes imitation.
    (c) Imitation occurs when one person has internalised the behaviour patterns of another.

4. Most children learn at school how the British electoral system works. Is this:
    (a) Informal learning
    (b) Modelling
    (c) Formal learning
    (d) An example of peer group influence?

5. Comment on the accuracy of the following statements:
    (a) Most people are uninfluenced by culture. Only intellectuals and 'arty' types take any real interest in it.
    (b) To speak of 'British culture' is meaningless because Britain has many different cultures, each with its own traditions, beliefs and values.
    (c) Culture is the unchanging heart of a society, that which is passed on from generation to generation.

6. Stereotyping is principally unfair because:
    (a) It ignores the justifications that may exist for a person's behaviour.
    (b) It disregards a person's individuality.
    (c) It encourages deviance.

4.2 Investigate threats to maintaining individual identity

In the previous Element we examined how an individual develops a sense of identity. In this Element we shall consider the ways in which this identity might be **threatened**.

In particular, we shall look at how certain events in a person's life and certain kinds of abuse can create stress and damage a person's sense of self-worth. We shall also examine how an individual might seek to cope in such circumstances, and at the ways he or she can be helped to do so.

Life stages/life events

It is important that you know the difference between life stages and life events:

Life stages Important stages in the development of the individual which are experienced by human beings in general and which occur in a predictable sequence and at predictable times. Examples of life stages include puberty and old age.

Life events Significant changes in a person's life which may occur through choice (such as marriage or moving house) or which may be unexpected (such as sudden bereavement or loss of employment). Unlike life stages, life events do not occur in a predictable sequence nor necessarily at predictable times, and they are unique individual experiences (everyone experiences puberty but only some people experience redundancy).

As the above definitions indicate, there is a difference between *life stages* and *life events*. Everyone passes through similar stages as life unfolds: adolescence, becoming an adult, entering middle age and so on. However, life events are unique individual experiences, though some (such as marriage) are more common than others (such as bankruptcy). Life stages are generally less stressful than life events. Each life stage usually involves an adjustment in our self-concept and sense of identity, but they are not generally traumatic experiences likely to induce extreme anxiety or physical or mental illness. Life events, however, sometimes do have such consequences.

Much research has been carried out into the effects of both positive and negative **life events**. (An example of a positive life event is promotion at work; bereavement is a negative life event.) In 1967 the American researchers Holmes and Rahe published a scale which attempted to measure the impact of life events. They examined the case histories of about 5,000 people and sought to identify those life events which commonly preceded the onset of illness or the exacerbation of existing illness. They then ranked the life events in order of stressfulness by asking 394 people to attach a 'stress value' to each event., The resulting scale is reproduced below.

Note that an individual may experience several stressful events at once: a pregnant woman may get divorced and lose her job. A rough indication of the amount of stress a person is under is given by adding together the 'stress value' scores of the events that person is experiencing (or has recently experienced) – the higher the score, the greater the stress. Of course the way an individual *responds* to stress will depend on a number of other factors, such as the individual's coping skills and the amount of support he or she receives from friends and family.

**Life events in order of stressfulness
(Holmes and Rahe 1967)**

Rank	Life event	Stress value
1	Death of spouse	100
2	Divorce	73
3	Marital separation	65
4	Jail term	63
5	Death of a close family member	63
6	Personal injury or illness	53
7	Marriage	50
8	Fired at work	47
9	Marital reconciliation	45
10	Retirement	45
11	Change in health of family member	44
12	Pregnancy	40
13	Sex difficulties	39
14	Gain of new family member	39
15	Business readjustment	39
16	Change in financial state	38
17	Death of a close friend	37
18	Change to a different line of work	36
19	Change in number of arguments with spouse	35
20	Large mortgage repayments	31
21	Foreclosure of mortgage or loan	30
22	Change in responsibilities at work	29
23	Son or daughter leaving home	29
24	Trouble with in-laws	29
25	Outstanding personal achievement	28
26	Wife begins or stops work	26
27	Begin or end school	26
28	Change in living conditions	25
29	Revision of personal habits	24
30	Trouble with boss	23
31	Change in work hours or conditions	20
32	Change in residence	20
33	Change in schools	20
34	Change in recreation	19
35	Change in church activities	19
36	Change in social activities	18
37	Small mortgage repayments	17
38	Change in sleeping habits	16
39	Change in number of family get-togethers	15
40	Change in eating habits	15
41	Vacation	13
42	Christmas	12
43	Minor violations of the law	11

Life events: effects on individual identity

Life events can affect an *individual* in a number of ways. Illness is itself a life event, but it appears that other stressful life events can themselves contribute to the onset of mental or physical illness, and this will be discussed more fully in the next Element. Life events can also affect an individual's self-concept, perhaps resulting in lowered self-esteem or sense of self-worth. A woman who undergoes a mastectomy, for example, may feel she is less attractive to her husband; a man who is made redundant may experience a feeling of uselessness.

It might be helpful at this point to return to the four main factors identified by Michael Argyle as contributing to the individual's self-concept (see page 76). These were:

The reaction of others
Comparison with others
Social roles
Identification

If we look at each of these in turn we shall see the potentially damaging effects that stressful life events can have on the self-concept of an individual.

• **The reaction of others** Our self-esteem is usually very dependent on reinforcement from others. We look to our spouse or partner for confirmation that we are attractive, to friends for confirmation that we are pleasant company, to workmates for confirmation that we are competent in our jobs, and so on. One consequence of a life event is often increased isolation, so that a person no longer receives such reinforcement. Unemployed people not only lose their regular daily contact with colleagues, but may also for financial reasons have fewer social meetings with friends. Someone who experiences a loss of mobility is likely to have fewer opportunities to meet other people.

The way that others react to an individual may also change as a result of a life event. People may shy away from someone who has recently served a term of imprisonment, or feel embarrassed about approaching someone they know to be suffering from a terminal illness. Sometimes the changed reaction of others is imagined rather than real: a man who has undergone disfiguring surgery may feel convinced that others are repelled by his appearance. The threat to that person's self-esteem, however, is no less real because of this.

• **Comparison with others** If the life event leads to greater social isolation, there is less opportunity to make comparisons with others. When comparisons are made, they may become less favourable. A woman who has always considered her marriage relatively happy when compared with the marriages of her friends and relatives will no longer believe this if her husband leaves her. A man who has always thought of himself as financially successful compared with his neighbours will cease to think this if his business fails. In such cases the individual's self-confidence and sense of self-worth are under threat.

• **Social roles** Life events can change the roles that an individual has, and this too can undermine the individual's self-concept. The onset of illness or disability, or admission to hospital, may mean a loss of independence and a new role as someone with an increased dependence upon others. Retirement or redundancy takes away an individual's occupational role and this may give the individual a feeling of diminished worth. When children grow up and leave home the role of a parent changes, and this may cause a parent to feel that her life has less meaning and purpose.

• **Identification** The life event may mean that certain models can no longer be identified with. To take an extreme case, a child whose father dies loses an important role model. Moving away from a close-knit community may mean that an individual no longer has a strong sense of identification with his neighbours. If identification with others decreases, an individual is likely to have increased feelings of isolation and insecurity.

Did You Know ?

A common factor in nearly all those who suffer from the illness anorexia nervosa is a distorted body image. That is, they believe that they look and are greatly overweight, when in fact they are severely and often dangerously underweight.

Effects of bereavement and loss

Particular effects upon the individual are associated with **bereavement**. Other, less obvious forms of loss often have similar consequences. Retirement, moving house, loss of a bodily function – these and other events can be followed by a period of grief, because as with bereavement an important part of the individual's life has been taken away.

Many writers have sought to describe the characteristic stages or phases of the grieving process. John Bowlby, for example, identifies the following four stages:

1. **Denial** Newly bereaved people may experience a sense of unreality and there may be a tendency to deny that the event has taken place, so that the bereaved person seems to continue behaving as if the death has not occurred.

2. **Sensation of loss** The bereaved person recognises the reality of the death and may feel despair, anger or frustration. They may have difficulty coping with ordinary everyday tasks.

3. **Restitution** The mixed emotions relating to the death are worked through. Here it helps if individuals are able to unburden themselves by talking through their feelings with friends, relatives or counsellors.

4. **Resolution** The individual comes to terms with the loss and with his or her own feelings towards it. There is a recognition that life must go on and relationships with others (from which the individual may have retreated) are likely to resume.

Although the reactions outlined above are common, it is important to recognise that each individual's experience of grief is unique. There is no set time for each of the stages and no clear-cut separation between them. Moreover, it is not certain that each stage has to be experienced by every bereaved person. However, it is generally accepted that achieving a healthy adjustment to loss takes time, and that grief needs to be 'worked through' in order for there to be a gradual coming to terms with what has taken place.

Effects of abuse

Experience of **abuse** can have serious psychological repercussions, especially if the abuse occurs during childhood. Abuse can take a variety of forms, including:

Physical abuse (when physical injury is inflicted)
Neglect (as when a child is not fed properly, or not kept warm)
Sexual abuse
Emotional abuse

Of these, emotional abuse is the hardest to define. It might occur for example if a husband persistently belittles his wife, or regularly and deliberately makes her feel afraid of him. Garbarino, Guttman and Seeley, in their book 'The Psychologically Battered Child' (1986) identify five forms of 'psychically destructive' behaviour towards children:

Rejecting: The adult refuses to acknowledge the child's worth or recognise the child's needs.
Isolating: the child is isolated from others and prevented from forming friendships.
Terrorising: the adult creates a climate of fear by bullying, frightening and verbally assaulting the child.

not physically

Ignoring: the adult often fails to respond to the child, and deprives the child of stimulation.
Corrupting: the child is compelled or encouraged to engage in deviant or anti-social behaviour.

Children who are victims of emotional or other abuse often experience problems of psychological development and adjustment. They may for example be withdrawn, anxious or aggressive, and experience behaviour problems and learning difficulties at school. In infants language development may be delayed.

Abuse of children can have lasting effects. Many adults who abuse children have themselves been abused during childhood. Their parents have given them a model of behaviour which they later imitate. Emotional abuse, for example, has been referred to as a 'family curse' (Covitz, 1986), passed on from one generation of the family to the next. Victims of sexual abuse often carry into adulthood a sense of guilt and shame, about the abuse itself and their inability to stop it. They may have a low opinion of themselves and have difficulty accepting that anyone else might like them or care about them, leading to problems in forming relationships.

Abuse of both children and adults often leads to diminished self-esteem. Feelings of worthlessness and powerlessness are common. Victims may consider themselves worthy of nothing more than the treatment they have received. The need for health and social care professionals to support and strengthen the self-image of clients who have suffered from abuse will be discussed more fully later in the Element.

Did You Know ?

It has been estimated that as many as 36,000 primary schoolchildren are being bullied in British schools each week. According to a children's mental health charity, many will be emotionally scarred for life. (Young Minds, 1994)

Coping with threats to self concept

Processes of coping: defence mechanisms

We have looked at some of the ways in which the identity and self-image of the individual might be threatened. In particular, the effects of life events and abuse have been examined. We shall now consider how the individual might seek to cope with threats of this kind.

People often attempt to avoid or lessen anxiety by adopting **defence mechanisms**. These reduce distress by distorting reality in some way: the individual defends himself against anxiety by deceiving himself about the reality of his situation. Defence mechanisms can be beneficial in the short term, by staving off anxiety until the person is better able to cope with it. In the longer term, however, they are unhealthy and undesirable. They involve self-deception and also postpone the inevitable: final recognition of the reality of a situation may be all the more traumatic if it is delayed for too long.

Anna Freud (1946) identified several defence mechanisms, some of which are outlined in the box below:

Defence mechanisms

Denial   Denying the existence of an unpleasant truth.

Repression   Pushing down into the unconscious thoughts that cause anxiety, so that they are 'forgotten'.

Regression   Mentally retreating to a period in our lives which we perceive to be safer.

Displacement   Directing our feelings not towards their real target but towards a substitute target. (For example, taking your anger at one person out on someone else.)

Rationalisation   Persuading yourself that something unacceptable or unjustifiable is acceptable and justifiable by finding an apparently rational explanation/justification for it.

Processes of coping: coping mechanisms

Unlike defence mechanisms, **coping mechanisms** are based upon an acceptance of reality and are conscious ways of trying to deal with anxiety in a positive and constructive manner. The suitability of particular coping mechanisms varies from individual to individual; indeed, what helps one individual to cope with stress may exacerbate stress in another. Nevertheless, some common coping mechanisms can be identified, and they will be outlined here.

Lazarus and Folkman (1984) distinguish between two kinds of coping:

Problem-focused coping
Emotion-focused coping

- **Problem-focused coping**   This involves viewing a situation rationally and objectively and deciding how best to tackle it. An individual may conclude that positive action can be taken to remove or lessen the anxiety. For example, somebody who feels isolated after moving house may decide to speak more to his neighbours. In some situations, obtaining more information may help an individual to feel more in control and lessen fear of the unknown. Research suggests for instance that hospital patients feel less anxious if their treatment is explained to them.

- **Emotion-focused coping**   This involves adjusting to a situation emotionally. A man whose wife is suffering from a terminal illness may be comforted by recalling past happiness, and may do his best to ensure that they enjoy their remaining time together to the full. A woman worried about her job may seek to give herself an emotional 'lift' outside working hours by socialising more with friends.

Protection and support: social networks

An individual can be helped to cope with anxiety and stress by receiving support from *others*. This support might be in the form of professional help provided by the health and social care services, or it might derive from **social networks**.

Social network   The set of informal relationships that an individual has, including family, relatives, friends, neighbours and work colleagues.

An individual's social network can offer practical support, for example by providing information or by suggesting alternative ways of coping with a problem. They can also offer valuable emotional support. If an individual's self-esteem has been low-ered, friends and family can help to raise it. They can help to put situations in perspective, so that sources of anxiety are seen as less threatening.

Although informal social support can be of great benefit, several life events (such as unemployment or loss of mobility) lead to reduced social contacts. In some cases, what has happened may cause the individual to shun the company of others. In such situations it is invaluable to have a caring network of friends and relatives, willing to make an effort to ensure that contact is maintained or increased.

Social support can also be obtained from formal, organised support groups. These enable individuals to share their anxieties with others who are, or have been, in a similar position. They offer an outlet for the open expression of feelings, provide practical information and are a source of general encouragement and advice.

(See also the section on self-help groups later in this Element and further discussion of social networks in the next Element.)

Professional support

Professional support can take a variety of forms, ranging from, in extreme cases, direct intervention (as when a child is taken into local authority care) to a simple willingness to listen to a client's anxieties.

A client who is experiencing stress or some other form of threat may seek help from a counsellor. Regardless of whether a professional counsellor is involved or not, some of the skills associated with counselling need to be possessed by the other health and social care professionals working with the client. There is a need to assess the client's ability to cope, and the support networks (such as friends and family) open to him, so that they can be utilised and where possible improved. Whatever the situation (be it bereavement, sudden loss of health or some other event or crisis), the particular psychological, emotional and social implications for the individual client must be considered.

Often the main priority is to help clients develop a more positive self-concept, so that they feel more confident about the future and better able to cope. This means talking through the client's problems, allowing and encouraging the honest expression of fears and emotions, and working towards practical and viable solutions. The professional needs to be an effective listener, giving the client time to unburden himself and responding in appropriate ways. (For more on the role of communication skills in health and social care work, see Unit 2.)

Such support can undoubtedly have a positive effect. Beverley Raphael (1984) studied two groups of widows, one of which received no intervention, while the other received regular support and the members of the group were encouraged to express their grief. She found that the widows in the first group showed more tendency to complain of excessive tiredness, depression and decreased work capacity. They also made more visits to the doctor and showed high incidences of such problems as sleeplessness, weight loss and poor appetite.

The client's family may also need support. The ill-health of a family member, for example, can be a stressful life event for the rest of the family. As well as involving them in the care of the individual who is ill, their own anxieties need to be understood and addressed.

Sometimes the problem is itself rooted in the family, as when a wife is the victim of marital violence. Here assistance can be afforded if the woman wishes to leave the family home (she might be given accommodation in a refuge). In some cases, however, the woman still cares for her partner and, if children are involved, may be reluctant to break up the family. It is then the role of care workers to encourage both partners to discuss their problems, in an attempt to save the marriage or relationship if this is desired. Where appropriate, specialist advice services (such as RELATE) can become involved.

Particular considerations apply when children are believed to be at risk. Often children are not in a position to seek appropriate help themselves (though the telephone helpline CHILD-LINE offers a valuable and confidential service). The role of those in a position to identify children who might be in need of protection is therefore important. These include teachers, social workers, health visitors and nurses working in children's wards and in obstetric units and accident departments.

The welfare of children is governed by the provisions of the Children Act (1989). The Act states that 'the child's welfare is paramount' and that the interests of the child must always come first when decisions concerning his or her welfare are made. It also emphasises the need for health and social care services to work in partnership with parents. Central to the Act is the belief that the raising of children is best carried out within the family home, with the State giving support when necessary, rather than intervention. Nevertheless, in extreme cases the child can be removed from the home.

If a child is reported to be at risk, the report must be followed up by the local authority's Social Services Department, which is under a statutory duty to make inquiries in order to determine whether or not some action to protect the child is taken. It may seek judicial authority for a range of actions, including short term emergency measures, supervision of the child at home or the permanent removal of the child from its parents. The child may be placed on the local authority's *At Risk Register*, and a health visitor or other care worker given the responsibility of working with the family and monitoring the child's well-being.

Self-help groups

People experiencing a problem or crisis in their lives often seek contact with others in a similar position. **Self-help groups** are the result of people who feel they have a similar problem meeting together to offer each other support and encouragement. They can be a valuable source of advice and information, and reduce the isolation often experienced by those under stress.

There has been a boom in the number of self-help groups over the last twenty years. Before the Second World War they were largely restricted to organisations for the blind and the deaf. In the 1950s a number of organisations were established by the parents of handicapped children, including the Spastics Society and MENCAP. Today these are large charities employing many full-time staff. The 1960s and 1970s saw the emergence of numerous smaller mutual aid groups, many linked with the growing women's movement and disability rights campaigns. Later there came community health groups, which bring together people from the local community to tackle health-related social and environmental problems. Projects such as the Waterloo Health Project in London and the Whiteway Health Project in Bath have focused on such issues as the take-up of welfare benefits, safe play spaces for children and support for isolated mothers. In 1983 over 2,000 self-help groups were identified in London alone. In 1991 it was estimated that there were as many as 50,000 groups in the UK as a whole, ranging from major national bodies to small support groups of half a dozen members.

Information as a source of support

Lack of **information** can be an important contributory factor in situations of stress and anxiety. Research has consistently shown, for example, that hospital patients who are given limited information about their illness and its treatment are more likely to become anxious and depressed, and often recover less quickly. Correspondingly, providing such information helps a client come to terms with his situation and often allays unnecessary fears.

Clients also need to be given information about the support available to them. Sometimes the range of support services is itself a source of confusion: the client can find himself confronted by a maze of agencies and services, encompassing the health service, social services, social security, voluntary organisations and the private sector. Here the assistance of the individual care worker, willing and able to guide the client and explain the options available, is invaluable.

In recent years an effort has been made to centralise the provision of health information, and many parts of the country now have centres offering health information services. Some form part of existing public library services, others are in hospitals or health centres. In some regions there are information phonelines and mobile information centres.

Self Check ✓ Element 2

7. Identify each of the following as either a life stage or a life event:
   (a) Changing school.
   (b) Winning a million pounds in a newspaper competition.
   (c) Middle age.
   (d) Puberty.

8. Comment on the following statements:
   (a) Life stages are major turning points in life, and are therefore usually more stressful than life events.
   (b) All life events are associated with anxiety.
   (c) Research suggests that the death of a husband, wife or partner is the most stressful life event an individual is likely to experience.

9. A child is repeatedly told by his mother that he is a disappointment to her and that she wishes he had never been born. Is this an example of:
   (a) Physical abuse
   (b) Neglect
   (c) Sexual abuse
   (d) Emotional abuse?

10. Comment on the following statements:
   (a) Defence mechanisms are always harmful because they are based upon evasion of the truth.
   (b) Defence mechanisms are an essential protection against anxiety and should be sustained for as long as possible.
   (c) Coping mechanisms are a particular kind of defence mechanism.

11. If somebody experiencing anxiety and distress receives help from friends and relatives, this is an example of:
   (a) Formal support
   (b) Self-help
   (c) Professional support
   (d) Help from a social network?

12. Which of the following is a self-help group?
   (a) RSPCA
   (b) RAC
   (c) Gamblers Anonymous
   (d) Tottenham Hotspur Supporters Association.

4.3 Investigate the relationship of social and economic factors to health

In this Element we shall examine social and economic influences upon health (see also Unit 3, Element 2). Initially we shall look at ways in which the ability to maintain good health and to cope with life events might be linked to income and wealth. The role that social support networks play in helping the individual to cope with life events will then be considered. Finally, we shall discuss the relationship between life events, stress and illness.

Health inequalities: income and social class

Those on low **incomes** are able to spend less on the maintenance of good health. It is not surprising then that many studies have shown a link between low income and poor health. These studies have often examined the health of people belonging to different social classes, using the Registrar General's classification, in which class is determined by occupation. (The Registrar General heads the government's statistical office and this classification is used extensively in government reports). See box below.

The Registrar General's social classification

Class 1   Professional occupations (e.g. lawyers, doctors)

Class 2   Semi-professions and middle managers (e.g. teachers, civil service, executive officers)

Class 3a   Skilled non-manual occupations (e.g. secretary, clerk)

Class 3b   Skilled manual occupations (e.g. plumber, electrician)

Class 4   Semi-skilled occupations (e.g. postmen, machine operators)

Class 5   Unskilled occupations (e.g. labourer, cleaner)

There is a close relationship between **social class** (as defined by occupation) and income/wealth. (Income is money received from such sources as wages and interest on investments, whereas wealth refers to capital assets such as houses and personal possessions.) Generally speaking, those from the lower social classes are likely to have lower incomes and less wealth than those from the higher social classes.

Note that the Registrar General's classification excludes those who are without an occupation. This means that many people from the groups listed below are not accounted for:

The elderly
The unemployed
Single parent families
The homeless
The sick and disabled

People in these social groups are often poor. Not all elderly people are on low incomes, but many are: in 1985, nearly a third of elderly people were living on or below the poverty line (using the supplementary benefit level), compared with ten percent of those below pension age.

Evidence firmly indicates that those who are in poorly paid occupations, or from one of the lower income groups listed

above, tend to be less healthy than members of higher income households. The findings of the Black Report (1980), based on research carried out in the 1970s, included the following:

- men and women of the unskilled manual class were two and a half times more likely to die before retirement than those in the professional class.
- the rate of reported longstanding illness among females in the unskilled manual class was two and a half times as great as that among females in the professional class.
- members of the lower social classes made far less use of preventive health services than members of the higher social classes.

Health inequalities: cultural explanation

Among the explanations for these inequalities considered by the authors of the Black Report was the cultural / behavioral explanation. This suggests that inequalities occur because those in semi-skilled and unskilled occupations have a greater tendency to behave in ways that are damaging to health than those in middle class occupations. They take less exercise, are more likely to smoke and their diet contains more fatty foods and less fruit and fibre. As mentioned above, they are also less likely to use preventive health services, such as immunisation and ante-natal care.

Health inequalities: economic explanation

However, the Black Report concluded that the most important kind of explanation was what it termed the materialist or structuralist explanation. This focuses on inequalities of wealth and income, and corresponding differences in working and living conditions. This Element is especially concerned with people's expenditure on health, and we shall now examine the effects of low income in more detail by looking at the following:

Diet
Housing
Exercise
Access to health services

Diet

The importance of *diet* to good health was investigated in Unit 3 Element 3. People on low incomes may buy less food than others, and they are also restricted in the kinds of food they are able to afford. Fresh, high protein food such as fish and meat tends to be expensive, while food of much lower nutritional value is often cheaper. There is also some evidence to suggest that the coping strategies adopted by parents on a low income sometimes include giving sweets and crisps to children. (Another coping strategy among adults is smoking, again damaging to health.)

Housing

Those on limited income often have to cope with poor *housing conditions*. The effects of damp and mould can lead to respiratory problems, especially amongst children. Other health problems associated with poor quality housing include inadequate heating, infestation, accidents and psychological stress.

The dangers to health are still more severe for those unable to afford a home at all. This is a growing problem in Britain. The number of families recorded by local authorities as officially homeless has risen from 53,000 in 1978 to 126,680 in 1989. Shelter estimates this to be around 363,500 individuals. As the local authority figures exclude certain categories of people, the real number is even higher. Homeless people suffer obvious health hazards in the form of lack of shelter, lack of warmth and difficulty in keeping clean. Minor illnesses such as coughs and colds occur more frequently and are more persistent.

Health problems can also arise in local authority hostels and temporary bed and breakfast accommodation. Living conditions are often unhygienic and limited cooking facilities can mean that families rely on poor quality take-away food.

Exercise

A brisk walk or a jog may cost nothing, but in practice limited finance can restrict opportunities to take *healthy exercise* in a number of ways. Deprived areas with a high concentration of people on low incomes often lack open spaces and other facilities. Children who live in high-rise blocks or houses without gardens are likely to spend less time in the open air. Many forms of exercise (such as badminton, tennis and weight training) do cost money – for equipment or the use of facilities – and this inevitably excludes those unable to afford the expenditure.

Access to Health Services

As noted earlier, those on low income tend to make *less use* of preventive health services. Research has found that the lower social classes make less use than higher classes of such services as cancer screening, family planning and maternity clinics, immunisation and dental services. A variety of explanations may account for this, including limited knowledge of the facilities that are available and the fact that social and economic problems such as poor housing and unemployment can have a generally demoralising effect, leading to apathy and lack of motivation. Limited income, however, undoubtedly plays a part. Some services may be difficult to reach without a car. Journeys by public transport, especially if a parent is accompanied by young children, can be difficult as well as expensive. In recent years there has been a growing call for more 'out-reach' services (such as mobile X-ray units), which take the service to the user.

Coping with life events

The capacity to cope with life events can be reduced if financial resources are limited. This situation may arise if a person already has a low income and limited wealth, or if the life event itself has economic consequences. Redundancy, retirement and the death of a family breadwinner, for example, can all lead to reduced economic circumstances.

A person on a low income may well be already under stress because of this, so a life event such as bereavement of loss of health only makes the existing anxiety that much worse. Lack of finance restricts the range of coping strategies available to such a person. She may feel in need of a break but be unable to afford a holiday, or wish to see more of her friends and relatives but be deterred by the cost of travelling to see them or meeting them socially.

In the case of those who unexpectedly find themselves on a low income, the burden of new financial worries adds to the anxiety caused by a stressful life event. They may have to cut back on 'treats' and activities they had previously enjoyed (such as visits to restaurants and cinemas), making the situation they now find themselves in still harder to bear. Such activities might in other circumstances have served as coping strategies, but limited financial resources prevent this.

The role of social support networks in coping with life event threats

We shall now consider the part that social support networks play in helping an individual to cope with life event threats. In Element 2 a social network was defined as the set of informal relationships that an individual has, including family, relatives, friends, neighbours and work colleagues. Research has shown not only that support from such a network can help an individual to cope in times of stress, but also that the absence of this kind of support can increase levels of anxiety.

Cohen and MacKay (1984) have identified three types of support that might be provided by a social network:

- **Tangible support** In the form of money, physical assistance etc. The effectiveness of this depends on the attitude of the recipient. If he or she feels inadequate or indebted, anxiety is only increased.

- **Appraisal support** Helping individuals put their situation into perspective and assisting them in coming to terms with it. Talking over a life event with somebody else may help to make it seem less threatening. Self-help groups provide appraisal support, encouraging those faced by a particular problem to believe that it can be ameliorated or overcome.

- **Emotional support** In the form of reassurance, sympathy, demonstrations of love, etc. As seen in the previous Element, life events often threaten a person's self-concept, and emotional support can be especially helpful in rebuilding damaged self-esteem

Coping with life events is more difficult without such support. Unfortunately, life events often lead to reduced social contacts. A person who becomes disabled, for example, may spend more time at home alone and relations with friends who are unsure how to respond to disability can become strained. In such situations the support provided by professional care workers becomes especially important.

Stress-related illness

Life events, as we have seen, are often stressful and this stress can lead in turn to **stress-related illness**.

Stress is a necessary and unavoidable aspect of life. If we were never faced by challenges and obstacles, we would soon lose all drive and motivation. Moreover, some stress (playing competitive sports, for instance) is pleasurable. It is also the case that a stressful situation which arouses anxiety in one person might arouse excitement in another: speaking in public, for example. The individual's perception of the situation, and the kind of stress experienced, is therefore all-important.

For the purpose of this Unit, we are concerned with negative rather than positive experiences of stress: levels of stress which exceed a person's capacity to cope and are therefore potentially harmful. In order to distinguish between a source of stress and the individual's reaction to it, the former is often referred to as a 'stressor'.

> **Stressor** An event or situation which threatens a person's well-being and gives rise to a stress reaction. Bereavement, loss of employment and sudden illness are examples of stressors.

Evidence suggests that there is a relationship between exposure to stress and certain kinds of illness. For example, some research studies have shown an increased rate of illness among those experiencing a higher number of stressful life events. Caution is needed here however as the illness may not be the direct result of stress but of behaviour caused by stress: a person who has suddenly become unemployed may be losing sleep or not eating properly, for instance. It is also possible that illness itself may make it more likely that the person experiences such life events as loss of employment and financial difficulties – here illness would be causing life events to occur rather than the other way round.

Did You Know [?]

'Sudden death syndrome' is a term used for deaths which occur within one year of retirement. Mortality statistics show that a larger percentage of people (mainly men) die suddenly within a year of retirement than would normally be expected.

It is clear however that bodily changes do occur as a result of emotional reactions to stress, and that these changes can in turn precipitate illness. Raised blood pressure and heart rate, increased secretion of hormones and the alteration of digestive functions can cause damage to tissues and organs of the body, especially if these body patterns are prolonged (as might be the case if a person suffers weeks or months of anxiety). If direct damage is not caused by these changes, they can still render the individual more vulnerable to infection and less able to recover from diseases.

Some of the main stress-related illnesses are listed in the box below. It is important to note that these illnesses are not *always* the result of stress – they can and do occur also in people who are not under any obvious psychological pressure.

Stress-related illnesses

Cardiovascular disorders
Heart disease
Raised blood pressure
Migraine headaches

Skin disorders
Neurodermatitis
Eczema

Respiratory disorders
Asthma
Hyperventilation

Gastrointestinal disorders
Ulcers
Colitis
Vomiting
Diarrhoea

Psychological and psychiatric disorders
Depression
Eating disorders

Heart disease and stress

The relationship between stress and illness can be illustrated by a closer examination of the case of **heart disease**.

There is much evidence to show that individuals exposed to excessive life event stress have an above-average risk of coronary heart disease. For example, people who have been exposed to catastrophic stresses (such as natural disasters or imprisonment in concentration camps) have shown a higher subsequent incidence of coronary heart disease – sometimes many years after the event – than matched groups of people who have not experienced such events. There is also clear evidence that stress can produce physical reactions which increase the likelihood of a heart attack. These reactions include raised blood pressure and increased blood levels of potentially harmful fats.

Two American cardiologists, Friedman and Rosenman, have sought to identify the major behaviour characteristics of the male who is prone to develop coronary heart disease. In a 1974 study they investigated why some people in stressful occupations seem to be more likely to suffer heart attacks. The incidence of heart attacks is notably high among high-ranking executives, who often work in a highly charged atmosphere in which they are regularly required to make major decisions. Friedman and Rosenman found that individual reactions to stressful situations varied, but tended to belong broadly to one of two types, which they termed Type A and Type B. Type A individuals were characterised by highly competitive behaviour, inability to relax or 'switch off' after work, impatience, restlessness and a tendency to do everything in a hurry and to worry about the passing of time. Type B individuals, on the other hand, were much more relaxed, not taking office worries home with them and generally calmer and less anxious in their approach to life. Type A individuals, the research showed, were much more likely to suffer heart attacks than Type B individuals.

Stress and lowered resistance to infection

There is also evidence to suggest that stress can affect the body's ability to resist viruses and infectious diseases. The immune system operates in a complex way to enable the body to protect itself against disease. When the body is under threat from an invading substance such as a virus, there is an increase in the cells that either contain or destroy other harmful cells or antibodies.

One research study (Kiecolt-Glaser et al 1984) took blood samples from a group of medical students one month before their examinations and again during examinations week. The students' levels of stress were also measured according to the Holmes and Rahe scale (see Element 2, page 78). The researchers found that activity of the natural killer cells (large white blood cells that destroy foreign cells) decreased between the first and second blood samples, indicating an increased susceptibility to illness. They also found that students with high stress scores on the Holmes and Rahe scale had lower natural killer cell activity than those with lower stress scores.

Stress and psychological/psychiatric disorders

Stress can also result in psychological and psychiatric illness. It is not surprising that stressful life events are associated with feelings of depression and anxiety, and sometimes these symptoms are severe enough to require clinical treatment.

Research in New York showed a correlation between the unemployment rate and the rate of admissions into psychiatric hospitals – as the former increased or decreased, so did the latter. Another group of researchers (Paykel, Prusoff and Myers, 1975) found that the incidence of significant life events during the preceding six month period was four times greater in suicidal patients than in non-suicidal patients. It has also been shown that patients hospitalised for depression are six times more likely to have suffered a recent bereavement. Other research has suggested a possible link between stressful life events (specifically, the loss of social support) and the onset of bouts of schizophrenia.

Did You Know ❓

Several studies have suggested that women's higher susceptibility to neurotic mental illness (such as depression) occurs as a result of the more stressful lives which women lead. Brown and Harris (1978) explain this in terms of the burdens of caring for others, lack of support and material disadvantage. Miles (1988) argued that an important factor is that women receive far less emotional support from their husbands than do husbands from their wives.

Self Check ✓ **Element 3**

13. How many of the following statements about the Registrar General's social classification are correct?
    (a) It places those who are unemployed in the lowest social class.
    (b) It places those in skilled non-manual occupations above those in skilled manual occupations.
    (c) It is based upon estimations of income earned.

14. The Black Report (1980) found:
    (a) That health differences could mainly be explained by cultural factors.
    (b) That cultural factors played no part in health differences.
    (c) That failure to use preventive health services was the main reason for poorer health among certain social groups.
    (d) That those in higher social classes enjoyed better health overall than those in lower social classes.

15. Comment on the following statements:
    (a) The diet of people on higher incomes is usually unhealthy because they buy too much food and over-eat.
    (b) Maintaining a healthy diet on a low income is not difficult because simple, nutritious food is cheap.
    (c) It is difficult to maintain a healthy diet on low income because lack of money restricts choice.

16. Which of the following statements is correct?
    (a) Financial resources are irrelevant to the ability to cope with life events unless the event itself causes a loss of earnings.
    (b) Limited financial resources can reduce the coping strategies available to a person who experiences a life event.
    (c) Life events are changes in an individual's personal life (such as divorce) rather than changes in financial circumstances.

17. Asthma can be a stress-related illness. Is it:
    (a) A cardiovascular disorder
    (b) A respiratory disorder
    (c) A gastrointestinal disorder
    (d) A psychological disorder?

18. Identify each of the following as behaviours associated with Type A or Type B individuals:
    (a) Anxiety about being late for appointments.
    (b) Unwinding at lunch times by taking a walk in the local park.
    (c) Accepting that a business project will take longer to complete than originally planned.
    (d) Fear of failure

Unit Test

Question 1
Cultural influences can affect the development of an individual's identity. Which ONE of the following is an example of cultural influence?

A Defence mechanism
B Population size
C Television
D Exercise.

Question 2
Consider the following statements:
Statement 1 Socialisation is a lifelong process.
Statement 2 The family is the first social group to which a child belongs.

Which combination of True (T) and False (F) best represents the two statements above?

A 1-T 2-T
B 1-F 2-F
C 1-T 2-F
D 1-F 2-T

Question 3
Which one of the following comments about an individual is an example of positive labelling?

A 'She's a juvenile delinquent.'
B 'She is from a good neighbourhood so we'll trust her.'
C 'What do you expect at her age?'
D 'A leopard never changes his spots.'

Questions 4–6
Social psychologists have divided the influences upon an individual's self-concept into four main categories:

A the reaction of others;
B comparison with others;
C social roles;
D identification.
Assign each of the following statements to one of these four categories:

Question 4
'He has always looked up to his grandfather and wants to be just like him.'

Question 5
'I have always been shy – not like the rest of my family.'

Question 6
'I have a busy life – I'm a mother, wife, teacher, daughter and general agony aunt.'

Question 7
The most important phase of socialisation occurs during which ONE of the following periods?

A Puberty
B Middle age
C Old age
D Infancy and childhood.

Question 8
The statement 'Men have always been better at Maths than women' is an example of which ONE of the following?
A Racial discrimination
B Stereotyping

C Social role
D Identification

Question 9
Consider the following statements:
Statement 1 A child imitating adult behaviour – e.g. 'dressing up like Mummy' – is exhibiting modelling behaviour.
Statement 2 Strong fears such as phobias can never be overcome.

Which combination of True (T) and False (F) best represents the two statements above?

A 1-T 2-T
B 1-F 2-F
C 1-T 2-F
D 1-F 2-T

Question 10
Which ONE of the following is an example of a life event?

A Middle age
B Bereavement
C Birth
D Adolescence.

Questions 11–13
It has been said that the grief associated with bereavement often has some or all of the following stages:

A Denial;
B Sensation of loss;
C Restitution;
D Resolution.

Imagine that the following observations have been made by a friend about the behaviour of a recently bereaved widow. Which stage does the widow seem to be experiencing in each case?

Question 11
'She's still not fully come to terms with what's happened but at least she's able to talk about it now.'

Question 12
'It suddenly seems to have hit her that he's gone.'

Question 13
'It's as if she's pretending to herself that it hasn't happened.'

Question 14
Which ONE of the following is a life stage?

A Emigration
B Divorce
C Adolescence
D Redundancy

Questions 15–17
Consider the following behaviour patterns:

A extreme competitiveness;
B compassion for others;
C able to relax at the end of the working day.

Select the behaviour pattern which is closely associated with:

Question 15
Type A individuals.

Question 16
Type B individuals.

Question 17
Neither of these.

Question 18
Mary has recently lost her husband, who was an engineer, and has herself just been made redundant.

Statement 1 Mary is in a vulnerable position because she is experiencing several stressful life events at once.

Statement 2 Mary's experiences could adversely affect her self-concept.

Which combination of True (T) and False (F) best represents the two statements above?

A   1-T 2-T
B   1-F 2-F
C   1-T 2-F
D   1-F 2-T

Question 19
A stressor is which ONE of the following?

A   Something which causes stress.
B   Someone who experiences stress.
C   A type of medication that alleviates the symptoms of stress.
D   An instrument for measuring stress.

Question 20
Which ONE of the following statements about stress is correct?

A   Stress is associated with a number of illnesses but it has no bearing on whether or not we catch infectious diseases.
B   All people show the same physical reactions to stress.
C   If an illness is to be caused by stress, the illness will show immediately.
D   The symptoms of stress can develop years after the stress has been experienced.

Questions 21–23
Listed below are some common feelings and experiences after bereavement:

A   Refusing initially to accept that the person has really died.
B   Receiving comfort and practical help from neighbours.
C   Receiving financial assistance from the State to help with funeral costs.
D   Drawing comfort from recalling happy memories.

Select the feeling or experience which is an example of:

Question 21
Emotion-focused coping.

Question 22
Defence mechanism.

Question 23
Social support.

Question 24
Alcoholics Anonymous is an example of which ONE of the following?

A   A community action group.
B   A subsidiary of the National Health Service.
C   A self-help group.
D   A defence mechanism.

Question 25
The At Risk Register is which ONE of the following?

A   A hospital list of patients whose illness may be life-threatening.
B   A local authority list of properties where housing conditions are a threat to the health of occupants.
C   A local authority list of children whose well-being may be in danger.
D   A government list of hospitals which may have to close if their financial situation does not improve.

Question 26
Consider the following statements:

Statement 1 A defence mechanism usually reduces stress by avoiding the truth in some way.

Statement 2 A coping mechanism may offer short-term relief but can never be more than a temporary, stop-gap solution.

Which combination of True (T) and False (F) best represents the two statements above?

A   1-T 2-T
B   1-F 2-F
C   1-T 2-F
D   1-F 2-T

Question 27
What is a social network?

A   A pressure group concerned with a social issue such as homelessness.
B   A voluntary organisation with branches in all parts of the country.
C   A diagram depicting an individual's family tree.
D   The set of informal relationships than an individual has.

Question 28
Research suggests which ONE of the following to be true?

A   Those on low incomes are more likely than those on higher incomes to suffer poor health.
B   Middle class people suffer more health problems than others because their lives are more stressful.
C   There is no connection between income levels and health.
D   Those in the highest social classes are more likely than others to die before retirement age.

Question 29
The Registrar General's Social Classification classifies people according to which ONE of the following?

A   Income
B   Educational qualifications
C   Occupation
D   The type of property they occupy.

Question 30
Consider the following statements:

Statement 1 People from the lower social classes tend to make less use of preventive health services than members of the higher social classes.

Statement 2 Exercise is free so is not thought to be a relevant factor in health differences between the social classes.

Which combination of True (T) and False (F) best represents the two statements above?

A   1-T 2-T
B   1-F 2-F
C   1-T 2-F
D   1-F 2-T

Question 31

It is sometimes argued that those in semi-skilled and unskilled occupations have a greater tendency than others to behave in ways that are damaging to health. Is this:

A   An economic explanation for health inequalities
B   A cultural explanation for health inequalities
C   A materialist explanation for health inequalities
D   A structuralist explanation for health inequalities?

Question 32

Which ONE of the following is NOT an example of a preventive health service?

A   A hospital casualty department
B   Immunisation
C   Cancer screening
D   Dental check-ups.

Question 33

A social support network is most likely to do which ONE of the following?

A   Help people from different parts of the country who are experiencing similar problems get in touch with each other.
B   Provide professional help and support to those in need.
C   Offer informal support to those in need.
D   Organise and co-ordinate the various sources of support available to a person in need.

Question 34

A neighbour organises a surprise birthday party for an elderly lady recovering after a car accident. This is an example of which ONE of the following?

A   Self-help
B   Emotional support
C   Professional support
D   Material support.

Question 35

Consider the following statements:
Statement 1 Research suggests that clients who are given information about their illness and their treatment often recover more quickly.
Statement 2 It is believed that those on low incomes often have less access to health services and to information concerning the availability of these services.

Which combination of True (T) and False (F) best represents the two statements above?

A   1-T 2-T
B   1-F 2-F
C   1-T 2-F
D   1-F 2-T

Question 36–38

Four important types of abuse are:

A   physical;
B   emotional;
C   sexual;
D   neglect.

Identify the type of abuse in each of the following cases:

Question 36

Bullying, belittling or ignoring a child.

Question 37

Inflicting bodily harm on a child.

Question 38

Encouraging a child to touch an adult in an inappropriate place.

Question 39

Victims of abuse who say they deserve the treatment they have received are showing signs of which ONE of the following?
A   Employing coping mechanisms
B   Denial
C   Diminished self-esteem
D   Regression.

Question 40

Consider the following statements:
Statement 1 Adults who abuse their children were often abused by their own parents.
Statement 2 The outward behaviour of abuse victims usually gives no indication to others that abuse is taking place.

Which combination of True (T) and False (F) best represents the two statements above?

A   1-T 2-T
B   1-F 2-F
C   1-T 2-F
D   1-F 2-T

Answers to Self-check Questions

1 (d)

2 (a) Classical conditioning.
(b) Operant conditioning.
(c) Operant conditioning.
(d) Classical conditioning.

3 (a) True
(b) False
(c) False Internalisation is associated with identification, not imitation.

4 (c)

5 (a) This is based on an extremely narrow understanding of what is meant by 'culture'. Nobody who lives in a society can avoid being influenced by an enormous number of cultural factors.
(b) This has an element of truth because Britain is a multicultural society. However, there are many cultural influences common to all, or almost all, of the population (such as the education system and the main television channels).
(c) It is true that some cultural traditions are passed on from generation to generation, but not true that culture is 'unchanging'. To take one example, popular entertainment has seen many changes over the last hundred years, including the arrival of cinema and television.

6 (b)

7 (a) Life event
(b) Life event
(c) Life stage
(d) Life stage

8 (a) Life stages *are* major turning points, but they are not 'usually' more stressful than life events. A major life event such as sudden bereavement is likely to be more stressful for most people than passing through a life stage.

(b) No – A positive life event is more likely to cause elation than anxiety.

(c) Yes – This is true.

9 (d)

10 (a) Defence mechanisms *are* based on an evasion of the truth but in the short term they can be beneficial. They are undesirable if sustained over a long period.

(b) No – See comment on (a).

(c) No – Check the definitions of coping mechanisms and defence mechanisms given earlier in the unit.

11 (d)

12 (c)

13 (b)

14 (d)

15 (a) This may *sometimes* be true but it is an exaggeration to say that it is 'usually' true.

(b) Misleading – Nutritious food is often more expensive than food of lower nutritional value.

(c) Yes – This is true.

16 (b)

17 (b)

18 (a) Type A

(b) Type B

(c) Type B

(d) Type A

Question	Answer	Question	Answer	Question	Answer	Question	Answer	Question	Answer
1	C	9	C	17	B	25	C	33	C
2	A	10	B	18	A	26	C	34	B
3	B	11	C	19	A	27	D	35	A
4	D	12	B	20	D	28	A	36	B
5	B	13	A	21	D	29	C	37	A
6	C	14	C	22	A	30	C	38	C
7	D	15	A	23	B	31	B	39	C
8	B	16	C	24	C	32	A	40	C

Unit Test Comments (selected questions)

Question 1
C The media are a very important cultural influence (see page 76).

Question 2
A Both statements are correct.

Question 3
B All four comments are examples of labelling, but only B is an instance of positive labelling. The other three make negative assumptions about the individual concerned.

Question 4
D Here the grandson identifies with his grandfather.

Question 5
B The individual's self-concept is influenced here by comparisons the individual makes between himself/herself and other members of the family.

Question 6
C The speaker is aware of having a number of different social roles.

Question 7
D Although socialisation continues throughout life, infancy and childhood is the most important phase.

Question 8
B In the statement both men and women are stereotyped.

Question 9
C Statement 1 is true. Statement 2 however is false because phobias *can* be overcome (see page 73).

Question 10
B The other three are life stages rather than life events.

Question 11
C Because the widow has not yet fully come to terms with her bereavement, she has not yet reached stage D.

Question 14
C The other three are life events.

Question 15
A This is a common characteristic of Type A individuals.

Question 16
C This is a common characteristic of Type B individuals.

Question 17
B This quality is not closely associated with Type A or Type B individuals, though of course this does not mean that either Type A or Type B individuals tend to lack compassion for others.

Question 18
A Mary is certainly experiencing several stressful life events – e.g. bereavement, redundancy, possibly financial difficulties. All of these events could also have damaging effects on her self-concept.

Question 20

D   A is incorrect because evidence suggests that stress can lower resistance to infection. B is incorrect because individual physical (and emotional) reactions to stress vary. C is incorrect because research suggests that stress-related illnesses can occur immediately *or* some time after the stress has been experienced.

Question 22

A   This is an example of denial, which is a defence mechanism.

Question 23

B   Here the comfort and help are provided by a social network.

Question 24

C   The work of Alcoholics Anonymous is organised by individuals who have experience of alcoholism themselves.

Question 25

C   See page 81.

Question 26

C   Statement 2 is incorrect because a coping mechanism can help an individual come to terms with a stressful situation in a lasting, positive way.

Question 27

D   See page 80.

Question 28

A   Evidence for this was for example provided by the Black Report in 1980 (see page 82).

Question 29

C   See page 82.

Question 30

C   Statement 1 was supported by the Black Report. As for Statement 2, although *some* forms of exercise are free others are not. Housing conditions (e.g. tower blocks) may also limit opportunities to take exercise.

Question 31

B   Differences in behaviour between people from different social classes are termed cultural differences (see page 82).

Question 32

A   A hospital casualty department treats health problems (e.g. those caused by accidents) *after* they have occurred and is therefore not a preventive health service.

Question 33

C   Answer A is a description of a self-help group rather than a social support network. Answer B is incorrect because the assistance offered by a social support network is not professional. A social support network *may* do what is described in answer D but C) is the better answer because C is a description of what all social support networks do.

Question 34

B   Is correct because the aim of the birthday party is clearly to help the elderly lady *feel* better.

Question 35

A   Both statements are correct.

Question 40

C   Statement 1 is correct. As for Statement 2, the outward behaviour of abuse victims *sometimes* gives no indication to others that abuse is taking place, but to say that this 'usually' occurs is misleading. Often there are indications – e.g. the abuse victim may be extremely withdrawn or exhibit disturbed behaviour.

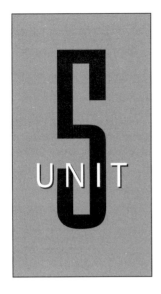

UNIT 5

Health promotion

Getting Started

In this unit we consider the following Elements.

Element 1	Prepare a plan for health promotion advice.
Element 2	Presenting health promotion advice to others.
Element 3	Different types of risks to health.

This unit covers 3 key areas.

- **Preparing a plan for health promotion advice** – The first element develops the framework required to be able to produce a *promotional plan*. It looks at mission statements, objectives, aims, target audiences. Also at how to reach the target audience and the resources that will be required to implement the promotional plan.

- **Giving and presenting health promotion advice to others** – The second element develops how to *present* health promotion advice. The key areas that will be examined are: **Smoking, Alcohol, Drugs, Substance Abuse and Safe Sexual Practices.**

- **Identifying different types of risks to health** – The third element looks at all the health areas in Element 2 and examines the *risks* to personal safety in relation to each one. Safety issues are examined in the home, at work, (including the Health and Safety at Work Act), as well as in the environment.

Useful Cross-references:

Unit 3 Element 1

Unit 3 Element 2

Aim   Long term result required at the end of the health promotion.

Analgesics   (pain killers) Drugs which influence parts of the brain which produce the feeling of pain.

Drug   A chemical which, when introduced to the body, affects the activity of the mind and body. Main groups of drugs are sedatives, stimulants, analgesics and narcotics.

Fad   An idea, plan or product which is popular for a brief time, before disappearing.

Fashion   Similar to a fad, but takes much longer to disappear. A fashion is often replaced by another fashion bearing some resemblance to the first.

Health   A state of 'well being', involving physical, mental and social aspects. It is more than the absence of disease or infirmity.

Mission Statement   A brief statement setting out the aims of the organisation.

Narcotics   Drugs which have a powerful effect on the nervous system. Where legally prescribed, only provided in small doses and under strict supervision.

Objectives   Key aspects that need to be completed to achieve the aim.

Preventative   An approach seeking to change attitudes and behaviour so that undersired outcomes are prevented from happening.

Proactive   An approach which takes the initiative and tries to decide what needs to be done in advance of certain (likely) outcomes actually happening.

Reactive   An approach which waits for certain outcomes to happen then reacts to them.

Sedatives   (depressants) Drugs which diminish feelings of anxiety and induce a state of relaxation.

Self-empowerment   An approach whereby the client is encouraged to take the actual decisions based on information given.

Stimulants   Drugs which induce a sense of alertness and reduce the feelings of fatigue.

Target Audience   The group which is the particular focus of the health promotion campaign.

Essential Principles

5.1 Preparing a plan for health promotion advice

This element, "Preparing a plan for health promotion advice", can be broken down into 5 sections as follows:

1. **What is health promotion?** This section looks at some general definitions and the relationship with health education.
2. **A framework for health promotion.** A generic framework for health promotional activities is developed.
3. **Approaches to health promotion.** This section looks at various approaches to health promotion with key activities.
4. **Why plan for health promotion?** In this section we look at the advantages and disadvantages of planning for health promotion.
5. **Key activities in planning for health promotion.** This section sets out fully the key stages in planning for health promotion and develops each one.

What is health promotion?

Although difficult to define, health involves a state of 'well being', involving physical, mental and social aspects. It is more than the absence of disease or infirmity. Some of the factors that effect one's health include the individual's life-style, housing conditions and financial situation. Other factors might include cultural backgrounds, the values and beliefs held, and social class membership. Still broader aspects involving the environment may also play a role, such as physical climate, educational opportunities, health care services available, and so on.

We now look at what **health promotion** is. Fundamentally it is about:

- Increasing health status of individuals
- Increasing health status of communities
- Increasing health status of a nation
- Increasing health status on a global basis

The World Health Organisation (WHO) define health promotion as:

> "The process of enabling people to increase control over, and to improve, their health"

It therefore includes having control over your *own* health (i.e. self improvement).

Health promotion also takes in **health education**. This is the process for giving out information to change people's behaviour or attitudes regarding health.

Promotion sometimes gets confused with the term 'propaganda' in a business, sales and marketing sense. Because of this, promotion is sometimes said by some people to be *inappropriate* for "the health industry". Nevertheless promotion is vital for the longevity of services in the future. This is because, in a more competitive environment, if your services

are unknown, then usage will inevitably be decreased. Of course it is important here to be clear about who the customer or client is. This is not always as simple as it seems.

A framework for health promotion

In general terms a **framework** for health promotion can be developed. Looking at health promotion, it can be broken down into 7 key activities, all inter-linked, as shown in Fig 5.1.

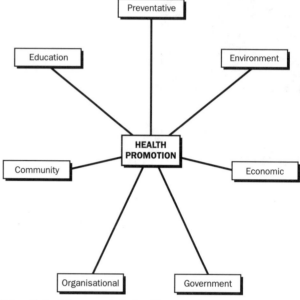

Figure 5.1   A framework for health promotion activities

Health promotion activities are **planned** activities and here we lay out a detailed way of preparing a health plan.

- **Environment** – This covers health aspects involving the home, work or public places as well as the environment in general, such as seas, rivers, land, rain, air etc.

- **Economic** – Influencing economic policies, e.g. by lobbying M.P.'s. The government's tax and spending policies can directly affect health issues, e.g. VAT on fuel in 1994.

- **Government** – Developing health policies which can filter down to all government departments, e.g. transport policy. An example of this might be encouraging more train usage and reducing road transportation. This may reduce the number of road accidents and the amount of harmful gases given off into the atmosphere, thereby reducing pollution related illnesses, e.g. asthma.

- **Organisational** – Getting organisations (businesses) ranging from very small to global companies to take on board health concepts. This might include reducing accidents by laying down a maximum number of hours it is possible to work without a break; encouraging smoke free areas within the organisation; etc.

- **Community** – Working with local communities to identify their own needs and develop action plans accordingly. (See the self empowerment approach in Element 2).

- **Education** – This can be broken down into 3 areas of health education:

Primary: – Preventing ill health arising by improving the general quality of life and therefore health

Secondary: – Preventing illnesses getting worse
  – Returning sick people back to health
  – Changing behaviour, such as stopping smoking

Tertiary: – Caring for permanent disabilities
  – Caring for handicapped people
  – Providing rehabilitation programmes

- **Preventative** – To prevent ill-health in the first place, for example by immunisation programmes for children.

Approaches to health promotion

Having established a general framework in the last section we shall move on to look at the various **approaches** to health promotion, including the *Preventative*, *Self Empowerment* and *Radical* approaches.

Top-down and Bottom-up approaches, fads and fashions are also explained in relation to a health promotional plan.

The Preventative Approach

The **preventative approach** is to fundamentally increase the *awareness* of a health issue, thereby changing attitudes and behaviour. The AIDS promotional campaign can be seen as such an example. It has taken many forms. One approach was to regularly publicise information about the number of people and the type of people (for example drug users) affected by the spread of the disease and the predictions for future years if present trends continue. It was hoped that by providing information of this kind it would encourage people to change their attitude to, and behaviour in, sexual relationships, eg. encouraging safe sex.

The preventative approach can be subdivided into three areas:

Primary prevention – This is the prevention of the spread of disease. An example is the immunisation programme.

Secondary prevention – This is finding the disease at an early stage and taking the appropriate action. An example is the screening for early diagnosis of cervical cancer.

Tertiary prevention – This is where a disease has had an effect and drugs are given to lessen the effects. For example giving drugs to a cancer patient.

Self Empowerment Approach

The **self empowerment** approach is one where information is given to the target audience or client-set for *them* to make their own decisions. Therefore the client-set need to be able to develop decision making skills. A possible outcome of this approach is that the decision taken may *not* be the one that the health promotional plan envisaged. Ideally, the plan needs to be flexible enough to be able to deal with this type of occurrence.

Radical Approach

The **radical approach** developed by Tones et al (1990) is that health promotion should start at the social, environmental and political level, rather than the individual level. The lob-bying of MP's to gain their support for health-related legislation would be an example of this approach.

Top-down and bottom-up

Should planning start at the top or the bottom? This is known as **Top-down** or **bottom-up** planning or promotion. The *top* being governmental and key decision makers. Or should you start with the *bottom*; i.e. the grass roots within a community or individuals at the workplace?

Fads and Fashions

Is the plan just a passing fad? A **fad** is an idea, plan or product which comes quickly but just as quickly goes (Fig. 5.2). An example is a gadget to help reduce weight loss, which is quickly disregarded, like the exercise wheel. This health "tool" was promoted by private companies in all forms of advertising, including the television and national newspapers. It very quickly became popular and just as quickly was disregarded. Many millions were sold, but few were used a short time after purchase.

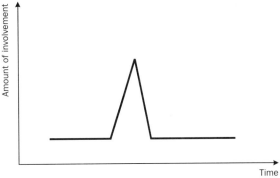

Figure 5.2   A fad

A **fashion**, as shown in Fig. 5.3, is something that comes as quickly as a fad, but takes longer to go. It might stay a year, or longer, and then be replaced by the next fashion. An example is the American-style *step classes*. Another example is *marathon running*. At its peak it seemed as if everyone between 16 and 60 (and older) was training for a marathon. Today, although far more popular than in the past, the craze of marathon running has reduced considerably. Of course there is nothing to say it will not become as popular again in the future! The general trend is for people to take more exercise and to consider health issues more seriously than in the past.

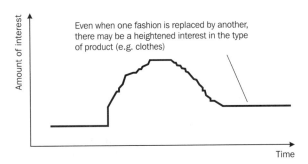

Figure 5.3   A fashion

Impact of a successful promotion plan

A successful promotion plan goes further than a fashion and changes *long term* opinions and behaviour on a given topic.

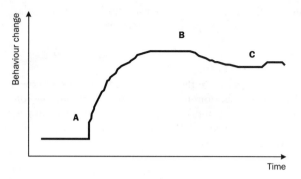

Figure 5.4 Successful promotional plan

The promotional plan to encourage condom use, is an example of a successful health promotion, which has had lasting affects on the targeted audience. In Fig. 5.4, point A is the *start* of the promotional plan; point B is at the *end* and a large change has been recorded. The important point is C, after the promotional plan has finished. The *long term* behaviour patterns have changed. Another example is the drinking and driving promotions. These are seasonal campaigns; however the amount of people who do not drink and drive at all, is now at much higher levels than in the past, i.e. people's long term behaviour has changed.

Why plan for health promotion?

It is worth considering here why we should *plan* for a health promotion. This is summarised now by looking at the advantages and disadvantages, as shown in Table 5.1.

Planning for health promotion

Advantages

1. Encourages you, and the team, to *think ahead*, at an early stage, thereby being able to react quickly when changes are required.
2. Can consider *reactions to the plan*, therefore can implement changes early on in the promotion (at the trial stage for example).
3. Good for *communicating to others*. Everyone should be moving in the same direction and be aware of the overall aims and objectives of the plan.
4. Helps *monitoring*, i.e. to know exactly where you are with the promotional plan.
5. Helps you set *budgets* accordingly.
6. Helps you set *milestones* and *targets*.
7. The programme can be *broken down* into more manageable smaller sub-units and linked to the resources available.
8. *Saves money*; this is achieved by reacting at the early stages rather than later when more people will be involved.

Disadvantages

1. Takes a lot more time at the beginning of the project.
2. Must be organised, or at least involve the key organisers.
3. Must find time to monitor progress, if the above benefits are to be achieved.
4. Must know *what* you are trying to achieve; some clear thinking has to take place and clear outcomes need to be agreed.
5. May involve additional people (therefore could slow process down and increase initial costs).

Table 5.1 Impacts of health promotion

Key activities in planning for health promotion

A **Health Promotion Plan** can be broken down into 8 *key activities* as follows:

1. Identify needs and priorities.
2. Set aims and objectives.
3. How to achieve the aims.
4. Identify resources.
5. Planning evaluation methods.
6. Set implementation plan.
7. Implement.
8. Re-evaluate.

This is a useful structure to develop any promotional plan. Here we look at the 8 key activities or planning stages in turn.

1. Identify needs and priorities

This is the starting point. The classic **needs analysis** is developed and consideration is given as to how proactive or reactive the plan should be. Priorities are considered.

What are the 'needs' of the people? The classic analysis of need consists of 4 types

1. Normative need.
2. Felt need.
3. Expressed need.
4. Comparative need.

Remember:

"Need, like beauty, is in the eye of the beholder"

- **Normative need** This is the *gap* between what 'an expert' believes is the standard and what is the actual situation. For example an expert may believe that 1,000 calories a day is an acceptable intake; if the client is actually receiving 700 calories a day, then a short-fall of 300 calories exists.

- **Felt need** This is what people 'feel' they require. Knowledge of a subject will affect what people feel they require.

- **Expressed need** This is what people 'express' that they need; i.e. 'felt need' is turned into a request or demand.

- **Comparative need** This is the *comparison* between different groups. People may develop 'felt' or 'expressed' needs because they have less than some other person or group.

Establishing needs is difficult. Even by asking people questions about their needs you may change their original felt, expressed or comparative need in the first place.

Proactive and Reactive

We have discussed top-down and bottom-up approaches. Another useful area is how **proactive** the health promotion campaign needs to be. For instance how much should we be involved in taking the initiative and deciding what needs to be done in *advance*? **Reactive** refers to reacting to situations *after* they occur. An example of acting *proactively* might be informing people at an early stage about a health issue such as AIDS, or *reactively* might be waiting for public demand to insist on knowing the 'facts', then reacting and passing on the information.

Promotional health questions that need to be considered

Other areas include:

- Who decides what the needs of a group are?
- What grounds are used to decide this?
- How are different needs prioritised? By whom?

2. Set aims and objectives

- **Mission and Values.** A **mission statement** is a short, and often one sentence, statement, formally setting out the purpose of the organisation. In many situations mission statements *are* used, and *departmental* missions are sometimes developed from the "master" *organisational* mission. Many health authorities have such statement's to show what the long term driving force is. This is sometimes followed by a statement of the organisation's **values**. This could include values such as including the client in all decisions made.

- **Aims and Objectives.** The **aim** is the long term result required at the end of the health promotion. It is important that the aims of an organisation and of a particular health promotional scheme clearly fit within the mission statement (assuming one exists) for the organisation and the values of that organisation, whether stated or implied. The **objectives** are key aspects that need to be completed to *achieve* the aim. The aim needs to be clear and concise and easily 'transportable' so that it can be used as a communication medium.

Objectives   Good objectives should follow the SMART principle.

- Stretching
- Measurable
- Achievable
- Realistic
- Time scales

The objectives also need to be *consistent* with the overall aim of the health promotion and the mission and values of the organisation or department.

The **hierarchy** of mission, values, aims and objectives is shown in Figure 5.5.

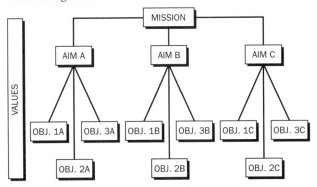

Figure 5.5   Mission, values, aims and objectives

All the aims of a company, organisation or government department should be in line with its mission and values.

The aims are prioritised into 3 key areas (called A, B and C) and each *aim*, in this particular example, requires 3 *objectives* to be met.

- **Aim A:** Objective 1A,   Objective 2A,   Objective 3A
- **Aim B:** Objective 1B,   Objective 2B,   Objective 3B
- **Aim C:** Objective 1C,   Objective 2C,   Objective 3C

All the activities of an organisation should be consistent with its underlying *values*.

3. How to achieve the aims

There are many ways to **achieve** a specific aim. These should be listed and recorded as part of the reason for choosing a particular approach, together with some explanation of why other approached were *not* used. This may be because of cost, unacceptability to client-set, too complicated, not measurable, or many other reasons.

Table 5.2 below indicates some of the skills and techniques which might help you achieve your aims.

Table 5.2   Means by which aims can be achieved

A main aim of many health promotion activities is to communicate effectively with a *target audience*. We now consider how we might achieve this particular aim.

- **Target audience**

It is imperative that your aims and objectives are very clear *before* moving on to define who the target audience will consist of. Table 5.3 gives some examples of types of target audience.

Examples of target audiences

Target Audience	Example
Adults	From 18+ yrs
Adolescents	13 – 17 yrs
Children	6 – 12 yrs
Pregnant women	2 months – 9 months of pregnancy
Smokers	over 5 cigarettes / day
Single women	not living with a spouse
Low income group	e.g. as defined by Government bodies
By Region	e.g. Merseyside
By Country	e.g. Wales
By community	e.g. East End of London
Age group	e.g. 40 – 49 year olds
Blood type	e.g. O RH POSITIVE
Illness	e.g. Lung cancer
Susceptible groups	Breast cancer, women of a certain age
Senior citizens	75+ age group
The list goes on	....

Table 5.3 Types of target audience

Suppose our target audience is *children* between 6 and 12 years.

Examples of ways to reach an audience of *children* to give effective health information:

1. Establish a national children's awareness day.
2. Create national cartoon character.
3. Use of media – Children's TV channels
   Radio – children's programmes
   Children's magazines, etc.
4. Leaflets to school (incorporating cartoon characters).
5. Talks / visits to schools with 'Question and Answer' presentations.
5. Competitions throughout schools and at home.
7. Use of well-known celebrities or sports personalities to enforce the message.
8. Reach children through parents, teachers, nursery nurses, etc.

Some standard ways have been listed of trying to influence / reach children, so that children are better acquainted with a health issue, e.g. smoking and its associated health risks.

4. Identify resources

It is important that, having agreed the aims and objectives and established the target audience, you identify the **resources** to be used in the health promotion. These resources could involve the following

- **People**   The number of people and skills necessary to achieve your aims and objective must be established. Are the people on the project to be full-time, part-time or voluntary workers?

- **Money**   How much money is required? Where will it come from: Government, local council, clients input, educational sources, voluntary groups etc? Has the financial pot got a limited time scale associated with it? Will sponsorship be required? Will local or national companies be involved?

- **Accommodation**   Where and what will be the accommodation for the people involved? What are the facilities required? Can other health authorities contribute, or a charity?

- **Materials and equipment**   This includes *published material*, such as leaflets, brochures, hand-outs, information sheets etc, and *audio-visual aids and teaching equipment* as shown in Table 5.4 below. This outlines the *internal resources* that an organisation would normally have at its disposal. *External resources* are ones that are available at a price from an outside body. The advantages and disadvantages of each medium is shown.

Medium	Advantage	Disadvantage
Internal resources:		
Promotional Video	Young Image	Audience concentration decreases quickly (unless very professionally made).
35mm slides	Colour, cheap	Old fashioned and slow, needs a presenter.
OHP	Easy	Basic Needs a presenter
Chalk and Talk	Developed at clients pace.	Lecturer style
White board	Easy to change	Not 'glossy', not transferable Lecturer style
Flip chart(s)	Easy to use	Lecturer style
Handouts	Easy to produce, and distribute.	Often not read, or only the first paragraph.
External resources:		
TV (national)	Wide audience; visual.	Targeting difficult and costly
Radio (local)	Cheaper than TV	No visual aid. Therefore it is difficult explaining things. e.g. how to put a condom on
Newspapers (national)	Daily; wide audience	Expensive. Difficult to target.
Audio/Video Aids	New concepts	Training required for full impact.
Video Wall (a bank of TV monitors in a display)	Visual impact. New ideas	Expensive; can only be shown in specific settings.

Table 5.4   Types of materials and equipment

Of course the resources you have identified must be consistent with the facts you have identified about your target audience. Let us continue our example where the target audience is *children* of a specified age range. It would be vital to be aware of the information available about the purchasing habits and concerns of children of a particular age and sex who are within the target audience. For example, a major report in August 1994 'Social Focus on Children' was published by the Central Statistical Office. Chart 1 tells us how much spending power children of various ages have. Charts 2–5 tell us the favourite readership items of boys and girls of various ages. Chart 6 tells us the concerns about the environment which children of different ages have.

Only by being fully aware of the characteristics of the target audience can you identify and select the resources most appropriate for use in your health promotion campaign. For instance, the average 1990's boy aged 11–14 reads Viz and The Sun; worries about *global* issues such as deforestation, polluted oceans and damage to the ozone layer; is concerned about litter and traffic fumes; has a little over £2.20 as pocket money; and so on.

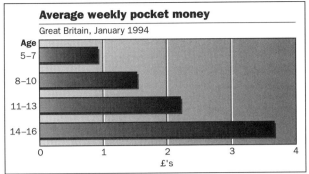

Chart 1.

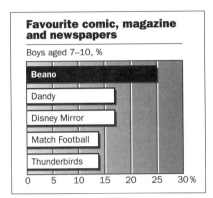

Chart 2.

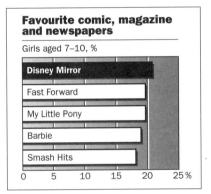

Chart 3.

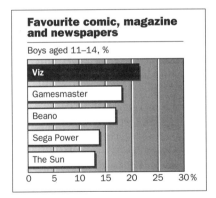

Chart 4.

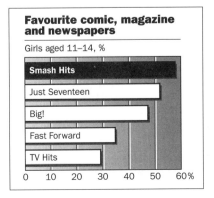

Chart 5.

Environmental issues seen by children as a problem: by age, 1993

England	Percentages		
	8-10 yrs	11-12 yrs	13-15 yrs
Local issues			
Litter	85	81	73
Traffic fumes	76	79	78
Danger to wildlife	79	76	68
Oil/sewage on beach	73	73	71
Factory pollution	72	74	69
Dog mess	74	67	61
Lack of trees/plants	59	65	57
Too much noise	39	30	23
Low-quality drinking water	18	23	23
Global issues			
Deforestation	90	89	91
Polluted oceans	88	90	93
Damage to ozone	79	89	91
Animal extinction	86	88	84
People not having enough to eat	86	83	83
People not having enough to drink	82	74	79
Global warming	53	77	86
Acid rain	64	66	77

Chart 6.

5. Planning evaluation methods

This section covers ways of **evaluation**, and considers trials and other issues that need to be considered *before* implementation takes place. The force field diagram technique is developed with an example.

The idea is to anticipate what might happen with your promotional plan *before* you put it into practice. You are evaluating 'before the event' as it were.

- **Force Field Diagrams** One way of trying to identify factors which will help or hinder your plan is to develop a **force field diagram** (Fig 5.6).

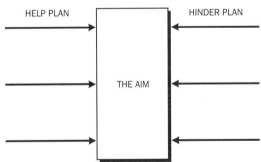

Figure 5.6 A force field diagram

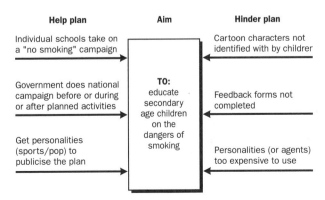

Figure 5.7 An actual field diagram

For example, you may wish to identify the factors you *expect* will help or hinder a campaign to reduce smoking by children or young adults (Fig. 5.7).

On this basis you can draw up a list of *activities* or *trial events* to test out some of these relevant factors before implementing the plan.

An example of actions that may need to be taken after the force field exercise has been completed.

- **Supporting helpful factors**
  1. Visit some schools to encourage them to associate with the scheme.
  2. Plan *local* activities around *national* campaign. Delay plan accordingly?
  3. Get sports personalities with reserves (in case some drop out). Ensure that these personalities are well known by the target audience (children aged around 14/15 years old.)

- **Avoiding hindrance factors**
  1. Test pilot cartoon character first (use national ones if appropriate).
  2. Give away free gift with every completed questionnaire form, or enter all completed forms into a prize draw.
  3. Select 6 key personalities and ask for quotations of fees charged, etc.

6. Set implementation plan

Now is the time to plan, in as much detail as possible, exactly what needs to be done and by whom. A large promotional scheme will need to be *broken down* into smaller, more manageable sub-components. Milestones will need to be set, and dates to achieve them will be necessary. An *action plan* will be necessary.

At an early stage in the scheme it is important to achieve commitment from all the people involved. Computer software planning packages may be useful to help run the scheme. Remember to include *feedback sessions* at all stages to be able to assess progress as the plan develops.

7. Implement

This is the stage when the planning stops (or part of it) and the *actions* are started.

Element 2 of this unit will consider in some detail the implementation of a number of health promotional plans involving smoking, alcohol, drug issues, and so on.

8. Re-evaluate

The last stage is the **re-evaluation stage**; it occurs *after* implementation has been completed and at regular intervals throughout the process as necessary.

Why evaluate?

It is important, *after* the campaign, to know the degree to which the original objectives were met. Or, if you are *mid-way through* the campaign, do the plans need to be altered; if so at what point and how, and what are the consequences?

Re-evaluation takes place for the following reasons:

- to inform others – to stop others reinventing the wheel.
- to reassess – for next campaign.
- to publicise successes (team building, motivation).
- to investigate unplanned outcomes.
- to give job satisfaction – it is a key way to allow people working on the plan to be aware of the final outcome and results.
- to assess the process and the methodology. This is not to start a witch hunt if, for instance, the promotion was not

as successful as originally planned, but to objectively review the process and methods used. With the benefit of hindsight, what would the team do differently if the promotion was just starting? These lessons may be transferable on to the next promotion.
- to get feedback from others. This includes those inside the team and outside the team (but within the same organisation) and, most importantly, the client(s).

The ways of assessing will differ, depending on the outcome that has been aimed at. For example a *behaviour change* will require *observation* to know if such a change has occurred. On the other hand *measurements* will be required to see if environmental changes have occurred, e.g. testing air or water pollution.

Self Check ✓ **Element 1**

1. What is the importance of Values, Mission, Aims and Objectives in relation to a Health promotional campaign?

2. Why is knowledge of the target audience so important?

3. How would you attempt to reach children (age 5 – 9 year olds) as the targeted audience?

4. Do you remember the SMART principle in relation to goal setting? Write down the key points.

5. Following the guidelines of this element a health promotional plan can be broken down into key activities. What are they?

6. The "Health of the Nation" document contains information on which topics?

7. What is the difference between Top Down and Bottom Up Planning?

8. Explain the key differences between the following three approaches to health care – the Preventative, Self Empowerment and Radical approaches.

5.2 Presenting health promotion advice to others

In this Element we look at *implementing* health promotion advice in a number of specific areas; such as smoking, alcohol, drugs, sexual practices.

In particular we consider 3 key areas.

1. **The nature, level and scope of the advice is clearly outlined to the target audience.** This section covers the do's and don'ts of giving health care advice. It continues with giving health advice to different targeted audiences on a range of health subjects.

2. **Recommendations on the ways that others could contribute to their own health.** Six key areas are discussed in general terms. These are exercise, diet, drugs abuse, accidents, personal hygiene and mental health.

3. **Style and format to reach your target audience.** Various ways are developed to reach each target audience. Likewise the style and the format of the materials and presentation methods are adapted to specific audiences.

The nature, level and scope of the advice and the target audience

In this section we will look at the do's and don'ts of giving health promotion advice.

The three targeted audiences focused on in this section are: Children, adolescents and adults.

Table 5.5 opposite outlines some *general* do's and don'ts.

Many examples of target audiences have been discussed in Element 1. Here we look at children, adolescents and adults health promotion areas to illustrate the differences between target audiences. This chart however does NOT cover the *methods* that should be used to reach these audiences.

How to get others to contribute to their own health

We shall concentrate on 6 areas as follows:

- Exercise
- Diet
- Drugs
- Accidents
- Personal Hygiene
- Mental Health

Exercise

The idea here is to encourage gently increasing **exercise** levels, up to a minimum of three times per week, for 20–30 minutes per session. This needs to be in addition to 'warm-up' and 'cool down' activities.

Other advice can include the following:

- Walk up stairs instead of taking the lift.
- Develop good posture during all activities including sitting and standing.
- Do some stretching exercises if you have to spend long periods in one position, e.g. on a long car or train journey.
- Join a sports club. Have some fun.
- Take time out for yourself. You deserve it. No-one else can look after you; you need to *want* to be healthier and to look after yourself both mentally and physically.
- Get off the bus or train one or two stops earlier and walk instead. It may save you money as well.
- Go for a brisk walk in the open air on a regular basis.
- Walk to the shops instead of taking the car where applicable.
- Think healthily
- Act healthily

Diet

The health advice regarding **diets** is to educate people to understand the make-up of the different foods we eat, e.g. some foods are better than others and each has its own different construction. (See Unit 3 for specific details).

With regard to **children** the approach is to encourage them to reduce their intake of fat and sugar and educate relatives, grandparents and friends to bring other alternatives to sweets and cakes when visiting children. The benefits of fruit should be encouraged. With regard to **teenagers,** diet can be related to exercise and personal appearance. If one feels good inside then it is more likely that they will look good on the outside. **Adults** need to understand about different foods and their benefits and when they should be restricted. It is useful for adults and teenagers to be aware that many people on diets never seem to be able to be happy with the results they obtain. Also to be aware that excessive dieting is as dangerous as being obese. Signs of anorexia and bulimia need to be watched for in extreme cases.

The way that food is prepared, handled and stored is also

The dos and don'ts when giving health promotion advice to individual clients

DON'T

Lecture
No one likes to be lectured to. It can be exciting, especially for teenagers, to do things which they have been told they are not allowed to do. Examples include not to drink, take drugs and smoke.

Give complicated messages
Trying to get 2 or 3 ideas over to the client at the same time in one short meeting may confuse the client. The use of health jargon terms may confuse clients. These are terms familiar to you but new to the client; this includes abbreviations (e.g. ENT, A&E). Likewise advising the client that they should stop smoking while sharing an ash tray with them may also confuse.

Never load your problems on the client
Or appear as superman / women. You are there to listen and to give guidance and support, not to worry the client regarding, for example, your staff shortage problems.

DO

Develop trust
Concentrate on developing good relationships, before preparing individual action plans. Be professional at all times. Be sure to know the field that you specialise in and know who the client should contact if other specialisms are required.

Give guidance and support
In a relaxed, fun, mature way, with lots of common sense. Ensure that the environment setting is correct for the meeting that is taking place.

Allow people to come to their own conclusions
Involve them in all aspects of their care and allow them to make their own choices, and decisions. Let them take responsibility for their own actions, which is important for long term success. Be aware that the clients' decisions may NOT be similar to yours.

Give options
Allow the client the time to digest advice given and always check for understanding. Allow individuals the opportunity to discuss further or seek clarification.

Get feedback
This can take many forms, verbal or written, direct or indirect. One way is to ask directly; e.g. What do you think of this idea, plan, suggestion? Of course you may only hear what the client thinks you want to hear! Remember when giving feedback that it should be non-judgmental and of benefit for the client's future development.

Plan
Do plan the client's visit or a meeting to obtain the optimum results. Recall the purpose of the meeting. What does the client want from the meeting? Are you sure? Check? What do you want? Do you need any promotional aids to assist you? How much time is available? Will all disturbances be minimised: telephone calls, personal interruptions etc.? Will another meeting be required? What is essential to be covered and what can wait if need be? How will the session end? Is your diary available to book a future session?

Table 5.5 Some points to remember when giving health promotion advice

very important. This is in relation to the amount of nourishment which remains in food after cooking and the prevention of food poisoning. An example of a good cooking habit is that *grilling* of food should be encouraged as opposed to *frying*.

| | Example of health advice to different target audiences | | |
Subject	Children	Adolescents	Adults
SMOKING	Explain dangers in children's terms. A quote from a six year old boy who, when asked about the dangers of smoking replied "your teeth and the inside of the body, goes black" might be used.	Bad breath, not good for relationships. Not 'cool' to smoke. Pop stars and sports stars are against smoking. Smoking affects performance. Where to go to get help.	Change habits to reduce smoking. Advice on how to stop, and where to get help. Facts and figures. Number of deaths. How your life deteriorates with smoking, e.g. can't climb stairs as you grow older; effects on pregnant women; impacts of passive smoking; etc.
DRUGS	Don't accept "sweets or presents" from strangers.	Drugs ruin your life. Drugs are not 'cool'. Do not mix with groups involved in drugs. Drugs make you spotty and unattractive, and affect performance.	Seek help. Dangers. Ruin your life, family. Beware of addiction to "milder" drugs e.g. sleeping tablets.
GLUE SNIFFING	Explain dangers. Teach how to say NO. Inform teachers, parents if someone invites you to sniff glue.	Don't mix with children that are involved in glue sniffing activities. Say NO! Definitely not 'cool'. Inform them of other activities available: Youth and sports clubs etc.	Inform parents of the signs to look for in their children and how to react if they suspect i.e. kind, caring approach, listen to your child's problem(s).
HIV/AIDS	Introduce to children as part of normal sex education. Explain how it can and cannot be caught.	Explain what it is. Inform about Safe Sex. Explain signs and symptoms and what to do. Talk about secure relationships.	How and where to get advice. What to do, etc. Give key facts, numbers and groups affected, etc.
ROAD SAFETY	Teach the Green Cross Code. Encourage children to pass their Bicycle Proficiency Tests. Wear visible (e.g. white) clothes at night.	How to help train younger children to always use the correct procedures. Don't Jay walk. Dangers and Deaths etc. "Wear something white at night" Cycling on the roads and the dangers associated. Pass a proficiency test and have bicycle regularly maintained.	Inform how to train your children. It is the parent's responsibility. What to do with children of different ages. Stress importance of setting a good example. Avoid speeding and drinking when driving.
FOOD	Use quotes/sayings such as "An apple a day keeps the doctor away". The bad effects of eating sweets and drinking cola. The "coolness" of other foods and drinks, e.g. Milk drinks, Fruit, Vegetables, Cereals. Encourage schools to only use healthy food for children.	Food and its effects on beauty and health. "What you eat is what you are". Fast food is not the best for your health and beauty, causes greasy hair and spots. Explain facts about anorexia, bulimia and avoidance mechanisms.	Information on Vitamins, Nutrients and Minerals. Explain good and bad cooking habits (i.e. don't overcook vegetables, use a small amount of water etc.) Dangers of sugars. Dangers of crash diets and how to be aware of what foods to eat and when.

Drugs

The recommendations on the ways that others could contribute to their own health in relation to **drugs** is firstly by *not taking* drugs wherever possible. If they are to be taken, it should be under the supervision or instruction of a qualified person like a doctor. The drugs should then be the weakest possible to achieve the end results, and for the least amount of time, so that addiction is prevented.

Existing drug users should be encouraged to go and seek professional help. Although many smokers, for instance, *have* given up smoking without this additional help.

Drugs include glue sniffing, smoking and alcohol abuse. See pages 102–107 for a fuller development of these topics.

Accidents

A large health concern is **accidents**. Individuals can help to *reduce* accidents by taking some simple precautions and being aware of where common accidents occur.

The key areas can be broken down into:

- Home
- Work
- Travel

Home – Consider electricity, gas and water utilities as potential killers. Treat all with care (see Element 3 for more details). An area of specific danger is the *Kitchen* and particularly the chip pan. In the *bathroom*, there is the danger for the very young and the elderly of drowning in bathwater. The old are also accident prone in relation to stairs, trailing leads, loose fitting carpets and wet floors, etc.

Fires are another important hazard and the installation of fire alarms and smoke detectors would reduce this risk if they were fitted.

Work – Risks arise from simple trailing leads, mechanical and electric equipment, hazardous substances, eye strain from excessive VDU operation, stress and mental illness.

Did You Know ?

The 'control of substances hazardous to health' regulations require employers to complete a risk assessment of all hazardous substances used in their workplaces.

Travel – When the weather conditions are poor there is a large increase in the number of accidents on the roads, especially during the rush hours to and from work. Driving too fast in poor visibility and wet conditions is a common reason for accidents. Road accidents have the largest accident figures, but railway lines and boats and aeroplanes all contribute.

Personal hygiene
Includes basics like:

- Washing your hand after going to the toilet; it is also important to wash dirty hands BEFORE using the toilet. This is to stop the spread of infection from the hands to the sexual parts.
- Clean teeth, in the morning, after meals and just before going to sleep.
- Personal hygiene is also very important in the preparation of food.
- Sexual practices, the use of condoms to help to reduce the spread of the HIV/AIDS virus and other STD's.

See Unit 3 for development of this topic.

Mental Health
Some key messages are:

- Look after yourself, as no one else can do this for you.
- Reduce stress. Understand when you are under stress. Do something about it. Reduce job related pressures. Relax.
- Be aware if others close to you are showing the signs of mental ill health; be available to listen to the persons concerns. Encourage the person to lead a healthy life style, including taking a lunch break, learning to switch off after work and at weekends, etc. Unemployed people are especially likely to suffer from stress. It is important to take up new activities and hobbies. Visiting libraries and other establishments, along with regular exercise, all help to relieve the stress.

A style and format to reach the target audience

Different **styles** and **formats** are required to reach different target audiences. The *same medium* like television, radio or newspapers can be used for different targeted audiences. This is because each has different sections or programmes geared for different audiences. For example, on television there are childrens programmes, teenage and separate adult programmes. This is true for other media (the Sunday Times for example has a separate cartoon section purely for very young children). This makes it easier to target selected audiences.

Some examples follow where the same medium can be used for different targeted groups. However as **segmentation** (the art of targeting different groups) continues, so different media have also specialised further. Newspapers, for example, cater for different sectors of the market. The Financial Times for the business community, while the Sun focuses on the mass market audience. Likewise TV now has children's TV, Sports channels, Women's programmes etc.

Some examples are given in Table 5.6 of *media* for reaching each of the three target audiences.

Children	Adolescents	Adults
Nursery and Junior School	School/Colleges	Workplace
Home	Home	Home
TV (children's) Cartoons	TV Teenage programmes	TV Adult TV Daytime TV
Children's video's	Video	Video
Cinema	Cinema	Cinema
PG films	15 films	18 films
	Video Game's and toys.	
Telephone support no's.	Telephone hot lines.	Telephone
Bill boards, (playgrounds)	Bill Boards (outside schools)	Bill Boards (shopping centres)
Children's radio	Radio (Youth programmes)	Radio (Adult)
Children clubs	Youth clubs	Day centres
Cubs	Scouts	Doctors surgery, clinics,
Sunday school	Community centres.	Church
Comics	Magazines (Soap, Film, Sports)	Newspapers (tabloid and non-tabloid)

Table 5.6 Methods of reaching 3 different target audiences

Style and **format** of presentation for any medium used is important in communicating with your intended audience.

Children	Adolescents	Adults
Fun and Friendly.	'Cool'. Young approach.	Factual. Humour.
Cartoon	Pop Stars	Actors
characters	Sports Personalities	
Short	Visual impact.	Accurate.
Colourful	New ideas; fast moving.	Clearly presented
Multi-lingual facilities required	Multi-lingual facilities required	Multi-lingual facilities required

---

Self Check ✓ **Element 2**

9. Make a table giving examples of health advice to different target audiences, namely *children*, *adolescents* and *adults*. Do this for each of the following subjects.

    (a) ALCOHOL CONSUMPTION

    (b) ACCIDENTS IN THE HOME

10. Consider three options that the Government could pursue to encourage greater usage of smoke detectors.

11. What legislation could be introduced to reduce the speed of cars on the road of England and Wales? (Under the belief that speed kills and increases the amount of gases in the atmosphere).

12. Which pressure groups may complain about the above schemes?

13. If a person in your group has a personal hygiene problem how would YOU deal with it?

14. Why should you NOT lecture to a client?

15. When giving health advice name 5 key factors that you should aim to achieve?

16. Why is it important to target different groups? What is the main problem with NOT doing so?

17. Explain how to reach different targeted audiences?

18. Name six areas in which a client could contribute to their own health.

19. What would you do if you noticed your client was suffering from stress? Would you have a different approach if it was YOU that was suffering from stress?

20. Identify three ways of reaching children as your target audience in a health promotion campaign.

21. Describe a feasible style and format for a promotion plan to reach adolescents?

22. Why is style and format important in a promotional campaign?

5.3 Different types of risks to health

In this element we will identify risks to health, their effects and the main ways of minimising the risks to health. The areas that are covered are:

1. The main risks to health associated with substance abuse; drugs, alcohol, solvent abuse, and smoking.

2. The main risks to health associated with unsafe sexual practices; sexual transmission of disease, including the HIV infection.

3. The risks to personal safety within the environment and ways of minimising the risks.

The main risks to health associated with substance abuse

This section will look at four key areas associated with risks to health

- Drugs
- Alcohol
- Solvent Abuse
- Smoking

Drugs

Drug users come from all walks of society. A popular image is of young "drop-outs" who turn to crime to sustain the habit, or put a drain on the health and social services. This group, however, is only a small proportion of habitual users.

One of the largest group of drug users are middle aged women whose dependency is on legally prescribed drugs, such as barbiturates and tranquillisers. The prescription of such drugs has dramatically decreased, but years of over-prescribing have left many people with a drug dependency problem.

Users of drugs often develop a *tolerance*. Tolerance means the way the body gets used to some kinds of drugs. To get the same affect, the body needs increasing amounts of the drug. Withdrawal symptoms include inability to sleep, nervousness, irritability, nausea, faints, delirium and, on occasions, convulsions which can result in brain damage. Sudden withdrawal can result, in extreme cases, in death.

People use drugs (including alcohol and cigarettes) for a range of reasons:

- out of curiosity
- pleasure
- to relieve stress, or to solve problems
- rebellion, or just because they are available
- boredom
- to be part of the group
- peer group pressure
- habit
- medical reasons

Drug use can be divided into three categories:

– legally approved drugs used in medicine;

– socially accepted drugs, such as alcohol;

– illegal drugs, not socially accepted, such as crack, cannabis, heroin.

The two main laws about drugs are **The Medicines Act** which controls the ways that medicines are made and supplied and **The Misuse of Drugs Act** which bans the non-medical use of certain drugs. The Misuse of Drugs Act places drugs into different classes. The penalties for offences involving a drug depend on its class. Class A drugs carry high penalties; Class C drugs lower penalties.

The main groups of drugs which affect the nervous system are:

1. sedatives
2. stimulants
3. analgesics
4. narcotics

1. **Sedatives (depressants)**. These diminish feelings of anxiety and induce a state of relaxatinn. *Examples* are alcohol, morphine and barbiturates (sleeping tablets), and tranquillisers, all of which can cause drowsiness, even in small doses.

Barbiturates: these are sedatives which are used medically to calm people down, as sleeping tablets and hypnotics. They come in capsule and powder form. Misusers swallow or inject themselves. Injecting barbiturates is one of the most dangerous forms of drug misuse.
Effects: these include nervousness, sleeplessness, irritability. Users tend to develop a physical and mental tolerance to these drugs and a sudden withdraw can kill.

Tranquillisers: these are prescribed by doctors to control anxiety, tension and to help people sleep. The drug is meant to be taken in pill form but misusers often inject themselves. e.g.; chlordiazepoxide, medazepam, diazepam and meprobromate.
Effects: they lower inhibition and can cause aggression and lessen alertness. If they are mixed with alcohol they can cause death. Dependency is common among long-term users. Once people stop taking this drug it can cause irritability, confusion and anxiousness and ex-users can find it difficult to lead a normal life.

2. **Stimulants**. These induce a sense of alertness and reduce the feeling of fatigue. *Examples* are caffeine in coffee, tea, cola and amphetamines (see below). They can become addictive.

Amphetamines: these were widely prescribed in the 1960's for depression and to people on diets to suppress their appetite.
Effects: amphetamines arouse the body, and give a sense of energy and confidence, followed by feelings of anxiety and irritability. High dosages can result in panic attacks. To maintain the effects regular users have to take an increasing dose. When users stop taking the drug they feel depressed and very hungry and their resistance to disease is lowered, which can have serious affects on their health and well being.

3. **Analgesics (pain killers)**. These have an affect on the part of the brain which produce a sense of feeling pain. *Examples* are paracetamol and aspirin.

4. **Narcotics**. Most are illegal drugs. They have a very powerful effect on the nervous system and are only prescribed under strict supervision and in small doses. (e.g. cocaine). *Examples* of illegal drugs are: cannabis, cocaine, heroin, opiates and LSD. An overdose causes unconsciousness, comas and can be fatal. They can be addictive and causes serious problems such as complete loss of psychological and physiological independence. They have become a serious problem in many countries. The dependent user often resorts to various methods, in particular crime, to obtain the drugs.

Cannabis: comes from the Cannabis Saliva plant which is often mixed with tobacco and smoked. It can be mixed with food and be eaten.
Effects: It makes people feel more relaxed and talkative. High dosages can cause feelings of anxiety, depression and panic. Cannabis is said to be addictive but, like tobacco, frequently inhaled cannabis smoke will cause breathing disorders, bronchitis and could lead to lung cancer.

Cocaine: is a powerful stimulant with properties similar to those of amphetamines. It is a white powder that is made from the leaves of the Andean coca shrub. It is an expensive drug that is injected or sniffed through a tube and absorbed into the blood supply. Another form of cocaine is **Crack** which has been treated with chemicals so that it can be smoked. It is cheaper than cocaine but more dangerous. The initial "high" is followed by unpleasant after effects, which encourage compulsive use.
Effects: Cocaine produces a feeling of well-being; it often reduces pain and gives an illusion of physical and mental strength. This can be helpful to people suffering from various physical problems. Recently there has been a growing pressure to legalise cocaine especially to those who need it to reduce pain and discomfort. As the drug wears off it can sometimes produce feelings of anxiety and panic; the effects tend to peak quickly and lessen rapidly. As a result the drug has to be taken more often to maintain the "high" feeling. Sniffing cocaine can destroy the membranes inside the nose; it can also, over the longer term, produce sickness, weight loss and sleeplessness.

Heroin: this is a white powder made from the opium poppy. It is injected, sniffed and smoked.
Effects: Opiates create a feeling of relaxation, warmth and contentment; heroin relieves pain, anxiety, stress and discomfort. It also depresses the brain activity and dilates blood vessels, hence the feeling of warmth; it also causes constipation. As the intake increases, the effects include sweating, chilling, aches, tremors, muscular spasms, sneezing and yawning. First time users often feel sick and vomit, especially if they have been injecting. Once physically dependent, the user needs more of the drug to get the same effect. The pleasure of use is replaced simply by getting hold of the drug. Once addicted the users are overcome with apathy; they often neglect themselves and others and havd a poor diet. Overdosing results in unconsciousness, coma, and death from breathing failure. The chances of death are increased if other drugs are involved.

Lysergic Acid Diethylamide (LSD) is a white powder that is often mixed with other substances and hs formed into tablets or capsules or supplied in sugar cubes or paper such as the Superman transfers which can be licked by children.
Effects: LSD depends on the user's mood. They often expe-

rience distorted vision and hearing and a feeling of being 'outside' the body. A "trip" begins an hour or so after taking LSD and lasts for around 12 hours depending on the dose. A bad "trip" can lead to depression, dizziness and panic attacks.

Magic Mushrooms: Some wild mushrooms can produce dreams or visions like Liberty Cap which contains hallucinogenic chemicals. It is difficult to tell the difference between Liberty Cap and the poisonous Amanita mushrooms.

Effects: the effects of taking magic mushrooms are very much like LSD, except the effects are quicker and do not last as long. They can also cause hallucination, vomiting and stomach pains. It is not illegal to pick wild mushrooms and eat them. But if you dry them and turn them into a preparation, then this could be an offence.

Ecstasy: This is a new drug with numerous street names (see chart below for just some of them). It comes in tablet or coloured capsules. It has become popular with the young and is found illegally at "raves" and discos.

Effects: ecstasy makes people very friendly and gives a feeling of having lots of energy. Depression follows once the effect of the drug has worn off. If it is taken in large amounts it can cause confusion, anxiety, paranoia and users can find it difficult to sleep. Girls find that it makes their periods heavier. It is especially dangerous for anyone who suffers from a heart condition or from epileptic fits. Studies have shown that long-term usage can cause certain brain cells and the liver to be damaged.

Addictive drugs

These are drugs that are habit-forming, affect the nervnus system and may result in an increased tolerance; hence these drugs need to be taken in a greater quantity to produce the samd effect and may cause withdrawal symptoms if they are not readily available.

The street names for many popular drugs are shown in the chart below. This is NOT a complete list as names vary in different regions and new names are always being used.

Drug	Street names
Barbiturates	Sekkies, Blues, Reds, Barbs
Tranquillisers	Downers, Eggs, Jellies, Benzos, Tranx
Amphetamines	Uppers, Speed, Sulphate, Whiz
Cannabis	Grass, Dope, Wacky Backy, Hash, Shit, Blow, Marijuana (Herbal cannabis)
Cocaine	Crack (treated cocaine)
Heroin	Smack, H, Skag, Junk
Ecstasy	E, Dennis the Menace, New Yorker, Rhubarb and Custard, Disco burger, Love doves
L.S.D.	Acid

Other drugs
Anabolic steroids

Used medically for growth defects and muscle wasting, anabolic steroids are used illegally by some, mainly young people, to produce a sudden increase in body size and weight. Some athletes have illegally used them to increase their strength and power.

Did You Know ?

There are three ways to take a drug. These are:
Swallowing: dissolves in the stomach then passes into the blood stream.
Inhaling: passes into the bloodstream from the lungs.
Injecting: passes straight into the blood stream.

Drugs are carried to the brain via the blood. The drug affects the brain and the messages being sent out by the brain. Different drugs affect the brain in different ways. Depressants slow down and stimulants speed up the working of the brain. Hallucinogens – cause hallucinations and visions.

Dangers associated with using illegal drugs

Illegal drugs are drugs used without a doctor's prescription. These include: Barbiturates, L.S.D, Amphetamines, cannabis, heroin and cocaine. The drug users that inject themselves are more at risk than other drug users, in particular drugs which are injected into the blood. This is because of the dangers of unsterilised needles which can result in blood poisoning, hepatitis and Aids. There is also no control over the quantity or quality of the drug being used; e.g., the quality can be altered by mixing the drug with impurities such as rat poison, or household cleaners (e.g. powders such as Ajax, Vim, talcum powder) which can cause serious side effects. The strength of the drug is unknown, therefore it is difficult to control the amount of drug being injected.

If a drug user becomes addicted to illegal drugs it can be hard to keep a regular job. The problems in earning money to keep up the habit, can result in stealing or prostitution to obtain money. Longer term problems can involve brain, liver and kidney damage. Drugs can also affect a person's personality and behaviour.

Other dangers include:

- having an accident while under the influence of drugs.
- making the drug user feel depressed and hopeless.
- causing unbalanced emotions and serious mental disorders.
- sickness and vomiting.
- girls can miss their periods.
- constipation problems are common with regular users.
- risk of catching an infection is greater, particularly ones which cause sores, abscesses, jaundice and blood poisoning.

Drug dependency

A person can become *dependent* on drugs in 2 ways. First an individual can get used to taking drugs and feel that they cannot cope with every day life without them; i.e. they become *psychologically dependent*. Second, if the body gets used to drugs, that is if a person feels physically ill without them, they become *physically dependent*.

An *addiction* can be defined as a state of periodic or chronic intoxication, i.e. a state of being poisoned, produced by the repeated consumption of a drug, which produces the following characteristics:

- an overpowering desire or compulsion to continue taking the drug and to obtain it by any means.
- a tendency to increase the body dosage, showing dependence on the effects of the drug.
- creation of an individual problem and, in the wider sense, a social problem.

Withdrawal symptoms

This happens when a person tries to stop taking habitual drugs; they become physically ill. This is the reason why it is so hard to stop taking drugs.

Drug treatment for addiction

Being *rehabilitated* (often in open centres) can take a long time. Some people manage to give up drugs for a while but return to the habit because they cannot resist the temptation. Some young people try drugs without developing a dependency on them. Many drugs can be bought from chemist shops, e.g. cough mixtures and laxatives. These drugs can still have a non beneficial effect on health, such as taking laxatives to control weight. People who do become dependent can find themselves with a very expensive habit, which can lead them into desperate situations such as crime. For a rehabilitation programme to be successful the drug user must be involved in all the processes of the programme for recovery, with the professionals and their family members being involved if possible.

Treatment and rehabilitation can be successful if the user is involved in the following:

- observation
- withdrawal of the drug in a drug dependency situation
- rehabilitation
- developing a sense of self worth.

One of the recent treatments is the *Harm Reduction Programme* incorporating the AIDS prevention programme. The program was introduced because of the growing incidence of HIV among drug injectors. The programme is intended to help drug-injected users to protect themselves and prevent the spread of the HIV virus. Many agencies work together, including the police, social workers and voluntary groups. The primary aim is to get misusers off drugs via a reduction of dependency on illicit drugs. By supplying *clean* drugs and needles, of a known dose, it has been argued that this would bring users in contact with the various services, and reduce dependency on illicit drugs. The purpose is to keep users alive and healthy until they themselves come to the decision to stop taking the drugs.

A user-friendly syringe and needle exchange service has been set up in certain areas of the country for drug injection users to exchange needles free of charge. The use of dirty, harmful street drugs can damage the drug-user's health. Many drug users are involved in drug pushing and other crimes to pay for drugs. As a result many are a burden on their family, the community, the law enforcement agencies, and other caring agencies. Often it is the *behaviour* of the drug users and not their knowledge of drugs, which is the problem. The organisers, with the help of drugs users, did NOT set up an educational programme to educate drug users about drugs. Instead, they set up a network of facilities and self-help services, which are accessible and where the drug user could gain the means to live a healthier and happier life.

Alcohol

Alcohol is the most socially accepted drug of our time, particularly in western societies. Drinking alcohol can be an enjoyable experience and in small quantities can be good for health. Alcohol is also a depressant, sedative and hypnotic (it produces sleep). It has a tendency to make people feel less inhibited than normal and reduces ones ability to concentrate, such as driving less effectively. The effects of alcohol begin quickly and can last for many hours, and into the next day. Nearly all the alcohol that is drunk is rapidly absorbed into the blood stream and is burnt up by the liver. It takes roughly one hour for the body to burn off the alcohol in one unit of alcohol.

After consuming 1 unit of alcohol the blood alcohol content increases by about 16mg of alcohol in 100ml of blood. Breath alcohol content increases by about 7mg of alcohol in 100ml. Legal limits for driving are: blood alcohol content 80mg of alcohol in 100ml of blood, or 35mg of alcohol in 100ml of breath content.

The legal limit for driving is three units of alcohol. It doesn't take many drinks to reach this limit

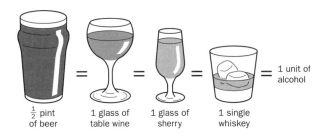

½ pint of beer   1 glass of table wine   1 glass of sherry   1 single whiskey   1 unit of alcohol

Figure 5.8

> ### Did You Know ?
>
> One pint of extra strong strength lager will put you over the legal driving limit. (It is valued at 6 units).

Young people are more affected by alcohol than older people.

> ### Did You Know ?
>
> Young drivers are 5 times more likely to have an accident after 5 units of alcohol than when sober.

Alcohol is the major cause of accidents. More than half of the people breathalysed are over twice the legal limit; 1 in 3 of the drivers in road accidents have levels of alcohol which are over the legal limit. Most drinking and driving accidents happen within 1 mile of the driver's home. If you drink in excess in the evening, you might still be over the legal limit the next morning and would fail a breathalyser test while driving in the morning. Alcohol misuse is a factor in deaths from falls, drowning, deaths in fires and suicides.

If men drink more than 21 units and women 14 units per week, on a regular basis, there is a *risk* of it damaging their health. Drinking more than 33 units for men, and 22 units per week for women, is almost certainly dangerous to health.

> ### Did You Know ?
>
> In 1992 over 600 people in the UK were killed in alcohol-related road accidents.

- **Women and drinking**. Women are more at risk from the harmful effects of drinking than men. One of the main reasons for this is the difference in the water content of the body. In women the water content is between 45–55% while in men the figure is 55–65%. Alcohol is distributed through the body fluids, therefore in men the alcohol is more diluted than in women.

  When women are pregnant or during breast feeding it is advisable not to drink alcohol as it passes into the blood stream, travels across the placenta to the baby. When breast feeding, alcohol can be passed to the baby through the breast milk.

EFFECTS OF EXCESSIVE ALCOHOL

1. Reaction time is decreased and efficiency of the brain is reduced.
2. Prolonged drinking can lead to physical dependency.
3. Digestive system is irritated which results in nausea, and a hangover, with the possibility of gastritis and peptic ulcers.
4. Accumulation of fat occurs in liver and can lead to hepatitis; this is an inflammation of the liver, and cirrhosis, which is a permanent scarring of the liver, and pancreatitis. It can contribute to being overweight. People who are diabetics are likely to have extra problems.
5. Problems with the nervous system, especially nerve pains in the arms and legs.
6. More young people are killed by alcohol related accidents (reckless actions) than by illegal drugs. Alcohol can cause accidents because it can affect a persons ability and judgement when driving, using dangerous machinery or when taken with various medications.
7. Can cause social problems at work, with family and friends.
8. Females are generally affected more than men by the same amount of alcohol consumed (see next section).
9. Depends on weight, sex, social setting.
10. Heavy drinking reduces resistance to infections.
11. Can lead to poor blood circulation and high blood pressure.
12. Skin blood vessels become dilated. The red nose of an excessive drinker is common.
13. Muscles experience fatigue and poor muscle co-ordination.
14. Many working days are lost because people have hangovers. Also many people turn up at wnrk but still feel poorly from the effects.
15. Sexual difficulties are common. This may be one of the underlying *reasons* for excessive drinking in the first place. Or the sexual problem could be a *result* of excessive alcohol.
16. Depression, and other psxchiatric and emotional disorders are common.
17. Cancer of the mouth, throat and gullet are possibilities with excessive drinking over a long period.
18. Malnutrition can occur at the same time as being overweight. This is because heavy drinkers get their energy from the alcohol instead of food, plus alcohol lacks the essential nutrients and vitamins that the body needs.

- **Government and alcohol**. The Government puts large amounts of duty on alcohol and it is common for regular increases to occur through the budgetary system. The Government also spends a small percentage of this money on health promotion.

  The government tries to limit alcohol abuse by:

  – prohibiting the sale of alcohol to under 18 year olds.
  – heavily taxing alcoholic drinks.
  – adopting further tax increases in the annual budgets.
  – custom controls.
  – using the breathalyser to catch drink drivers, particularly common around the Christmas festive season.

- **Alcoholics**. Alcoholics can be helped by various organisations such as Alcoholics Anonymous (and so can their family). Also additional help is available via special hospitals and clinics.

There is however some evidence that a *small* amount of alcohol can be good for health. This is in the region of one (or two) small drinks a day. This is because a small quantity of alcohol could lead to less cardiovascular disease in light drinkers than in non-drinkers. Alcohol prevents the action of platelets in the blood (concerned in clotting); as a result blood is less likely to become 'sticky' and the blood vessels are more likely to stay open'.

Solvent abuse

Solvent abuse refers to a variety of substances which are inhaled; they include glue, paint thinners, aerosols, petrol, butane gas and cleaning fluids. Many glues and household products contain many chemical solvents to stop them solidifying. Fumes from the solvents are breathed in; these fumes affect the brain and gives a temporary pleasant feeling, which can result in delirium and unconsciousness. The sensation is similar to drunkenness with a reduction in anxiety, and memory impairment. Some people increase the effects by inhaling from the inside of a plastic bag placed over their head. The dangers of suffocation from this method are very apparent and some abusers have died from this. Solvent abuse such as glue sniffing can become addictive and is a dangerous habit; people have died from glue sniffing, often from choking on their vomit.

Did You Know ?

Many people have died from their *first* attempts of solvent abuse because they have squirted aerosol gases directly into their mouths, so freezing their air passages.

Many accidentally injure themselves because they are using the solvents in unsafe places such as railway lines or in unsafe building to be out of public view. Heavy solvent misuse can cause lasting damage to the brain. Long term misuse of cleaning fluids and aerosols have been known to cause damage to the liver and kidneys.

Some of the reasons why young people abuse solvents:

- to be part of a group
- cheap and easy to obtain
- seek attention
- escape from problems
- rebellion
- boredom/curiosity

Note that for some teenagers it can be a passing phase and the person will grow out of it.

Possible *signs* of someone abusing solvents are:

- a chemical smell on the breath
- traces of solvent on clothing
- empty containers like tins and aerosol
- not eating and loss of body weight
- slurred speech
- persistent irritable cough

- sores around the mouth and eyes
- mood swings, irritability and moody
- a sudden and uncharacteristic decline in school performance
- onset of truancy

Many of the above symptoms could also be associated with many other causes other than solvent abuse and therefore it is important that a child is not wrongly accused.

It is *not* against the law to take solvents, but the effect on young people can result in possible conviction for public order offences such as threatening behaviour or breach of the peace. It is an offence for shopkeepers to sell solvent based products to anyone under 18 years old, if they know or have reasonable cause to believe that the products are being abused and not used for their normal purpose.

If a parent suspects their child of substance abuse, it is important to talk and to listen to the child in a respectful way, to find out the following:

1. Are they abusing solvents?
2. How long has it been going on?
3. How regular?
4. Who else is involved?
5. Why have they turned to solvent abuse (search for the deeper reasons)?
6. When do they abuse solvents?
7. Where do they go to abuse solvents?
8. Where do they get the solvents from?

All this information may not come out in one session. Therefore it is important that trust is built up in the relationship. Find time to LISTEN to the person. Do not expect immediate results; the aim should be for long term behaviour changes.

Smoking

> ### Did You Know **?**
>
> Smoking is the most important cause of preventable disease and early death in the UK. In 1991
> - 32,169 people in England died of lung cancer, 81% were caused by smoking.
> - 25,511 people died from chronic bronchitis and emphysema and other smoking diseases.
> - Over 140,000 people died from coronary heart disease (CHD)
> - The risk of dying from CHD is $2\frac{1}{2}$ times greater in smokers than in non-smokers; and $3\frac{1}{2}$ times greater for heavy smokers.
> - If smokers suffer from high blood pressure or high cholesterol, there is an 8 fold increase in the risk.

All forms of smoking are bad for health; smokers are at a greater risk from illness and early death than non smokers. It increases the risk of heart disease, while stopping smoking reduces the risk. Lung diseases (especially bronchitis and lung cancer) and osteoporosis in older age are very common among smokers. The younger people start smoking, and the more cigarettes they smoke, the greater the risk. Smoking is responsible for over 111,000 deaths in England each year, and 1 in every 5 fatal heart attacks is related to smoking.

It is illegal to sell tobacco to children under sixteen years of age. However, surveys show that nearly 85% of tobacconists would be willing to sell cigarettes to children obviously under age.

> ### Did You Know **?**
>
> Over 11 million smokers in Britain have stopped in recent years; 9 out of 10 have done so without medical assistance. However ...
> 29% of women and 31% of men in the UK still smoke cigarettes.
> Around 25% of boys and girls smoke regularly.
> Smokers often think that the risks to health are lower than they really are.

Smoke from tobacco contains over 4,000 different chemicals. The three which affect the body and cause disease are nicotine, carbon monoxide and tar. Each will be discussed now.

1. **Nicotine.** This is a powerful and fast acting drug that can be addictive. When tobacco smoke is inhaled, nicotine is absorbed into the bloodstream and in 7 to 8 seconds the effects can be felt in the brain. The effects on the rest of the body are many and complex. Nicotine stimulates nerve impulses in the central nervous system and the autonomic nervous system, and in large amounts nicotine can inhibit them. The immediate effects of nicotine from smoking are:

   - increase in blood pressure
   - increase in the heart rate
   - increase in hormone production
   - changes in blood composition
   - changes in metabolism
   - constriction of small blood vessels under the skin.

The effects of nicotine on mood and behaviour depend on the following:

   The strength of the cigarette(s)
   The number of puffs and how deeply they are inhaled
   How long the person has been smoking
   Their smoking habits
   The situation they are in at the time
   The smokers general constitution.

2. **Carbon Monoxide.** This is a poisonous gas and is found in relatively high concentrations in cigarette smoke. It combines readily with the haemoglobin, the oxygen carrying substance in the blood, to form carboxyhaemoglobin. Carbon monoxide combines more readily with haemoglobin than oxygen does, hence up to 15% of a smokers blood can be carrying carbon monoxide around the body instead of oxygen. Reductions in oxygen supplies can cause problems with growth repair and the exchange of essential nutrients. Carbon monoxide is harmful during pregnancy as it reduces the amount of oxygen being carried to the uterus and foetus.

   Carbon monoxide can affect the electrical activity of the heart. Smoking can also encourage fatty deposits to form on the walls of the arteries. This can lead to the arteries becoming blocked, resulting in circulation problems and heart disease.

3. **Tar.** Cigarette smoke when inhaled is condensed and around 70% of the tar in the smoke is deposited in the lungs. Research seems to indicate that the substances are thought to cause cancer, damage the lungs, causing narrowing of the bronchioles and the ciliostasis.

   In the UK cigarettes have a tar branding, according to the amount of tar they yield. This is either: low, low to middle, middle to high.

Even when tar is reduced many of the other harmful substances are not, such as nicotine and carbon monoxide.

The main diseases caused by smoking are:

- **Heart and circulation**
  Coronary Heart Disease (CHD)
  Atherosclerosis, the build-up of fatty deposits and the loss of elasticity in the artery walls. This can lead to a variety of diseases including strokes, peripheral vascular disease and gangrene.

- **Cancers**
  mouth, nose and throat
  larynx
  oesophagus
  lung and bronchus
  pancreas
  bladder
  kidneys
  cervix
  Leukaemia

- **Lung disease**
  damage and loss of efficiency in the lungs
  chronic bronchitis and emphysema
  recurrent infections in the lungs and airways

- **Other related disorders**
  shortness of breath
  coughs, sneezing
  ulcers in the stomach and duodenum (peptic ulcer)
  effects on fertility
  defective vision (tobacco amblyopia)

Women and Smoking

As a group, women took up smoking in large numbers later in the 20th century than men. Hence the long term effects of smoking in woman are still emerging. Lung cancer is rising as a cause of death and in Scotland it has already overtaken breast cancer as the major cause of cancer deaths in women.

- Can effect fertility
- Increases the risk of spontaneous abortion and other complaints during pregnancy
- Low birth weight babies under 2.3 kgs (5 lbs)
- Prenatal mortality – death of a foetus after 26 weeks of pregnancy and the death of a new-born child during the first weeks of life
- Increases risk of cervical cancer
- Accelerates the onset of the menopause
- Associated with osteoporosis (brittle bones)
- Results in 1 in every 5 coronary heart deaths in UK
- Smoking and taking oral contraceptives increase the chance of having a stroke by 10 times compared to non-smokers not using oral contraceptives
- Lung cancer for woman is the commonest form of fatal cancer in Scotland
- Women tend to smoke more when under pressure
- Death rates from lung cancer for woman were less than half those for men in 1992. Men tend to smoke in relaxed circumstances
- Women smokers tend to feel less confident and more dependent on cigarettes compared to men
- Women smokers tend to see themselves as suffering from more stress than men

Many health campaigns promote the idea that smoking makes you less desirable and attractive than non-smokers.

This is particularly aimed at girls, many of whom think it makes them appear older. They think it is cool and sophisticated. Smoking is generally decreasing, but at a slightly lower rate for females than males.

Health promotion advice helps females to handle stressful situations rather than smoke. Women are encouraged to work on their self esteem and confidence and to look at the reasons *why* smoking increases their self esteem and confidence.

Young people and smoking

Young people smoke for a range of reasons. 25% of boys and girls are regular smokers by the age of 15.

Why young people smoke

- Smoking is associated with adulthood.
- Tobacco promotion; the youth are exposed to it in many forms.
- Peer group pressure; increases the likelihood of smoking
- Parental attitude; children whose parents don't mind if they smoke are more likely to be smokers.
- Children who smoke are twice as likely to have parents, brothers or sisters who smoke.
- To experiment with cigarettes.

Passive smoking

This is breathing in other people's cigarette smoke or smoke from the burning end of a cigarette. The latter is known as *side stream smoke* whereas *main stream smoke* is that exhaled by a smoker and inhaled by another person. Passive smoking can cause irritation to the eyes, nose and throat, dizziness and sickness, as well as a stale smell of smoke left on clothing of all the people in the close vicinity of smokers.

Did You Know **?**

That there is an increased risk of 10 – 30% in contracting smoking related diseases for non smokers as a result of passive smoking over long periods.

Passive smoking can affect the health of the whole family especially babies and children, and particularly affects the ears, nose and throat, causing chest infections like bronchitis and pneumonia. Some doctors and dentists have refused treatment to smokers. More and more public places are becoming non smoking areas. Some airlines have a no smoking policy on ALL their aeroplanes for journeys under 2 hours, because of the concerns of passive smoking.

Giving up smoking

When smokers give up, their risk of getting lung cancer or heart attack diminishes so that after 10-15 years an ex-smokers risk is only slightly higher than someone who has never smoked. Research have shown that many people have stopped smoking without too much difficulty and many have found it easier than they expected. There are many aids on the market to help giving up smoking including patches that are put on the arm.

Most people can cope better with the withdrawal symptoms if they *understand* what is happening and can develop strategies to overcome any problems. Successful strategies include trying to understand why and when the person smokes and what type of smoker the person is. For example some people smoke when they are concentrating while others when they have nothing to do with their hands. Some people always smoke after a meal; others while they are drinking alcohol. Some people smoke at regular intervals throughout the whole day while others smoke more at certain times. Getting the person to understand all these and other reasons for smoking will help in the withdrawal process. The main withdrawal symptoms are cravings, increased appetite, anxiety, irritability, coughing, mouth ulcers, light headedness and tingling sensations.

Did You Know **?**

That cigarette sales in Britain have fallen by 25% over the last 10 years.

The main risks to health associated with unsafe sexual practices

Good personal, sexual practices can actively promote well-being and health. Sex has, however, always had certain risks associated with it. These include unplanned pregnancy and sexually transmitted diseases, especially the HIV virus which can cause AIDS. (See Unit 3.2) One of the safest ways to avoid infection is to stay with one non infected partner; another is to practice safer sex, as discussed later in this section, and by avoiding unprotected casual sex, multiple partners and to use a condom. Condoms not only help protect against pregnancy, sexually transmitted diseases, HIV, but could also protect against cancer of the cervix. Sexually transmitted diseases (STD's) are passed from person to person during sexual intercourse.

HIV and AIDS

Acquired Immune Deficiency Syndrome (AIDS) is caused by a virus called Human Immunodeficiency Virus (HIV), a disease which interferes with the body's normal immunity to disease. The HIV virus enters the bloodstream, attacks and destroys the body's defence supplies, hence the body is vulnerable to attack from a range of infections which can result in a serious illness and eventually cause death. Such infections are called *opportunistic infections*. There can be lengthy periods between being infected with HIV and the development of the conditions which constitute AIDS.

The AIDS virus is in a group of viruses called *lentivirianae* of which only a few species are known. The AIDS virus infects white blood cells in the lymph nodes and in the spleen. It also infects cells throughout the brain. (Any anti viral agent that only prevents multiplication of the virus must be continued for life. Any agent which destroys all cells containing the virus would also destroy brain cells).

In 1990 trials of a vaccine began, but it will be many years before the results are known. There are many problems associated with trying to create a vaccine for AIDS. A vaccine uses an altered version of the infecting virus, and this infection stimulates the body to make antibodies to it without causing infection. A problem with AIDS is that the virus destroys the immune system which produces the antibodies in the first place.

The virus has been detected, in varying degrees, in the blood, semen, and vaginal fluids. To become infected by the virus, a person must be infected by a person who is already HIV positive.

HIV Transmission

HIV is *transmitted* in three main ways

* through unprotected sexual intercourse (anal or vaginal) passed on in an infected person's blood, semen or vaginal fluids.
* by injecting drugs, using shared needles and equipment.
* from an HIV positive mother to her unborn child or at the time of birth.

There are other ways that the HIV virus can be transmitted:

* by blood products e.g. Factor 8 (haemophiliacs) and by contaminated blood transfusions which happened before the risks were known. Since October 1985 UK blood donations have been screened and blood plasma products are specially treated. (Being infected by blood products is still a problem in certain countries.)
* by blood to blood contact, for example through open wounds.

There are no immediate symptoms when a person first becomes infected with the HIV virus. The only real way of knowing is by a blood test that produces a positive result. Shortly after infection, the virus can cause illness similar to glandular fever or influenza which lasts for a short time. This is often followed by a period in which no symptoms appear and may last for months to years, but a person can carry the virus and pass it on to other sexual partners. Symptoms include weight loss, fever, diarrhoea. The symptoms vary from person to person depending on the infections they catch. Swollen glands, profound fatigue, unexpected weight loss, fever, nightly sweats, prolonged shortness of breath, a dry cough, skin disease and infection by a large variety of bacteria e.g. tuberculosis or pneumonia. The disease can be fatal even without any visible symptoms.

A person with AIDS is vulnerable to infections because an AIDS sufferer's natural immune system can no longer work properly. The AIDS virus cannot survive for long outside the human body. It cannot be spread by coughing or sneezing, and it cannot be caught from lavatory seats. It is not a contagious disease; neither can it be caught by every day casual contact by skin, like shaking hands, hugging or caressing.

The virus is *not* known to have been passed on in public places, e.g. by using cafes, restaurants, cinemas, theatres or swimming pools. However it is advisable to avoid sharing razors or toothbrushes. There have been alleged cases of patients contracting HIV from dentists in the USA. This is thought to be via the instruments not being sterilised and autoclaved in the correct manner.

AIDS is one of, if not the most, serious medical problems in recent history. Methods of controlling the spread depend on *prevention* such as safer sexual practice because as yet no cure has been found.

Safer sexual practice

The body fluid, semen, contains a great concentration of HIV virus in an infected person. Safer sex involves doing whatever *prevents* semen entering their partners's body. Hence penetration of the penis in the vagina or anus is high risk. Using condoms correctly can reduce the risk of becoming infected with HIV and other sexually transmitted diseases. Condoms with a water based lubricant can reduce the risk.

Condoms can tear, split or drop off; they are not a guarantee against HIV. There is no risk in partners caressing each other. Individual and mutual masturbation is safe as long as contact between semen, genital fluids, cuts and sores are avoided. The basic principle is self protection and not allowing these fluids inside oneself.

HIV Testing

Where the body is infected by the HIV virus, it reacts by producing antibodies. An HIV test can tell whether the body has been infected by the *virus*. It does not tell if one has got AIDS, neither can it predict when or whether a person will go on to develop AIDS.

If the test does not find the HIV antibodies in the blood, then the person, probably, has not been infected with the virus. However it can take from two to six months (and in some cases even years) for the antibodies to develop after a person has become infected with the virus.

If a person has a negative result, this does not mean that they cannot be infected in the future if they put themselves at risk. If the test *does* find the antibodies to the virus in the blood, then the person does have HIV, not AIDS. But an infectious person can pass the virus on to other people, through sexual contact or blood, even though the person may look, and feel, fit and well.

Many babies who test positive initially, do so because they reflect the mothers antibody status. This does not mean that they have AIDS.

Did You Know **?**

That the World Health Organisation estimate that 8 – 10 million adults and ½ million children in the world are infected with the HIV virus.

The risks to personal safety within the environment and the ways of minimising risks

This section will cover the risks to personal safety and looks at three areas:

- Home
- Work (includes the Health and Safety at Work Act, 1974, revised).
- Environment

Home

Most accidents happen in the **home**. Around 5000 deaths are recorded each year as a result of accidents in the home; most if not all are preventable. To appreciate the dangers of the home, 1 in every 10,000 persons in the UK will die as a result of accidents in the home each year.

Fire is a major cause of death in the home. This is usually through careless handling of fires, through cooking, and smoking. Under 5's are involved in a larger percentage of accidents, mainly poisoning and burns. The elderly: 75 + year old women account for nearly 76% of all home accidents via falls, burns and scalds. Over half the people killed by fire each year are over 60 years old.

Falls are mainly caused by slipping or tripping on wet or well polished floors, poor lighting, or because of trailing flexes.

Other ways to reduce accidents in the home include:
- *Scalds* – Always take care when handling hot liquids. Pots and pans on cookers should always be turned inward. If possible use a cooker guard, especially with young children. Always cover hot water bottles and look for signs of 'clumsiness' via ageing regularly.
- *Cuts* – Mainly caused by carelessness when using knives, glass etc; always wear gloves when picking up broken glass. Glass doors can be dangerous to children or people slipping. Cover with special clear plastic sheeting to pre-

vent injury against falls. Make sure there are no loose rugs near glass doors.
- *Smoking* – Do not smoke in bed; always extinguish cigarettes and pipes when finished.
- *Cooking* – Accidents are one of the most common causes of fire; never leave pans unattended especially chip pans. Never fill more than half full with fat; if it does catch fire, turn off heat, cover with damp towel or lid and leave for at least 30 minutes.
- *Back injury* – Mainly caused by lifting incorrectly.
  Always – bend knees when lifting
  place feet slightly apart
  keep arms close to body
  keep back straight
  brace abdominal muscles before the lift
  use thigh muscles to provide power
- *Harmful substances* – Everyday household cleaners, chemicals etc can be potentially hazardous if certain safety precautions are not followed. Most substances such as cleaners, medicines, have instructions on the containers, which describe the handling, dosage and disposal of the substance.
  Harmful substances especially for toddlers
  Turpentine and turpentine substitutes.
  Caustic soda,
  Paint strippers,
  Paraffin,
  Alcohol based solvents,
  Bitrex added to chemicals makes them taste bitter
  (Tesco plan to add this to household products).

Harmful substances need to be stored, handled, and disposed of safely, examples are given in Table 5.7 on page 111.

- *Fire* – Install smoke alarms and follow safety tips.
- *Home security* – Install window, door locks and alarm if possible, door chains, ask callers for identification, do not keep keys on chains behind doors.

Looking at safety, room by room, in the home
Kitchen – Must have dry hands before using electricity, watch flex's, kettles, irons etc. especially where young children are about.
Garden – While lawn mowing one should wear protective shoes and gloves. Watch that flex does not get under blades. Do not switch on power while the machine is connected; *switch off* before repairing, ensure regularly maintained. Use safety switches/circuit breakers while working with electricity in the garden.
Bedrooms – Electric blankets (generally) don't tuck in wired area; check blanket is laid flat. Have it checked annually. Not appropriate for those likely to be incontinent or who lack sensation.
Sitting rooms – Overloading by using adapters; keep flexes short, otherwise could trip over them.
Bathrooms – 3 pin electricians sockets should never be fitted (only 2 pin shaving, low voltage sockets) and could provide pull cords. Portable appliances like hairdryers should never be used.
Hallways and Stairs – Badly fitted or worn carpets in these areas are particularly dangerous as are polished floors and loose mats. Always keep these areas clear of obstructions as they will be required as an escape route in an emergency.

Electricity in the home

To avoid electrical hazards, switch off electricity at mains before doing any repair work.

Substance	Storage	Handling	Accidents and treatment	Disposal
Bleach disinfectants	Keep out of reach of children. Keep upright in a cool place. Never remove label or put substance in another container (e.g. pop bottle).	Follow instructions. Do not mix with other fluids.	Wash off eyes and skin with running water. If swallowed, dilute the chemical by drinking plenty of water. Do not make the person vomit. This will only harm the mouth for a second time.	Pour down drain with lots of cold water.
Insecticides	Keep out of reach of children. Keep in labelled containers.	Follow instructions, wear protective clothing, boots and gloves. Wash hands after use. Keep children and pets away from the treated area. Cover food.	For weed killers which are petroleum based, or products which are acid or alkaline (Caustic based), milk should be drunk. Always take the container to hospital with the patient.	Carefully store in sealed containers, preferably in special drums on authorised council tip sites.
Drugs	Keep out of reach of children. Use sealed cap containers. Keep in locked cupboard.	Follow instructions carefully. Do not take more than recommended dosage.	Overdose – always take container to hospital with patient (with any remaining tablets).	Use before expiry date, return to Pharmacy or flush down the toilet all unused medications.
Aerosols	Keep out of reach of children. Protect from sunlight.	Do not spray near naked flames or people's faces. Keep away from asthmatics.	If handled correctly they should be safe. If they explode they can do damage to the body; seek medical assistance straight away.	Do not pierce or put on a fire, as it may explode.
Compressed gas	Store below 50°C.	Change gas outside when empty. Do not use near naked flames.	Seek medical assistance straight away.	Do not pierce or put on a fire, as it may explode.

Table 5.7 Useful information on harmful substances

When you purchase electrical goods check that they conform to approved safety standards; and ensure that there is a *B.E.A.B. Safety label* attached. This means that the goods have been careful tested for safety and conform to approved British Standards. Plugs should have a B.S. 1363 number on them. Likewise an ASTA mark (approved Association Short circuit Testing Authorities) should be looked for. Avoid buying electrical goods from car-boot sales! See Figure 5.9 on how a 3 pin plug is wired.

Most appliances need to have an earth wire. This allows the current to flow to earth and not to a person if there is a fault in the appliance. It therefore acts as a safety valve. Some appliances are insulated so that if any electricity escapes it will pass to the plastic which is around the appliance.
Electric shock – is the result of coming into contact with high or low voltage.
Low voltage – As a result of a person coming into contact with a household electricity supply – such as cutting through lawn mower cable. **Do not touch the person.** Switch off the electricity supply or break the contact between the person and the low voltage using a dry wooden pole, d.g. brush handle, to push the person's limbs away from the electricity. Do not touch the person, as you may still receive a shock.

In general, injuries resulting from worn or overloaded circuits or absence of proper earthing are common.

Do you know how to switch off the electricity supply?
High voltage – If a person is still in contact (e.g. electricity pylon) with the high voltage, **do not touch the person.** Call the police. A high voltage can spark across several metres distance. Do not go near the person until it is safe.

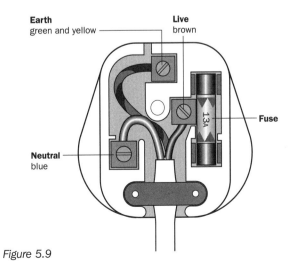

Figure 5.9

Gas in the home
When gas can be smelt

- Put out naked lights, cigarettes etc.
- Do not strike matches.
- Do not switch electrical lights or plugs *on or off* (can cause a spark).
- Open windows and doors to let gas escape.
- Check gas appliances to see if any have been left on and if pilot lights have gone out.
- Turn off gas supply. Do you know how to switch off gas supply at the meter?
- Call the gas board. The emergency number should be kept handy, or otherwise look under Gas in the telephone directory.

Did You Know ❓

- Gas board officials have the right to enter any building to inspect its supply of gas and gas appliances.
- Gas appliances should be fitted and serviced by official gas service persons (not unauthorised persons).
- It is an individual's responsibility to make sure that a gas appliance in their home is not dangerous.
- It is an individual's responsibility to turn off the supply of gas if there is a suspected leak and report it to the gas board.

Gas must not be turned on again until the leak or appliance has been repaired. Natural gas is not poisonous, but gas fumes from fires and heaters are as they contain carbon monoxide, which in appliances must be properly ventilated; flues, chimneys etc must be cleared regularly so as not to become blocked. Water heaters and gas boilers should be serviced yearly. Over 50% of gas accidents are caused by faulty second-hand appliances. These should be checked by an expert before purchase.

Water

Water spillage is a common reason for accidents; wipe up water on the floor or stairs immediately.

Do you know how to switch off the domestic water supply?

Reporting accidents – to police, fire, ambulance

Stay calm, and give the details of accident, and the precise place of the accident, injuries sustained, treatment given, witnesses, and substance taken (if applicable). Give containers etc. to emergency services when they arrive.

First aid

Do give First Aid treatment if required BEFORE the emergency services come. It may be too late if you wait.

Make sure you have learnt how to give necessary First Aid.

Work

Another key area that accidents occur is the **workplace**.

Did You Know ❓

Over 600 people die every year and around 260,000 people are injured from accidents at work.

The **Health and Safety at Work Act** was introduced so that employers and employees were both aware of their legal responsibilities while at work (see Table 5.8).

Health and Safety at Work Act 1974 (Revised)

(Not domestic servants in private homes)

This act covers all working people, i.e. employers, workers and the self employed. Its aim is to protect people at work and the general public who may be affected by work activities. It states the general duties of employers, workers, and manufacturers of equipment and chemicals.

If a person is injured while employed they may be able to sue their employer in the court for compensation for their injuries.

Duties of employers

Main duties of employers are listed below. The purpose of all these regulations is to make sure that employees have good conditions for working in.

Employers must:
- provide a safe workplace without risk to health. Dangerous machinery must be properly guarded, serviced and maintained regularly.
- make sure that machines and chemicals are used, stored and transported safely and without risks to health. (safety procedures must be followed).
- provide good welfare facilities. Workplace must be adequately heated, ventilated and well lit. (minimum temperature 16°C)
- provide wash rooms and toilets.
- make sure the workplace is not overcrowded each person must have about 3.5m³ of space.
- make sure the workplace is kept clean.
- provide safe entrances and exits. Also stairs and gangways must be kept clear from obstructions.
- provide fire precautions which must be up to approved standards. Fire alarms and extinguishers must be checked regularly and fire exits clearly signed and kept clear.
- provide clear instructions for the procedure in event of fire; this must be clearly displayed and fire skills should be practised.
- make sure that employees are provided with information, training and supervision which is necessary to ensure their health and safety.
- make sure that employees know how to do their job, how to operate machinery properly and are made aware of potential dangers.
- make sure that employees know the accident procedure and where the First Aid Box is kept.
- provide a written safety policy and make sure that it is brought to the notice of all employees. If 5 or more people are employed a prepared written statement must be given about their general policy, organisation and arrangements about health and safety at work (which must be revised and up dated on a regular basis).
- make sure that their firm's activities do not place the health and safety of any of the general public at risk. Dust fumes, waste produce must be controlled so as not to cause damage to people or the environment.

Duties of employees

Employees must take reasonable care of their own safety. If they disregard the safety rules and contribute to an injury to themselves, they may only get a reduced amount of damages awarded by the court.

Employees must:
- take reasonable care of their own health and safety, and of that of other people who work with them.
- co-operate with the employer in matters of health and safety.
- not interfere with equipment which is provided for health and safety.

Table 5.8 Health and Safety at Work Act, 1974

Many diseases can be caused by working in bad conditions. Disease of the respiratory system can be caused by working in hazardous conditions e.g. near to broken asbestos or inhaling dust etc. Pollutants like various dusts in the work environment have caused many people to have serious health problems. Exposure to dust causes damage to air passages. Abrasive action of dust particles leads to infection, and the development of lung abscesses which results in a lack of blood flowing through the lungs at each cycle. All this may result in stress on the heart, and cause heart failure.

Some common work-related diseases such as asbestosis, silicosis and emphysema will be reviewed now.

Asbestosis – is caused by continuous inhalation of dust and fibres of asbestos, which causes a type of pneumoconiosis (lung disease). Certain workers were exposed to asbestos in the building industry, and in asbestos factories, before safety regulations which restricted the use of asbestos were introduced. Demolition workers are still at danger from asbestos.

Silicosis – is a kind of pneumoconiosis, and is caused by inhaling silica dust, mainly from rock and fine sand (masonry and quarrying.) The silica particles collect in the lungs and become surrounded by scar tissue made up of dead cells. The lungs then become still so that it is hard to breathe. As a result the disease silicosis may develop. Correct breathing apparatus must be worn, and perhaps a mask or face shield. Work involving silica is often carried out in the presence of water, which reduces the amount of dust in the air.

Emphysema – is the abnormal presence of air in tissues or cavities of the body. The body is affected in the following ways:

1. The efficiency of gaseous exchange is much reduced.
2. Overdistension of the alveoli, whereby they rupture and fuse together and form abnormal air spaces.

Symptoms are breathlessness and cyanosis (skin turning blue), often the result of bronchitis which is caused by irritative particles in the bronchial tubes which in turn become infected with bacteria. There is no cure for emphysema due to damage done to lungs being irreversible. It is strongly advised not to smoke, as this irritates the condition. Antispasmodic drugs can be taken to ease the condition.

Environment

We shall examine hazards to personal health in the **environment**, looking at air pollution, smog, traffic fumes, CFC's, acid rain, noise, land and water pollution as well as radiation.

Pollution is the presence in the environment of substances in the wrong amount at the wrong place at the wrong time.

Air pollution

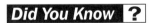
Did You Know ?

Each day we breathe in 14,000 litres of air.

Smoke consists mainly of tiny particles of carbon and tar. It is produced in power stations and homes. Smoke is controlled by the Clear Air Acts of 1956 and 1968. It was the 1968 Act which created smokeless zones. (London, 1952, around 4,000 people died from smoke and fog which produced a poisonous smog). Since the Acts were passed London receives much more sunlight. The Acts have stopped deadly fogs, but

not pollution by sulphur dioxide and nitrogen oxides. Smoke particles may reduce photosynthesis in plants which can result in mutations in various organisms.

Smog

Irritates the eyes, lungs and damages plants. It is produced when sunlight and ozone (Oz) in the air act on the oxides, nitrogen and unburned hydrocarbons released from vehicle exhausts (called photochemical smog). Smog and fog together used to affect many British cities before the clean Air Acts.

Traffic Fumes

Car exhaust fumes contain about 1000 toxic elements, including poisonous gases such as carbon monoxide and nitrogen oxides (which can produce smog) resulting in a reduction in the oxygen carrying capacity of the blood. This can be harmful, especially in people with heart disease or anaemia. Petrol which contains lead can affect the brain and nervous system, especially in children; it affects their ability to concentrate and learn. Lead mixed with petrol is claimed to improve the performance of cars (which is debatable). By law, in Britain, lead in petrol has been reduced from 0.4 to 0.15 grams per litre. Also lead free petrol is now available at a lower price than leaded petrol. In the USA a reduction in lead in petrol was matched by a fall in the levels of lead in people's blood. Other sources of lead pollution can be found in lead pipes and in some canned foods. Diesel produces less air pollution, but is linked with an increase in asthma sufferers.

Chlorofluorocarbons (CFC's)

CFC's are gases which can easily liquefy when compressed; often used in refrigerators, aerosol cans and plastic foams. CFC's react with ozone (Oz) about 25km above the earth. This reaction damages the ozone layer, which causes problems since the ozone filters out most of the ultraviolet radiation in sunlight.

Scientists have discovered 'holes' in the ozone layer which appear each spring. If CFC's continue to destroy the ozone layer this will allow more ultraviolet (UV) radiation to get through, which could cause cancers, damage to crops, and could also interfere with the oxygen cycle and weather patterns. Some industrial countries have agreed to reduce production of CFC's. Chemical industries are trying to produce substitute substances which are not as harmful to the ozone layer.

Acid Rain (sulphur dioxide and oxides of nitrogen)

Acid rain results from the burning of coals, oils, and natural gases from power stations, industrial plants, vehicle engines and domestic use. Oil and coal contain sulphur. When they are burned they release sulphur dioxide (SO_2) into the air, sulphur dioxide dissolves in rain water and forms an acid. When it falls it causes serious damage to forests, crops and aquatic ecosystems.

Noise Pollution

Recommended upper level for noise at work is 85 decibels. Sound is measured in units called decibels by using a sound/decibel meter: 1 decibel (dB) is the smallest amount of sound that can be detected.

Did You Know ?

People who live near airports are 8 times more likely to suffer from mental stress.

People may not be able to hear sounds at high frequencies. But noise above 90 decibels causes stress and can cause arteries to constrict and put strain on the heart.

Domestic noise can be caused by noisy neighbours, playing music too loud, wearing walkmans for long periods at a time, etc.

Land Pollution

This is the accumulation of industrial and urban waste (scrap metal and plastics etc). Industry produces chemical waste, some of which is highly toxic. This waste is controlled by *The Control of Pollution Act* and *Deposit of Poisonous Wastes Act*. Dumping is only allowed on licensed sites.

Water Pollution

This is caused by effluents from 3 main sources.

1. *Domestic*
   - Sewage (treated); if not treated can cause cholera and typhoid.
   - Organic pollutants.

2. *Industrial*
   - Toxic wastes which have not been treated.

3. *Agricultural*
   - Inorganic or organic fertilisers and pesticides are often washed off the land by irrigation or leaching.
   - Pesticides accumulate in the tissue of organisms, in particular towards the top of the food chain.

Nitrates and phosphates from farm land and sewage in water can cause excessive growth of microscopic green plants (algae) which can result in a serious oxygen shortage in the water (eutrophication). Sometimes the amount of nitrates getting into the drinking water can be dangerous, especially to babies and young children. The maximum laid down by the European Union is 50mg per litre.

Radiation

This can cause cancers such as leukaemia. It exists in the environment naturally. Nuclear power is a source of energy; its waste products are radioactive. Radioactive waste is produced in large quantities at nuclear power stations, much of which can remain active for thousands of years. It is very difficult to dispose of safely. The storage of this waste causes much concern. It is often stored in containers in the sea or on land. High-level radioactive waste is dumped at sea in lead and concrete containers. Medium and low level radioactive waste is usually buried underground.

The accident at Chernobyl, 1986, caused increased radioactivity in more than 20 countries and at distances over 2000 kilometres from the plant. Sellafield in 1983 discharged radioactive waste and polluted beaches and sea in the area. Nuclear power stations do not, however, release potentially harmful gases such as sulphur dioxide.

People working at nuclear stations, plus people who work in hospitals, and dental nurses involved in taking X-rays, are monitored to check the amount of radiation which they are exposed to. There is growing concern about the risks to humans, animals, water and land from radioactive contamination.

Each person in Britain receives about 2 milli-sieverts (mSv) each year from natural sources. By law a person should not receive more than 50m (Sv) each year. Around 1–3% of all cancers and 0.1–2% of genetic deformities might be due to the effects of radiation.

Self Check ✓   Element 3

23. What is a drug?

24. What are the key reasons that people take drugs?

25. There are four main types of drugs that affect the nervous system. What are they?

26. What are the THREE ways to take drugs?

27. Name THREE ways in which accidents in the home could be reduced?

28. How many units of alcohol are there in a pint of 'normal' beer?

29. In 1992 how many people were killed by alcohol related road accidents. Was it over: (A) 60 (B) 300 (C) 600.

30. List THREE ways in which the government might seek to reduce alcohol consumption?

31. What is solvent abuse?

32. What are the three main chemicals which affect the body and cause disease by smoking?

33. What risks are there to women smokers rather than men smokers?

34. What is passive smoking?

35. What causes the AIDS virus?

36. How is AIDS transmitted?

37. If someone had a drug overdose and you rang the emergency services, what information would you give them?

38. What should you do and not do if you smell gas in the home?

39. Why was the Health and Safety at Work Act introduced?

40. What are CFC's?

Useful addresses (with telephone numbers)

Action on Smoking and Health (ASH)
109 Gloucester Place
LONDON W1H 3BH
0171 935 3519

Cancer Link
17 Britainia Street
LONDON WC1X 9JN
0171 833 2451

Health and Safety Executive
Public Enquiry Point
Room 014
St. Hugh's House
Stanley Precinct
Bootle
Merseyside L20 3QY

AA (Alcoholics Anonymous)
PO Box 1
Stonebow House
STONEBOW
York YO1 2NJ
01904 644026

Families Anonymous
650 Holloway Road
LONDON N19 3NU
0171 281 8889

SCODA (the Standing Conference On Drug Abuse)
1 Hatton Place
LONDON EC1N 8ND

Institute for the Study on Drug Dependence (ISDD)
Address as for SCODA
0171 430 1993

Re-Solv. (the Society for the Prevention of Solvents and Volatile Substance Abuse)
30A High Road
STONE
Staffordshire ST15 8AW
01785 817885

Unit Test   Answer all the questions

Question 1
Which one of the following is NOT part of the framework for health promotion?

1. Government
2. Environment
3. Economics
4. Lecturing

A   1
B   2
C   3
D   4

Question 2
1. Top-down Approach is a planning approach which starts from the top and then involves people at a lower level.
2. Bottom-up Approach is looking at middle management and pushing ideas up to key decision makers.

Which option best describes the two statements

A   1. True   2. True
B   1. True   2. False
C   1. False   2. True
D   1. False   2. False

Question 3
1. A FAD is an idea or scheme that comes quickly and reoccurs on a regular basis?
2. A FASHION is something that comes quickly but takes longer to go. It might stay a year or longer.

Which option best describes the two statements?

A   1. True   2. True
B   1. True   2. False
C   1. False   2. True
D   1. False   2. False

Question 4
Which of the following are advantages in planning for health promotion?

1. Allows time to consider reactions before implementing the plan.
2. Good for communicating the plan to others.
3. Allows there to be lots of meetings.
4. The programme can be broken down into manageable sub-units and linked to the resources available.

A   1 & 2
B   3 & 4
C   1, 2 & 3
D   1, 2 & 4

Question 5
A Health Promotion Plan can be broken down into 8 key activities as follows:

A   Identify needs + priorities.
B   ....
C   How to achieve the aims.
D   Identify resources.
E   Evaluation.
F   Set implementation plan.
G   Implement.
H   ....
Insert the correct statements for (B) and (H) above.

1. Set aims + objectives

2. Re-evaluate.
3. Develop a Mission Statement
4. Consider next programme

Choice
A   B1   H2
B   B3   H4
C   B2   H2
D   B2   H4

Question 6
One would recommend a TRIAL takes place because ...

1. it saves time and money rather than doing the complete promotional plan.
2. it is a way of evaluating the outcome of a particular course of action.
3. it involves the whole community.
4. the target audience can then be determined.

Choice
A   1 only
B   1 and 2
C   3 and 4
D   4 only

Question 7
Statement 1
Felt need – this is what people 'feel' they require. Knowledge of a subject will affect what people feel they require. *Expressed need* – this is what people 'express' that they need i.e. – *felt need* is turned into a request or demand.

Statement 2
Comparative need – this is the comparison between similar groups, which are at similar levels of health promotion *Normative need* – this is the gap between what 'an expert' believes is the standard and what is the actual situation.

Which is True?
A   Statement 1 T   Statement 2 T
B   Statement 1 T   Statement 2 F
C   Statement 1 F   Statement 2 T
D   Statement 1 F   Statement 2 F

Question 8
Resources can be:
1. People
2. Time scales
3. Financial
4. Materials and Equipment

Choice
A   1, 2 & 4
B   1, 2 & 3
C   1, 3 & 4
D   2, 3 & 4

Question 9
A **force field diagram** can be used for the following:

1. looking at the factors that will help the plan.
2. looking at the factors that may hinder the plan.
3. as a diagram showing key activities with time scales associated with each activity.
4. as a device that could be used to aid team working

Choice
A   1 & 2 & 3
B   2 & 3 & 4
C   1 & 3 & 4
D   1 & 2 & 4

Question 10
Computer software planning packages may be useful to help run a promotional scheme.

Is the statement: TRUE or FALSE?

Question 11
After a campaign has been completed a re-evaluation should NOT then be undertaken.

Is the statement: TRUE or FALSE?

Question 12
Team working is NOT an activity associated with promotional plans?

Is the statement: TRUE or FALSE?

Question 13
Feedback should be included at all the key stages of a promotional plan

Is the statement: TRUE or FALSE?

Question 14
From each of the lists below pick two correct answers

In giving health promotion advice to others:
DO
(i)   Develop trust
(ii)   Give guidance and support
(iii)   Give many options
(iv)   Lecture – where required.
DON'T
(i)   Involve the client in aspects of health care
(ii)   Get feedback
(iii)   Give complicated messages
(iv)   Appear as superman/women.

Which one is correct?
  DO   DON'T
A(i) & (iv) (i) & (iv)
B(ii) & (iii) (ii) & (iii)
C(i) & (ii) (iii) & (iv)
D(ii) & (iv) (ii) & (iv)

Question 15
The three statements below are targeted to three different groups regarding Drugs.
                          DRUGS
(i)   Don't accept "sweets or presents" from strangers.
(ii)   Drugs ruin your life. Drugs are not 'cool'. Do not mix with groups involved in drugs. Drugs affect personal appearance.
(iii) Seek help. Dangers: ruins your life, and your family. Beware of addiction to "milder" drugs, e.g. sleeping tablets. Look for signs in others.

Which answer best represents the groups targeted by each statement?
A (i) Adults   (ii) Adolescents   (iii) Children
B (i) Adolescents (ii) Adult   (iii) Children
C (i) Children   (ii) Adolescents   (iii) Adult
D (i) Children   (ii) Adult   (iii) Adolescents

Question 16
Which one of the following is NOT part of the make up or characteristic of foods:
Vitamins, Minerals, Fats, Carbohydrate, Carbon Monoxide, Fibre, Salts, Proteins and Water.

Is it
A Vitamins
B Minerals
C Carbohydrates
D Carbon Monoxide

Question 17
People use drugs (including alcohol and cigarettes) for a range of reasons including:

1. out of curiosity
2. pleasure
3. to relieve stress
4. rebellion
5. boredom
6. to increase their cash flow
7. to be part of the group
8. habit
9. to help them get a job

Which statements are fundamentally incorrect?
A   1,3,9
B   6,9
C   2,6
D   4,5,6,7,8,9

Question 18
1. *Sedatives* (depressants) diminish feelings of anxiety and induce a state of relaxation.
    Examples are alcohol, morphine and barbiturates
2. *Stimulants* induce a sense of alertness and reduce feelings of fatigue.
    Examples are caffeine and amphetamines

Are the Statements TRUE (T) or FALSE (F)?
A   1T   2T
B   1F   2F
C   1T   2F
D   1F   2T

Question 19
1. *Analgesics* have an effect on the parts of the brain which produce a sense of feeling pain. Examples are cocaine and heroin.
2. *Narcotics* have a very powerful effect on the nervous system and are only prescribed under strict supervision and in small doses. Examples are Cannabis, and LSD.

Are the Statements TRUE (T) or FALSE (F)?
A   1T   2T
B   1F   2F
C   1T   2F
D   1F   2T

Question 20
Drugs can only be taken in the following ways:
(i) *by swallowing* which dissolves in the stomach then passes into the blood stream.
(ii) *by injecting* which passes straight into the blood stream.

Is the whole Statement TRUE or FALSE?

Question 21

Is this statement TRUE or FALSE?

Drugs are carried to the brain via the blood. The drug affects the brain and the messages being sent out by the brain. Different drugs affect the brain in different ways. Depressants slow down and stimulants speed up the working of the brain. Hallucinogens cause hallucinations and visions.

Question 22
Examples of drugs are:

1. Aspirin
2. Cocaine
3. Steroids
4. Vitamins

Which statements are TRUE?

A   1 & 2
B   1 & 2 & 3
C   1 & 2 & 4
D   2 & 3

Question 23
Effects of excess alcohol are:

1. Reaction time is decreased and efficiency of the brain is reduced.
2. Digestive system is irritated which results in nausea and a hangover with the possibility of gastritis and peptic ulcers.
3. The blood vessels of the skin become pale and contract.
4. Poor co-ordination results.
5. Somewhat unpredictable, depending on the individual's weight and sex

Which statements are correct:
A   1,2,3
B   1,3,5
C   1,2,4,5
D   2,4,5

Question 24
The government tries to limit alcohol abuse by:

1. prohibiting the sale of alcohol to under 25 year olds,
2. heavily taxing alcoholic drinks
3. custom controls to prevent illegal imports
4. using the breathalyser to catch drink drivers

Which is correct?
A   1 & 2
B   3 & 4
C   2 & 3 & 4
D   2 & 4

Question 25
Smoking is the third most important cause of preventable deaths in the UK. Stopping smoking has a neutral effect on heart disease.

TRUE or FALSE?

Question 26
Possible signs of someone abusing solvents are:
 (i) a chemical smell on the breath and traces of solvent on clothing
 (ii) persistent irritable cough and sores around the mouth and eyes
(iii) increase in rate of weight gain
(iv) mood swings and irritability

A   (i) & (ii) & (iii)
B   (i) & (ii) & (iv)
C   (ii) & (iii) & (iv)
D   (i) & (iii) & (iv)

Question 27
Personal solvent abuse is:

A   An illegal offence for everyone
B   An illegal offence for the under 16 year old's
C   Not an illegal offence
D   An illegal offence for the over 16 year old's

Choose one of these possible answers

Question 28
Which one of the following answers best fits this statement?

For shopkeepers to sell solvent based products with rea-sonable grounds to suspect the products are being abused:

A   It is an illegal offence
B   It is an illegal offence to sell to under 16 year olds
C   It is an illegal offence to sell to over 16 year olds
D   It is not an illegal offence

Question 29
Some women smoke for the following reasons:

 (i) to control nerves
 (ii) influence of advertising
(iii) increases the chances of getting pregnant
(iv) thought to control weight

Which is INCORRECT:
A   (i)
B   (ii)
C   (iii)
D   (iv)

Question 30
The problems associated with smoking in females are:

 (i) Can affect fertility and increases risk of cervical cancer
 (ii) Accelerates the onset of the menopause and is associ-ated with osteoporosis
(iii) Smoking and taking the pill increases ones chances of heart disease and having a stroke
(iv) Smoking and taking the pill increases ones chances of getting pregnant

Which is INCORRECT:
A   (i)
B   (ii)
C   (iii)
D   (iv)

Question 31
Acquired Immune Deficiency Syndrome is caused by a virus called Human Immunodeficiency Virus which interferes with the body's normal immunity to disease.

TRUE or FALSE?

Question 32
In general the Health and Safety at Work Act 1974 mainly covers:

A   Working people
B   Managers
C   Safety issues in home and office
D   General public

Question 33
If a chip pan catches fire the immediate thing to do is to turn off the heat and ...:

A   throw water on it.
B   cover with damp towel or lid and leave for at least 30 minutes.
C   take the chip pan out into an open area (like the garden, or a balcony)
D   call the fire brigade

Question 34
Chlorofluorocarbons (CFC's) are gases which can easily liquefy when compressed. They are often used in refrigera-tors, aerosol cans and plastic foams. They damage the ozone layer so that ultra-violet light causes more skin damage than it used to.

TRUE or FALSE

Answers to Self-check Questions

1. All these aspects should be consistent with each other. The *Mission Statement* will briefly summarise the *Key Aims* of the campaign, which themselves will be consistent with a set of *Values* underlying the campaign. The *Objectives* are milestones or targets to be achieved along the way in order to fulfill the Mission Statement and meet the stated Aims.

2. Without such knowledge you will be unable to identify the resources and strategies needed to reach the target audience with the intended message.

3. Through activities that 5–9 year olds' actually do, using types of media and messages which they are used to receiving and which make sense to them. Children slots on TV and radio, children videos, primary school teachers, parents etc. See also charts 1–6 on page 97.

4. See page 95.

5. See page 94 for 8 key activities or stages.

6. See page 95.

7. Top-down starts by targeting the message at the top (key) decision makers, who filter the message to those 'below'. Bottom-up starts by targeting the message to those at the grass-roots.

8. *Preventative approach* seeks to increase awareness, thereby changing attitudes and behaviour.
   Self empowerment approach allows those in the target audience to make their own decisions after being given the relevant information.
   Radical approach is one in which health promotion starts at the social, environmental and political level, rather than at the individual level. For example, MPs might be lobbied to support legislation to make certain actions illegal or subject to greater penalty than before (e.g. compulsory seat-belts, tighter alcohol limits for drivers, etc.)

9. Many types of answer along the following lines would be acceptable here.

	Children	Adolescents	Adults
Alcohol Consumption	Drink milk	Drinking reduces performance	Excessive alcohol can wreck families; 20% of all divorces are related to abuse of alcohol.
Accidents in the home	Don't put anything, including fingers, into electrical sockets.	Untidy bedrooms are an accident hazard. They also give a bad impression to your friends.	Never leave a child in a bath unattended. 10% of all child deaths in the home involve drowning in baths.

10 Here are three options. Of course many other options could be presented.
   1. Reduction of VAT on smoke detectors.
   2. Insistence that all new properties have this equipment fitted as standard.
   3. Promotional campaign explaining the danger from house fires and the effectiveness and low cost of smoke detectors.

11 Here are just some possibilities.
   1. Reduced speed limits on all roads; enforced by speed camera surveillance.
   2. Increased use of 'sleeping policemen' in residential areas to encourage people to reduce speed.
   3. Dramatic increase of petrol prices (e.g. increasing excise duty on petrol).
   4. Promotion of fuel benefits to drivers of reducing speed and getting more miles per litre, etc.

12. Oil companies, oil companies' shareholders, road haulage association, AA, RAC, specific individual rights groups, etc.

13. The easiest thing is NOT to do anything, but this doesn't help the individual. You might try to establish if the individual is aware of the problem, perhaps by talking about personal hygiene in general. You might also check whether the individual is fully aware of personal hygiene solutions – e.g. washing regularly etc. This would be a 'self empowerment' approach. If the problem is more serious, a more direct 'authoritative' approach might be necessary.

14. This may be seen as patronising and may be counterproductive, making the client determined to resist your advice because of a dislike of the method of your aproach.

15. These might include: (i) developing trust
   (ii) giving guidance and support
   (iii) providing accurate information
   (iv) allowing individuals to reach their own conclusions
   (v) seeking feedback.

16. It allows you to focus on the needs and characteristics of that group (e.g. children aged 10–14). Otherwise the message may be too general and presented in ways (and using media) which fail to make sense to that group.

17. See page 101.

18. Various possibilities e.g. diet, exercise, taking prescribed drugs, avoidance of accidents (home/work), personal hygiene, mental alertness, etc.

19. Listen to the client: provide information on identifying stress symptoms and on stress avoidance measures. Self-empowerment approach: encourage client to develop his/her own action plan to overcome stress. If you were the sufferer, seek someone in whom you could confide/discuss, with experience/expertise in stress related issues. Build time into your own programme which is specifically ear-marked for 'relaxing' activities, etc.

20. Many possible answers, e.g.
   (i) Use media identified as being widely accessed by children of that age and sex (see charts 1–6, page 97).
   (ii) Use personalities admired by children of that category (pop stars, athletes, etc).
   (iii) Use appropriate school networks (e.g. teachers, parent-teacher groups, . . .) etc.

21. Many possible answers; see, for example page 102.

22. Because certain styles and formats are better able to get the message across to various target groups.

23. See page 102.

24. See page 102.

25. See page 103.

26. See page 104.

27. Many possibilities. For example: avoid loose or slippery floor fittings, remove trailing leads, use smoke detectors, turn pan handles inwards when cooking, avoid smoking in bed, etc.

28. 2 units (6 units in strong lagers).

29. Over 600.

30. Many possibilities. For example: heavier taxing of alcoholic drinks, more breathalyser tests of drivers, raising age-limit for purchasing drink, etc.

31. See page 106.

32. Nicotine (addiction), carbon monoxide (poisonous gas) and tar (can cause cancer).

33. Many possibilities. For example: low birth weight babies, acceleration of onset of menopause, increased risk of spontaneous abortion, higher incidence of cervical cancer, increased risk of heart disease (when also taking oral contraceptive), osteoporosis (brittle bones)

34. Breathing in of other people's cigarette smoke.

35. See page 109.

36. See page 109.

37. Any information on the type of drug and amount involved, time of overdose, etc. Keep container and any remaining tablets/liquid for inspection on arrival, etc.

38. See page 112.

39. To increase the protection of people at work and the general public insofar as they are affected by working activities. To make employers, employees and the self-employed aware of their duties and responsibilities.

40. Chlorofluorocarbons. Used in refrigerators, aerosol cans and plastic foams. Damage ozone layer when they are exposed to the atmosphere.

Answers to Unit Test

Question	Answer	Question	Answer	Question	Answer	Question	Answer	Question	Answer
1	D	8	C	15	C	22	B	29	C
2	B	9	D	16	D	23	C	30	D
3	C	10	True	17	B	24	C	31	True
4	D	11	False	18	A	25	False	32	A
5	A	12	False	19	D	26	B	33	B
6	B	13	True	20	False	27	C	34	True
7	B	14	C	21	True	28	A		

Unit Test Comments

Question 1
The seven interlinked activities which form the framework for health promotion are Government, Environment, Economics, Organisational, Community, Education and Preventative – not 'lecturing'!

Question 2
Bottom-up Approach starts with the grass roots within a community or individuals at the workplace.

Question 3
A fad is a 'one-off', not something which recurs regularly

Question 4
Having lots of meetings is not, by itself, an advantage.

Question 5
All plans need 'aims and objectives' (B1) and after implementation must be 're-evaluated' (H2).

Question 6
A trial run will be on a smaller scale and can avoid costly mistakes later, thereby saving time and money. It is also a way of checking whether the intended outcome of a particular course of action is likely to occur.

Question 7
A comparative need involves different groups.

Question 8
Time is not a resource: it is a constraint.

Question 9
Answer C is part of an action plan, not a force field diagram.

Question 10
Computers can keep track of complex schemes involving many activities.

Question 11
Re-evaluation is valuable at the end of a campaign to learn lessons for future planned events.

Question 12
The effectiveness of the implementation of most plans will depend upon many people being committed and involved, with high morale.

Question 13
Without feedback you will be working in the dark.

Question 14
Giving many options may confuse the client; lecturing clients may annoy them and result in resistance to your advice. On the other hand clients should be involved in as many aspects of their health care as possible and feedback from the client is most important.

Question 15
(i) clearly involves advice to children in dealing with strangers; (ii) involves aspects which might 'appeal' to adolescents; (iii) highly factual and matter of fact – likely to appeal to adults.

Question 16
Carbon monoxide is a toxic gas, found for example in cigarette smoke.

Question 17
Expensive drugs will reduce cash flow and hinder getting a job.

Question 18
All aspects of these statements are true.

Question 19
Examples of analgesics are paracetamol and aspirin, not cocaine and heroin.

Question 20
Drugs can also be taken in by inhaling (e.g. smoking).

Question 21
All aspects of this statement are true.

Question 22
Vitamins are not drugs.

Question 23
Blood vessels become reddened, not pale.

Question 24
The prohibition is only to those under 18 years.

Question 25
Smoking is actually the first and most important cause of preventable death in the UK. Stopping smoking will reduce heart disease.

Question 26
A loss of weight, not increase, is likely to occur as they neglect their general welfare and diet.

Question 27
Personal solvent abuse is currently legal; it is a relatively new offence and the law has not yet caught up.

Question 28
The sale of solvent based products to likely abusers is illegal.

Question 29
There is no evidence or widely held perception that smoking increases the chances of getting pregnant.

Question 30
The combining of smoking with the contraceptive pill does not increase the chances of becoming pregnant.

Question 31
All aspects of the statement are true.

Question 32
The Act is mainly for working people.

Question 33
A and C would cause further danger to your person; D would take too long to be of immediate help.

Question 34
All aspects of the statement are true.

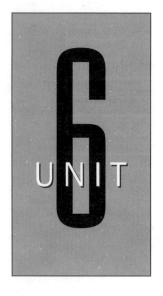

UNIT 6

Structure and practices in health and social care

Getting Started

Unit 6 consists of 3 Elements as follows:

> Element 1 Investigate the structure of health and social care provision.
>
> Element 2 Investigate the impact of legislation and funding on provision and priorities.
>
> Element 3 Investigate ways in which services within health and social care operate

In this unit we will be looking at the **delivery** of health and social care in the United Kingdom in relation to organisational structure. How the delivery is funded will be considered, including systems and services that go to make up the framework of health care provision.

Element 1 takes a brief historical perspective before looking at the current system and structure of health and social care in the UK.

Element 2 looks at funds to operate the system and at how the voluntary system operates alongside the statutory services. A wider perspective then examines the factors affecting priorities in the Health Service, such as the state of the economy. Lastly the impact of legislation is reviewed.

Element 3 looks at the services operating in the health and social care system and at developments in community and hospital health provision, social work, and health education. The strategies for service delivery are then explained, including the holistic, intervention and preventative approaches among others.

Cross-references:
Attitudes and other social influences on behaviour (Unit 1, Element 1)
Communication with individuals (Unit 2, Element 1)
Promoting communication within groups (Unit 2, Element 2)
The development of Care Plans (Unit 7, Element 1)
Approaches within Care Plans (Unit 7, Element 3)

Duty Where a local authority *must* provide a service.

Holistic Whole person approach to health.

Internal market The seperation of *purchasers* of health care from *providers*. Providers compete with each other for the 'custom' of purchasers, who have the responsibility of seeking out the best possible deal for the patients they represent.

Power Where a local authority is permitted to provide a service, but may choose whether or not to do so.

Primary health care Usually refers to care in the community.

Providers NHS Trust hospitals, District Managed Hospitals, Private Hospitals.

Purchasers District Health Authorities, GP Fund Holders and private patients.

Secondary health care Usually refers to care provided by hospital staff in a hospital context.

Statutory provision Legally required by Act of Parliament.

Welfare state Those services which are organised, purchased or provided by the government.

Essential Principles

6.1 Investigate the structure of health and social care provision.

In this Element we look at:

1. The framework for the current system of health and social care provision.
2. The roles of key personnel in caring for different client groups.
3. The processes by which users gain access to provision.

The framework of the current system

At the present time health service workers at all levels are involved in massive changes. This includes the way in which services are planned, delivered and financed. There is also considerable change in the information systems and paperwork methods used. However, since its formation in 1948, the National Health Service has been in constant change (see historical perspective below)

Historical perspective

- In 1942 the Beveridge Report stated that there should be: 'comprehensive health and rehabilitation services for the prevention and cure of disease and restoration of capacity for work, available to all members of the community.'

- 5th July 1948 the National Health Service (NHS) was formed.
  The responsibility for the nations health from 1948 to 1974 was shared by:
  - Local Executive Councils (GPs, etc.)
  - Local Authorities (ambulance, home health support services etc.)
  - Regional Hospital Boards (hospitals).
  It was costly and bureaucratic to run.

- In 1974 the NHS was re-organised and the majority of services were placed under the control of Local District Management Teams, Area Health Authorities (AHA) and Regional Health Authorities (RHA).

- In 1983 the Area Health Authorities were replaced by the District Health Authorities (DHA)

- In 1985 the health service supervisory board (which dealt with objectives and resources) and NHS management board (which dealt with how policies were applied) were set up.

- In 1989 the Government's White Paper 'Caring for People' and the resulting Community Care Act (1990) put forward ideas about caring for people within the broader community.

- In 1989 the Government's White Paper 'Working for Patients' led to major reforms in the organisation and management of the NHS itself. These were outlined in the 'National Health Service Act' 1990, and set up an 'internal market' in health care. The main idea being to decentralise decision making involving the allocation of resources to a more local level and to introduce more competition into health care provision. This was to be achieved by making a clear distinction between pur*chasers* of health care and *providers* of health care (see below).

- In 1991 the Patients Charter was drawn up by the Department of Health. It outlined what people can expect as a right from the Health Service (See UNIT 2).

- In 1993 the Patients Charter was extended to include what people are entitled to expect from their General Practitioner (GP).

The Present Situation

The Secretary of State for Health and the Department of Health are directly responsible for the organisation and finance of family practitioner committees, GP services and 14 Regional Health Authorities (RHA's) in England. However the strategy is for the number of RHA's to be reduced. The RHA's are responsible for 192 District Health Authorities (DHA's) which provide a range of services for people living in each district, mainly by *purchasing* health care for its population. Each DHA has an associated Community Health Council (CHC) attached to it. The CHC represent the views of the general public on local health services.

The structure of the NHS is as shown in Fig. 6.1.

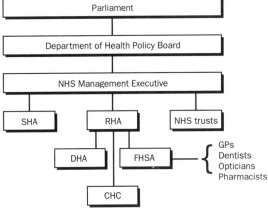

Key
SHA = Special Health Authorities
RHA = Regional Health Authorities
NHS = National Health Service
DHA = District Health Authorities
FHSA = Family Health Service Authorities
CHC = Community Health Council

Figure 6.1 Structure of the NHS

Parliament has the final say on all NHS matters, in theory anyway. The Secretary of State for Health chairs the Department of Health Policy Board (see diagram) and heads a department of more than 5,000 civil servants. This board determines the overall strategy for the NHS. The board includes 'captains' of industry and the top personnel from the health service. The strategy is put into effect by the NHS Management Executive; again people from outside the health service are included on this committee.

The NHS has been organised as a geographically-based administrative hierarchy. The country is divided into regions, each with a Regional Health Authority (RHA). Each region is then divided into districts, each with a District Health Authority (DHA). The DHAs have been responsible for local management and finance of a range of hospital and associated services within their district. In the new NHS structure, the relationship between RHA and DHA has remained largely intact, but the role of the DHA has changed (see below). General Practitioner (GP) services continue to be organised within another distinct hierarchy under the guidance of the Family Health Service Authorities (FHSA) but with a new, more independent element of GP fundholders.

- The 14 RHA's (in England) distribute funds to the DHA's, FHSA's (Family Health Service Authorities), GPFH's (GP Fund Holders) and confirm that funds are being spent wisely. The RHA are also the referees in disputes between purchasers and providers.
- The DHA's manage hospitals and GP's that have *not* opted for fund holding status. However their main role is now to assess the health care needs of the population within their district and to *purchase* the necessary health services from providers.
- NHS trusts run self-governing hospitals, and report directly to the Department of Health NHS Management Executive. They are **providers** of health services. They earn their income principally from contracts with DHA's and GPFH's, who are the **purchasers** of health care for their local population.
- The 90 FHSA's in England provide information on local health services, handle complaints, and ensure that GP's and dentists, pharmacists and opticians do their work and get paid.
- Special Health Authorities (SHA's) include the Health Education Authority (HEA), and the famous London teaching hospitals. SHA's are not part of the main NHS structure and therefore report directly to the NHS Management board.
- CHC's are a statutory group who in fact have very little finance from the RHA's, or power; they rely on persuasion as their key method of influence. The CHC's represent the consumers interests and provide information and advice to the public.
- Under the NHS and Community Care Act 1990 the DHA, Social Services and FHSA must all work together to produce an **annual plan** to meet the health care needs of the people in their area.

Did You Know **?**

- Public spending on NHS – over £34,000 million in 93/94; second only to Social Security.
- NHS employs over 1 million persons (not counting GP's); over $\frac{1}{2}$ are nurse-related. Largest employer in UK.
- 8 million in-patients (hospital) each year.
- 20 million people attend outpatient, accident and emergency services each year.
- Around 200 million GP visits each year, 30 million dental visits.
- Over 435 million drug prescriptions dispensed each year (7 per member of UK population).

The health and social care service consists of statutory, voluntary and private provision, which combined should meet the needs of the clients. **Statutory provision** is state funded and is an obligation by law, while a **statutory organisation** is one established by legislation. **Voluntary provision** is funded by charities and non-profit making agencies, while **private sector care** is mainly profit making. Each will be reviewed in turn.

Table 6.1 outlines the main purchasers and providers within the new health care arrangements.

Providers	Purchasers
NHS Trust hospitals District managed hospitals Private hospitals	District Health Authority (DHA) GP Fund Holders (GPFH) Private patients

Table 6.1 Providers and Purchasers

Note that in Table 6.1 we have included the private sector. The 'purchasers' will include private patients paying directly for treatment or, more usually, through health insurance schemes. The 'providers' include private hospitals which may offer services to NHS patients. Equivalently, NHS hospitals may offer services to private patients. Some exchange between the public and private sector has occurred previously but its extent is expected to increase.

Statutory Provision

Social services departments have a responsibility, by law, to protect vulnerable groups of people and to provide services for them. Statutory responsibilities are changed from time to time by Acts of Parliament.

Voluntary Provision

A definition of the **voluntary sector** is that it covers bodies which engage in activities that are *not* carried on for profit and are *not* provided by a local or public authority. A voluntary sector organisation can be defined as non-statutory and provides services to, or acts in the interest of, any client group or groups. It is free from certain legal duties and is not set up by law. In practice, there is no clear-cut boundary between the voluntary and public sector, as they are both represented on joint consultative committees, etc.

Voluntary organisations are enormously important in supplementing the services of the statutory health and social service organisations.

Did You Know **?**

Many voluntary organisations receive some of their income from public funds.

Some voluntary organisations receive much of their funding from the government. This could limit them in expressing their views in a forthright manner, particularly when they have opposing views to those of the Government.

Voluntary organisations can be assessed in the following ways:

- Scale
- Main purpose
- Client groups
- Fund-raising activities

- **Scale.** The size and range of the voluntary organisation can be:

  - *Local*: Local voluntary organisations are set up by local people for a particular scheme or need (e.g. under 5's groups)

- *National:* national voluntary organisations are usually a central organisation with local branches across the country. (e.g. Dr Barnardo's)
- *Regional and city based groups:* these are smaller versions of the above e.g. East of England arthritis association.
- *Support groups or societies:* are usually set up for a particular condition (such as a specific skin condition like eczema.)
- *International:* international voluntary organisations operate on a world scale, and are funded by many sources (OXFAM, Save the Children, etc)

- **Main purpose.** Voluntary organisations are set up for a number of purposes, including:

  - Providing services and care *not* provided by the existing systems.
  - Fund raising (A large amount of time is often spent on this activity).
  - Counselling services.
  - Providing skilled help by trained personnel.
  - Increasing public awareness in relation to health care.
  - Enabling people to define their own health needs – via self help/mutual help groups.
  - Representing *users* and providing information and booklets etc.
  - Representing *carers* and providing courses and seminars for carers.
  - Representing *volunteers* working with sections of the community who might feel alienated.
  - Collaborating with health authorities to provide services.
  - Promoting and sponsoring research.
  - Campaigning.
  - Acting as advocates for change; putting pressure on public authorities to try and influence policy-making.
  - Experimenting with pioneering new forms of care.

- **Client Groups:** Voluntary organisations are becoming extremely specialised in their area of interest (e.g. particular attention is now being paid to confusion and dementia in the elderly).

  Here is a list of some of the client groups:

  - child care services
  - family care schemes
  - elderly people
  - dementia sufferers
  - people with mental illness
  - people with learning difficulties
  - people with drug and alcohol related problems.
  - people with progressive illnesses and chronic health problems
  - AIDS/HIV sufferers.

Did You Know ❓

Voluntary services are used to fill the gaps in the existing services.

Many of the established social services were originally set-up and run by volunteers – where there was a need. One of the rules of the voluntary services is to make sure that the people in need *make use* of the state services which are available. Many voluntary organisations work in co-operation with the local and central authorities to improve the services offered to the public. This helps to ensure that people in need do *not* get overlooked. Some voluntary staff are paid for their services and clients can, if they so wish, make a donation for services received from voluntary organisations.

- **Fund raising activities.** Voluntary organisations raise money from a range of sources including:

  - direct from the public, through collections, donations and subscriptions
  - grants from government
  - other bodies, e.g. the European Social Fund
  - skilled work done by professional volunteers to supplement their activities
  - work contracted out by local authorities, etc.

Traditionally the voluntary sector depended on grants from central and local government which made them vulnerable. Today, voluntary organisations are funded in many ways, one of the most important is from the health and social welfare agencies who *contract out*; such as a local authority which enters into an agreement to pay for services. Voluntary bodies suffer from financial problems, caused by the 'care gap' which is the actual difference in cost between *providing care* and the *benefit* received from the state by the client (like income support to people who live in care). To keep the placements, additional money is provided by local and health authorities. This is known as planned 'deficit' funding.

Some voluntary organisations active in community health services:

- **College of Health.** Founded in 1983 to promote self care; provides preventative health information and education on health matters, to help people make the best of NHS and alternative therapies.
- **Action on Smoking and Health** (ASH) founded 1971
- **British Diabetic Association** (BDA) founded 1934
- **Chest Heart and Stroke Association** (CHSA) founded 1899
- **Queens Nursing Institute** (QNI) founded 1887; administrates trust funds education
- **Accept National Services.** Founded 1975 to promote education, training, preventative measures, treatment and research connected with alcohol, tranquilliser and drug misuse. Runs special centres and day units.
- **Marie Curie Memorial Foundation.** Founded 1948 for the welfare of cancer patients.
- **National Society for Cancer Relief** (NSCR). Founded 1911.
- **Macmillan Nurses Hospice.** Care and homecare in patients own home.
- **Family Planning Association** (FPA). Founded 1930.
- **National Association for Maternal and Child Welfare** (NAMCW). Founded 1911 for education.
- **British Association for Services to the Elderly** (BASE). Founded 1974.
- **Association For All Speech Impaired Children** (AFASIC). Founded 1968.
- **Community Health Group for Ethnic Minorities.** Free 24-hour interpreter and translation services (20 languages).
- **Citizen Advice Bureau** (CAB). Gives advice on health and other matters.

Private Provision
Private health care is an alternative to the National Health

Service (NHS). There are basically three types of private provision:

- private insurance cover
- fees's for services
- premiums to medical organisations.

More and more organisations provide private health care as a perk of the job. It offers the client more control over the timing of their treatment and an opportunity to avoid the waiting lists.

The *agencies* which provide private medicine range from:

- Profit making organisations, such as American Medical International (AMI).
- Provident organisations (such as BUPA) which are theoretically non-profit making but often have subsidiaries which are profit making.
- Charitable organisation (e.g. church run hospitals)

In Britain the 3 main private companies are:

- British United Provident Association (BUPA)
- Private Patients Plan (PPP)
- Western Provident Association (WPA)

There has been a recent expansion in the number of people taking out private medical schemes; this has been actively encouraged by the Conservative government.

The private sector treats proportionately fewer children and older people. The private sector tends to avoid complicated 'high tech' operations and tends to focus on routine surgery.

The Government has tried to encourage the private sector by giving tax relief (in 1989) on private health care insurance to the over 60's. The highest rate of increase in private health care has been in the number of private and residential nursing homes. Since 1979 they have increased by fivefold. The growth was encouraged by changes in supplementary benefit regulations. In the early 1980's local authorities provided 70% of residential places for people aged 65 years and over. The community care legislation of 1993 enabled monies that were held by social security to be transferred to local authorities to *purchase* residential and nursery home care from private and voluntary sector providers. This does not apply to placements in the local authority homes. If local authorities want to carry on running their own residential services, they must meet the full cost themselves.

Did You Know ?

There are regional imbalances in private provision. There are six times as many private beds per head of the population in the Thames Region and Southern England, as in the Northern Regions.

Provision in Northern Ireland, Scotland and Wales

In Northern Ireland, Scotland and Wales the structure of the Health Service is different from England. Each country has their own Secretary of State who is responsible for health services. There are no Regional Health Authorities (RHA). In Northern Ireland the four Health and Social Services Boards also look after personal social services. Wales has 9 District Authorities and 8 FHSA's. Scotland has 15 Local Health Boards which combine the role of District Health Authorities (DHA) and FHSA's.

Basically:

DHA = Local Health Boards.
CHC = Local Health Councils

The Main Social Services

Social services are provided by the state through central government departments and local authorities. They are provided to help those who have a need, and not necessarily those in need of money. The state has many *statutory* services. Together they are referred to as the *Welfare State*.

- State Earnings Related Pension Scheme (SERPS) and widow pensions
- National Insurance (compulsory – provides partial cover during periods of non-earning, e.g. unemployment).
- Income Support – payments to people not in full-time work and on a low income to guarantee a certain minimum income; discretionary payment for cases of special hardship have been removed.
- Personal Social Services – run by local authorities and voluntary organisations.
- Family Credit – extra financial help claimed by family heads in work but on a low income.
- Child Benefit – universal payment made to families with 1 or more children.
- Education Service (state schools) – since 1988, education establishments have been allowed to become autonomous (opted out) with control over their finances.
- National Health Service
  Family/Personal
  Doctors, Dentists, Opticians, Pharmacists
  Hospital services
  Community Health Service

The roles of key personnel in caring for different client groups

The roles of key personnel can be categorised into three broad areas: **Primary**, **Secondary** and **Tertiary** health care.

Primary Health Care

This generally refers to care in the community provided by staff that are mainly allocated to GP's practices and Health Centres.

Examples of **primary health care** teams include:

Primary health care team

Social workers
GP's
Health visitors
Community nurses
Midwives
Community midwives
Receptionists
District nurses
Practise nurses
Marie Curie nurses
Chiropodists
Community psychiatric nurses
Community physiotherapists
Occupational therapists
Physiotherapist
Community dieticians
Residential care staff
Day care staff
Domiciliary nurses
Speech therapists
Counsellors
Other community workers are: Dentists, Opticians and Chiropodists

Secondary Health Care

This is generally provided via hospital staff. The client can be an inpatient or an outpatient. Hospital staff may also visit patients in their own homes, which is part of community care.

Examples of **secondary health care** teams include:

Secondary health care
Consultant
Senior registrar
Registrar
Senior house officer
House Officer
Anaesthetist
Registered general nurse
Health care assistant
Psychiatrist
Psychologist
Physiotherapist
Occupational Therapist
Radiographer
Hospital social worker
Dietician
Pathology laboratory staff

Tertiary Health Care

This is provided by institutions for long term care.
The key workers that will be examined under **Tertiary Health Care** are:

- Social workers
- Care workers
- General Practitioner's (GP's)
- Hospital and Community Nurses
- Personnel in professions complementary to medicine

Social Workers

We will look at **Social Workers** in relation to social services and social work departments. For over 50 years there has existed a systematic training for social workers. However, there still exists today a confusion and vagueness over the role of social work and social workers.

The main sources of professional qualifications are a new jointly recognised professional qualification, the Certificate of Qualification in Social Work (CQSW) and the Certificate in Social Services (CSS). These qualifications are *generic* in type, i.e. provide a more general education and training as opposed to the previous *specialist* training qualifications like mental health officer or children's officer. The departments that social workers work for, are accountable to local committees with elected members and are run by Directors of Social Services for social work.

Many social workers are involved in **casework**; this involves intensive work to help particular individuals cope with their problems. Social workers also arrange for the necessary services to be provided to clients. Social work teams cover geographical patches. Social workers can often be attached to primary care teams.

Services are grouped into districts and broken into *area based* levels. Area teams have consistent features such as intake duty systems, sub-teams based on communities and client specialism. They provide services such as home care or group work.

Social workers mainly work with people in their own homes and in the community. 'Community work' in this context means working with groups of people, encouraging self-help and community developments (e.g. setting up groups,

associations, etc). Social Work Departments have organised services which respond to the needs of *specific* client groups. Such as:

- families, children and young people.
- elderly people, disabled people.
- clients with learning disabilities and mental illness.
- offenders, who are not part of the probation service.

Care Workers

This section will look at, **care workers** and their role.

1. *Informal carers.* A 'carer' is someone who looks after another person. The Carer's National Association (leaflet number 2 1989) defines care workers as people, other than paid workers, who are looking after a relative or friend who, because of disability, illness or old age, cannot manage at home. The 1990 Community Care Act defines an *informal carer* as a person who is not employed to provide the care in question.

> ### Did You Know ?
>
> There are six million carers in the UK, of which three and half million are woman.

One in every 5 households contain someone who is providing care for a person who cannot manage without help. Carers are mainly aged between 45–65 years of age. One in every 5 people in this age group have a caring responsibility.

Two Acts of Parliament have been passed which take into account the needs of carers. The first of these Acts was *The Disabled Persons Services, Consultation and Representation Act of 1986*. This states that local authorities have a duty to inform the disabled person and their carer of the services available to them. The second act was the *Community Care Act 1990*; this was a result of the Government's White paper 'Caring for People' 1989. The objective of the Act is for local authorities to provide services to allow people to remain at home, to provide assessment of need and give support to carers.

2. *Care Workers.* Care workers are *employed* by local social services, health boards, voluntary organisations and private care agencies. They are responsible for providing appropriate personal and domestic assistance, such as home care assistants, etc.

One of the main functions of a care worker's role is to make sure that those cared for feel supported and are not ashamed of any need or inadequacy that may be present.

A constant part of the role of the care worker is to understand the needs of their client in relation to the *changing system of benefits*, such as the changes in benefit for seriously disabled people. These were introduced in April 1993 in relation to the D.S.S. community care legislation; monies that are paid to clients now became part of the cost of their care. Care workers also need to understand statutory benefits, such as Income Support and the Social Fund which can be used to meet the needs of the client. Care workers must know enough to put the client in touch with sources of information and advice to help the client in claiming benefits. Care workers may also have a responsibility for ensuring that their clients have their physical needs catered for, perhaps even the collecting of the client's pension.

Some Community Workers / Services

- *Incontinence Services.* Some health authorities have a laundry service attached to the home help service

- *Meals on Wheels.* Administered by social services department (usually delivered by volunteers)

- *Home Helps.* Mainly provide a cleaning service, also washing and shopping (some areas free of charge)

- *Care Attendant Schemes.* Usually trained helpers to help the disabled or elderly to live in the community (but not designed to provide the level of care required to live independently at home)

- *Education.* For the chronically sick and disabled.

- **General practitioner's (GP's)**

GP training involves 5/6 years as an undergraduate followed by 3 years of supervised practice. GP's are a vital resource within the NHS. GP's provide health care to the patients on their list.

People *register* as patients with a local doctor (GP). The main function of a GP is to detect signs of illness, diagnose and treat if possible, often by prescription medicines. Alternatively the GP may refer to other health specialists, e.g. hospital to see a consultant for an X-ray or to other relevant agencies such as counselling services, social services, etc.

Apart from diagnosis and treatment, many GP's run various *clinics*: e.g. anti-natal, well-women/men clinics, preventative medicine sessions. Other services offered include:

- Immunisation
- Health check ups
- Family planning

Some GP's are involved in the General Practice Fund Holding System (GPFH).

- the amount of money the GP receives will be agreed between the GP and the Regional Health Authority.
- the funding takes into account the number of patients registered at the practice, their special needs, the proportion of elderly, etc. If the practice overspends, the patients will still get their treatment.
- the GP will use the funds to *purchase* services for the patient. This will give the GP greater flexibility (shorter waiting lists etc). Of course a possible disadvantage is that GPs may choose the cheapest means of provision rather than the 'best'.
- The practice can use any savings from the fund for their patients benefit, e.g. employ nursing staff, use better equipment, premises, etc.

Doctors in Hospitals

```
Hierarchy of hospital doctors

Consultant
Senior registrar
Registrar
Senior house officer
Junior house officer
All qualified doctors
```

A consultant has a team of doctors working for him/her. In most hospitals medical students accompany a consultant on his ward rounds. Consultants are *responsible* for their patients (even if they are not present, e.g. at an operation). They delegate responsibility to the operating team, etc.

Hospital and Community Nurses
- **Nurses in hospital**

There used to be State Registered Nurses (SRN) or Enroled Nurses (EN – have a shorter training). There are now conversion courses to transfer between the different parts of the register and from Enroled to Registered nurse. Many hospitals have introduced *primary nursing*, i.e. patients have their own nurse, who is mainly responsible for their care. Nurses work alongside doctors and not for them. Nurses do not report to doctors; they also, like doctors, have their own nursing hierarchy.

- *Charge nurses* (run major wards)
- *Registered Nurse* (RN) (qualified, 3 years training)
- *Student Nurses*
- *Ancillary staff* (not trained nurses)

There are also Registered Mental Nurses (RMN) and Registered Sick Children's Nurses (RSCN).

- **Nurse Education and Training**

The name given to the change in nurses education and training is *Project 2000*. It is called this as health care professionals are looking towards the year 2000 and society's changing needs, such as a growing elderly population, the need for care in the community and the increasing number of people with a mental illness or a handicap living in the community. As a result there has been an increase the number of *community nurses*. The chart shows some changes envisaged or underway under Project 2000 for nurses.

```
Nursing

Past situation

Enroled Nurses frustrated at lack of progression.

Low pay, even with many years of experience.

High levels of frustration among all nurses; pressure of work etc.

Nurses do not have enough time to spend with patients.

There are many unqualified staff with lots of experience and skill, but no way of progression.

Future

A single nurse training for all.

Clinical grading of pay and responsibility scales (for nurses who want to work directly with patients).

Reward unqualified care staff with a career structure and introduce progression via National Vocational Qualifications (NVQ).

Nurse education to be brought closer to the training of other caring professions, and involve working more closely with other caring professions.

Train new health workers, e.g. health care assistants to work for registered general nurse.

Attract more men into nursing.

Encourage people with different qualifications to enter nursing.
```

Students are no longer seen as an additional pair of hands. This has resulted in changes in training; 20% of time is now spent on the ward. Students in the past have had too much responsibility and this was one of the reasons for a high drop out rate among students (in the region of 35% per year).

Did You Know ❓

On average 60% of all Student Nurses leave each year. 90% of nurses are female; 50% of nurse managers are men.

- Many female nurses leave to have families and do not return.
- Many nurses are being encouraged to return to nursing by offering refresher courses.
- Staff with under 5's need child care at work; there is a need to introduces workplace crèches.
- P/T work in nursing usually has low status; there is a need to introduce flexibility in working hours, including senior posts.

District Nurses

These are qualified nurses with additional qualifications who mainly provide home nursing care, which involves much work with the elderly. They also treat people who visit the doctors surgery; in particular, people who have been discharged from hospital.

District nurses carry out a wide range of practical nursing care arranged by GP's and social workers, home help and family members. They are attached to GP practices, but employed by the District Health Authority. A great deal of assistance is given by nursing assistants (auxiliary nurses). District nurses are involved in planning nursing care and arranging duties. The district nurse reports to a nurse manager within the DHA, and also works on health education and prevention.

Other Nurses

- *Practice Nurses* – employed by general practitioners. Most of their work is done in the treatment room; most of their salary is recoverable from family practitioner committees.
- *Specialist Nurses* – advise on diabetes, incontinence etc; based in hospitals, specialist clinics and in GP surgeries.
- *Marie Curie Nurses* – found in most health authorities. They provide support for terminally ill cancer patients in their own homes. Arranged by own GP or district nurses.
- *Nurse Practitioners* – few in number; they have extended training and perform many tasks normally carried out by doctors.
- *Sick Children Nurses* – qualified with additional training; they are trained to understand the special needs and problems from birth through to adolescence.
- *Health Visitors* – trained nurses with additional qualifications; they have professional independence. They do not wear uniforms or carry out hands-on nursing. Their prime purpose is in preventative medicine via health education, much of which is directed towards infant and family health advice and also the elderly. The health visitor takes over the care of the mother and baby from the midwife and makes regular visits to the family at home or at a clinic, until the child starts school. They advise on breast feeding, immunisation, family planning, etc. They work mainly with individuals, visiting people at home, at a health clinic or

GP clinic, or work with support groups, e.g. trying to prevent child abuse. They work closely with GP's, District Nurses and other professions and agencies such as Social Workers.

Some health visitors are involved in *specialist* roles like working with the terminally ill, diabetics, tracing various contacts (e.g. infectious diseases) and liaising with the hospital services (e.g. paediatrics and geriatrics).

- *Community Midwives* – qualified nurses with additional midwifery qualification. They are practitioners in their own right, and prescribe drugs with a doctors sanction. Their role is to provide care throughout pregnancy, during childbirth and including postnatal care. They work in hospital obstetric units and in the community, often being attached to GP surgery and health centres.
- *Community Psychiatric Nurses (CPN)* – the majority have a hospital base and support patients by visiting them in the community, after they have been discharged from hospital. Some health authorities have an open referral system, i.e. if a person feels in need of help they can contact a CPN directly. CPN may also work in group practices at GP surgeries. CPN may work with people who have mental illness in general, or with sub-specialists, such as child, adolescent psychiatry, psycho-geriatric.

Other Hospital Staff Services

- *Dieticians*: give advice on diet; e.g. as regards obesity, diabetes, heart disease, kidney problems, etc.
- *Medical social workers*: advise patients on benefits and services; arrange provision after discharge.
- *Physiotherapists*: use exercise and manipulations to help prevent the disabling effects of illness.
- *Radiographers*: take X-rays.
- *Speech Therapists*: speech and language therapists offer assessment, treatment, advice and counselling to people of all ages with a communications disorder and related eating or swallowing problems. Most services operate on an open referral policy.

Personnel in professions complementary to medicine

- **Alternative Medicine** An alternative approach to health care lies *outside* the orthodox health care system. There are three types of alternative therapies: Physical, Psychological and Paranormal.

  Physical therapies include naturopathy, which is based on the premise that substances accumulating in the body as a result of wrong habits, particularly dietary ones, are the underlying cause of all diseases. The list in this category is long and includes: Herbal remedies, Aromatherapy, Homeopathy, Osteopathy, Chiropractice, Acupuncture and Reflexology. All of these are different physical therapies.

  Psychological therapies include counselling services and humanistic psychology which is popular in the UK.

  Paranormal therapies include spiritual healing within the spiritualist movement. Many of the above are used in conjunction with existing orthodox methods by clients. However each needs to be assessed on its own merits. Alternative (complementary) medicine has often used a more *holistic* (whole person) method of treatment, by looking into the clients life style, diet and overall activities *before* attempting to prescribe any form of treatment. There are over 30,000 complementary therapists in the UK.; around 2,500 are medically qualified.

The medical profession remains sceptical about the value of alternative/complementary medicine, mainly because it is perceived to be non-scientific. But many doctors refer their clients to complementary practitioners such as:

Osteopaths
Acupuncturists
Hypnotherapists
Chiropractors
Herbalists

Clients often turn to complementary medicine with chronic conditions for which orthodox medicines offer little relief, such as allergic conditions, back pain, migraines, arthritis and illnesses such as cancer.

The processes by which users gain access to provisions

This section explains the processes by which users **gain access** to provision of health care. This includes:

- Referral through professionals.
- Private self-referral.
- Compulsory referral.

Referral through professionals

Referral through professionals would normally be via the local doctor (GP) but could be via the health service, magistrates, the police, or from school via the head teacher, etc. The local GP will write a letter referring the patient/client to the relevant outpatient clinic. The patient/client will then be contacted by the hospital/clinic and given a date for an appointment to see a specialist, usually a consultant. If it is necessary for the client to be admitted to hospital, the specialist will refer them; on admission, they will then become an *in-patient*.

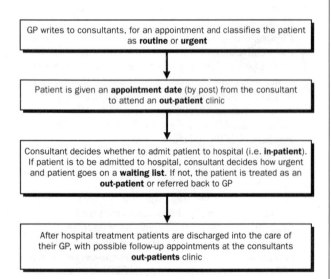

Figure 6.2 GP Referral flow chart

Other Referral through professionals types

- *Health service referral*, via GPs, nurses, health visitors; e.g. requesting a place for an elderly person in an elderly persons home.
- *Magistrate referral* of under 14's after having appeared in court.
- *Police referral* of under 14's who the police are concerned about; e.g. have given 'warnings' to them which have made no difference to their behaviour.
- *School referral*, via the teacher, head, or education welfare dept, due to behaviour problems at school.

Various other services could also refer, e.g. citizen's advice bureau's, probation service, solicitors, etc.

Private self-referral

An individual (or a family member) can contact social services by letter, telephone or by visiting an area office. Another method of **private self-referral** is via neighbours or friends. This might occur where such people are concerned about a situation, e.g. children left alone, elderly neighbour, etc.

Compulsory referrals

A person considered a danger to himself or society at large can be **compulsorily referred** into hospital. Initially, they can be retained against the clients wishes for up to 28 days. This is for observation and assessment, including whether there is a need for retention beyond this period. The *Mental Health Act 1983* outlines conditions for detention. After the 28 days, the next stage is for six months, then one year. There is also a 72-hour option for emergency admissions or detention of a patient already in hospital.

Self Check ✓ Element 1

1. Who stated in 1942 'comprehensive health and rehabilitation services for the prevention and cure of disease and restoration of capacity for work, available to all members of the community.' Was it:
   (A) Wilson
   (B) Beveridge
   (C) Thatcher
   (D) Benn

2. What is the relationship between RHA's and DHA's?
   (A) The RHA reports to DHA's.
   (B) The DHA reports to RHA's.
   (C) RHA's and DHA's both report to the Health Executive
   (D) There is no relationship between the two.

3. Purchasers include which of the following:
   (A) DHA
   (B) GPFH
   (C) FHSA
   (D) Hospital Trusts

4. Providers include which of the following:
   (A) DHA
   (B) GPFH
   (C) FHSA
   (D) Hospital Trusts

5. The CHC is a provider of health services
   True or False?

6. The Department of Social Services is a purchaser of health care.
   True or False?

7. Distinguish between primary, secondary and tertiary health care.

8. Identify five members of a primary health care team.

6.2. Investigate the impact of legislation and funding on provision and priorities

This element looks at the following

- Sources of funding
- Factors influencing priorities
- The role of legislation in influencing provision and priorities
- The impact of funding

Sources of funding in health and social care.

To run the health and social care service system, large amounts of funds are required. The various sources of funds include:

- Central government
- Local government
- Registered charities
- Commercial organisations

Central Government

Did You Know ?

The NHS is funded in the main (approximately 82%) from general taxation and National Insurance Contributions (14%); the remainder comes from fees for dental treatment, prescriptions etc.

The NHS received £34.4 billion in 1994 (total). Over the last decade the amount of funds received for the NHS as a percentage of the total government budget has increased from 10% to 13%.

The role of **Central Government** in relation to the NHS is to:

- Provide 'adequate' resources to NHS
- Use legislation to promote health (e.g. seat belt law)
- Look into the consequences of taxation, low / high taxes on alcohol, tobacco, etc.

Politics is mainly about setting priorities.

There are many *advantages* to funding the NHS in this centralised way. These include:

- a relatively cheap way of funding the NHS. There is less need for extensive invoicing of bills and preparation of contracts, i.e. less bureaucracy than in a market system.
- easy to control, from a national viewpoint at least; it is easy to cut or increase funding when required.
- easy to administer; the funding is simply transferred from central Government to lower tiers in the NHS hierarchy.
- this method is seen as 'fair' by many people
- it is the existing 'tried and tested' system.

Disadvantages of such centralised funding may include:

- unresponsive to social demands for increases in public spending on health.

- limits individual choice in health care provision.
- creates a non-competitive environment.

Did You Know ?

The paperwork and administrative procedures needed in the more 'market' based system of health care in the U.S. is very costly. U.S. administrative costs take up 20% of total health revenue; UK administrative costs are currently around 5% of total health care spending.

The UK spends about 6% of its National Income on health care, compared to over 8% in most other advanced countries.

Local government
Local government's role is to:

- Provide education for children and help to make decisions about their health.
- Provide housing; there is a direct correlation between poor housing conditions and poor health.
- Provide leisure facilities; useful to encourage better health of the nation, e.g. reduce stress by exercising.
- Maintain safe environment (free from pollution, minimise accidents, injuries, etc.)

The local authorities have a *responsibility* to provide certain services for people living in that area. This can be broken down into essential services and other services:

- **Essential services:**
  Housing
  Education
  Refuse collection

- **Other services:**
  Street lighting
  Parks – maintenance
  Noise control
  Libraries
  Recreational services

Local Government is the main providers of the home care services. The service costs around £300 million per year to run. Some local authorities have been 'rate capped' and have had grants reduced as a punishment for 'over-spending'. Take one example of expenditure by care groups for Social Services in a *local district*, namely Westminster, London. The total expenditure, estimated for 1993/94, is £66.1 million. A third of this is apportioned to the elderly and another third to children and families, while the remainder is split between 7 care groups.

Local authority spending on health and social services is funded in several ways: through central government grants, the council tax, business rates and via charges for specific services. Around two-thirds of all local authority expenditure on health care is via central government grants. Only 2% of the total expenditure on personal social services is raised via fees and charges.

Registered charities
Many **registered charities** exist in the UK. Some are household names like:

- Dr Bernardo's
- National Children's Homes (NCH)
- Shelter
- Samaritans

Charities work with the voluntary sector, as described in Element 1. Charities are organisations whose application for charitable status satisfies the Charity Commissioners in England, or the Inland Revenue in Scotland or Northern Ireland.

The key areas they must conform to in order to receive charity status must include at least one of the following:

- Relief of poverty
- Advancement of education
- Advancement of religion
- Advancement of purposes beneficial to the community.

Charities fill the *gaps* in the welfare state and are actively encouraged by the present conservative government.

Registered charities benefit from government legislation in the following ways:

- claim tax relief and other relief
- receive covenants at beneficial rates
- apply for grants from charitable trusts

Other sources of funds in this field include donations to charities or to the NHS directly.

Did You Know ?

That the 'Moonies' (the religious group based in America), are a registered charity and that Amnesty International (the group that looks into world-wide abuse of prisoners) cannot obtain registered status.

Commercial organisations

Private sector organisations such as companies, partnerships and sole traders have a role to play in health care. They are normally set up to provide profits for the shareholders or owners and are not involved with the provision of community health services.

Many of the largest UK companies are members of the *Per Cent Club*. The members give no less than 0.5 per cent of their UK generated pre-tax profit to charity and community affairs. From membership of this club, BT gave £14.6 million in 1992/93. Work in the community covers six main areas:

People in need
Economic regeneration
People with disabilities
Education
Environment
Arts

Many people who cannot get services under the NHS decide to go *private*; e.g. chiropodist, physiotherapy, counselling, domiciliary nursing services, and alternative treatments such as acupuncture, homeopathy and hypnotherapy are often purchased privately.

Some district health authorities make use of private agencies when they are short staffed, to cover sickness, holidays, etc. They also employ many private sector organisations in food, cleaning and the provision of manufacturing equipment, etc.

Often health authorities and the private sector collaborate on joint ventures, e.g. in health education programmes for

employees, staff training, health promotion, and screening services. Some private commercial companies fund, directly or indirectly, the health service or charitable organisations for the following reasons:

- general ethos of 'doing good' or putting something back into society
- shows them as a caring company
- creates public sympathy for their overall causes
- good advertising (may be cheaper than other methods)
- makes employees with private company 'feel good' about the company.

In the UK, around 14% of health care was privately funded in 1994. The percentage is much higher than this average figure in certain types of care, e.g. in long term care of the elderly, abortions, and non-emergency surgery.

Private financing takes two forms. First, people can subscribe to an insurance scheme (e.g. BUPA) which pays for health care when the subscriber needs treatment. Second, people can pay directly for health care as they receive it.

Did You Know ?

The UK figure of 14% of health care being privately funded compares with 60% US, 28% Australia and Japan, 26% France, Canada and the Netherlands, 22% Italy, 8% Sweden.

Other funding methods

Possibilities include:

- introducing charges for certain activities, e.g. non urgent services, such as minor surgery for cosmetic reasons.
- excluding some services from the NHS. This is known as negative funding. It may include not providing the service at all, or allowing the waiting lists to grow to lengths that encourage clients to find alternative methods (e.g. to obtain the same services by going private).
- encouraging sponsorship; one idea is allowing advertising inside all NHS buildings.

These are just a few of the many ideas being considered to increase funds for the NHS.

Factors influencing priorities in health and social care

This section will analyse three key areas:

- state of the economy
- availability of scarce resources
- political priorities

The state of the economy

In good times, in theory anyway, more money would be available to spend on the areas the government regards as most important. In 1978/79, 10% of the total public expenditure was used for health; this percentage has slowly risen (not evenly) to 13% in 1994.

In *real* terms (after taking inflation into account) the amount of money spent on health has increased year on year from £21bn (at 1993 prices) rising to £36bn as forecast for 1994/95 at those same prices. See Table 6.1

Year	Expenditure on health £bn (real terms as in 1992/93 prices)	Health as % of total public exp.
1978/79	21	10.0
1984/85	26	10.9
1988/89	29	12.1
1992/93	33	13.4
Forecast		
1994/5	36	unknown

Table 6.1   UK Health spending

Source: Adapted from HM Treasury, Public Expenditure (HMSO, London 1994).

Other general economic factors which may influence health expenditure include:

* the Public Sector Borrowing Requirement (PSBR). This is the *excess* of government spending over tax revenue. At £46bn in 1994, the government is anxious to reduce its value and thereby keep government spending under control.
* the inflation rate; a lower inflation rate means costs of health provision grow more slowly, but so too will government grants, etc.
* level of employment; high levels of unemployment are associated with deteriorating levels of health and greater health/social security needs.

As we can see from Figure 6.3, those Regional Health Authorities (RHA's) with the highest unemployment rates are those which issue the most prescriptions per year. This indicates that rising unemployment is associated with increasing ill-health, putting greater strains on the NHS budget.

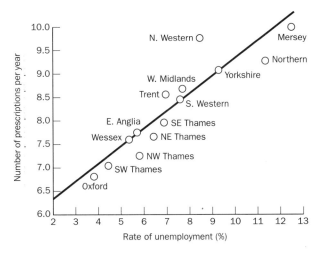

Figure 6.3

Availability of scarce resources
Resources used in Health Care activities can be:

- land/building
- personnel
- equipment
- medications
- finances

A *resource* is an item that can be used and has a worth.

* **Land and buildings** – These are a scarce resource in highly populated town centres. There has been a general policy to reduce the number of key-sited central city hospitals and replace them by hospitals in outer city areas.

* **Personnel** – A lack of personnel can be a major problem. Many trained specialists are attracted overseas by larger salaries and better life styles and this can cause a drain on the NHS resources. Examples of personnel resourcing problems occur if there are too few radiographers during a period of icy weather when many people slip over and need X-rays. Likewise a shortage of consultants for particular ailments will cause long delays.

* **Equipment** – Problems may arise from a shortage of expensive equipment, like dialysis machines and incubators for babies, or small but important items like needles. A shortage of any equipment can be vital. Of course stockpiles of equipment scattered around hospitals will be wasteful of needy finances that could be used elsewhere.

* **Medications** – A lack of medicine can also be vital. This could be influenza vaccine required by the young, the elderly and the weak *before* an attack of an influenza virus projected for the country. Information as to likely epidemics normally becomes well known and many people of all ages start requesting vaccinations of this type, causing an additional drain on resources.

* **Finances** – Budgets are set and adjusted regularly, for example where a short-fall in money receipts compared to the amount expected occurs. Lack of funds will affect the complete system, from *capital* projects like 'losing' a new hospital or new equipment to *current* projects such as reducing the number of beds on a ward within a hospital.

The ageing UK population is placing great strain on health care resources. Whereas 13% of the UK population was over 65 years in 1971, by 1991 the figure had risen to 16%, and it is still rising. As can be seen from Fig. 6.4, the greatest expenditure per head on health care is needed at birth and for age groups beyond 65 years, and especially for the very elderly (85 years +).

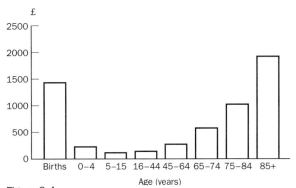

Figure 6.4

Did You Know ?

Only 1.4% of the UK population was aged over 80 years in 1951. By 1991 that figure had risen dramatically to 4.5% of the population being over 80 years.

Political priorities

The government sets out its priorities within its *manifesto* and *policy papers*. It then gets elected (or re-elected) into office and can try to achieve some of the pledges it made to the electorate. These priorities and action plans are *NOT* set in stone, and rarely have specific plans or dates of achievement attached to them. This clearly gives the government of the day considerable discretion as to the precise policies it pursues.

Recent Conservative manifestos have included ideas such as:

– to extend patient choice
– to delegate responsibility to where the service is provided
– to secure best value for money, (by allowing hospitals to apply for self-governing trust status, and set up GPFH status for doctors)
– putting patients first (see Patients Charter, Unit 2)

It is within this framework that a range of changes have been introduced into the Health Service over the last decade.

As a statement of political priorities, the 'Health of the Nation' White Paper in 1992 is perhaps the clearest available statement (see Table 6.2 and 6.3). The goal of the government is to secure continual improvements in the health of the population:

1. By adding years to life: i.e. increasing life expectancy and reducing premature death.
2. By increasing the quality of life and minimising illness.

The White Paper identified five key areas as priorities for action: cancer; heart disease and stroke; mental illness; HIV/AIDS and sexual health; and accidents. *Main targets* were set for each of these areas (see Table 6.2).

Coronary heart disease and stroke
Targets
• To reduce death rates in the under 65 age group for both coronary heart disease (CHD) and stroke by 40 per cent by the year 2000 (from a 1990 baseline).
• To reduce death rate for CHD in people aged 65–74 by at least 30 per cent by the year 2000 (from a 1990 baseline).
• To reduce death rate for stroke in people aged 65–74 by at least 40 per cent by the year 2000 (1990 baseline).

Cancer
Targets
• To reduce the death rate from breast cancer in the screened population by at least 25 per cent by the year 2000 (1990 baseline).
• To reduce the incidence of invasive cervical cancer by at least 20 per cent by the year 2000 (1986 baseline).
• To reduce the death rate for lung cancer under the age of 75 by at least 30 per cent in men and by at least 15 per cent in women by 2010 (1990 baseline).
• To halt the year-on-year increase in skin cancer by 2005.

Mental health
Targets
• To improve significantly the health and social functioning of mentally ill people.
• To reduce overall suicide rate by at least 15 per cent by the year 2000 (1990 baseline).
• To reduce the suicide rate of severely mentally ill people by at least 33 per cent by the year 2000 (1990 baseline).

HIV/AIDS and sexual health
Targets
• To reduce the incidence of gonorrhoea by at least 20 per cent by 1995 (1990 baseline) as an indicator of HIV/AIDS trends.
• To reduce by at least 50 per cent the rate of conceptions among the under-16s by the year 2000 (1989 Baseline).

Accidents
Targets
• To reduce the death rate for accidents among children aged under 15 by at least 33 per cent by 2005 (1990 baseline).
• To reduce the death rate for accidents among young people aged 15–24 by at least 25 per cent by 2005 (1990 baseline).
• To reduce the death rate for accidents among people aged 65 and over by at least 33 per cent by 2005 (1990 baseline).

Source: The Health of the Nation, Cm 1986, 1992, pp 18–19.

Table 6.2 Health of the Nation: Main targets

The 'Health of the Nation' White Paper also identified *risk factor targets*, i.e. specific ways in which some of the causes of the illnesses identified in the five 'main target' areas could be tackled.

Diet and nutrition
Targets
• To reduce the proportion of men drinking more than 21 units of alcohol (roughly 10.5 pints of beer) per week, and the proportion of women drinking more than 14 units per week, by 30 per cent by 2005 (1990 baseline).
• To reduce the proportion of obese men and women in the 16–64 age group by 25 per cent and 33 per cent respectively by 2005 (baseline, 1986/7).
• To reduce the average percentage of food energy derived by the population from saturated fat by at least 35 per cent by 2005 (baseline, 1990).
• To reduce the average percentage of food energy derived from total fat by the population by at least 12 per cent by 2005 (baseline, 1990).

Smoking
Targets
• To reduce the proportion of men and women smoking cigarettes to no more than 20 per cent by the year 2000 – a reduction of around a third (baseline, 1990).
• To reduce the consumption of cigarettes by 40 per cent by the year 2000 (baseline, 1990).
• To reduce the prevalence of smoking among 11–15 year olds by at least 33 per cent by 1994 (baseline, 1988).
• To reduce smoking among women at the start of pregnancy by at least 33 per cent by the year 2000.

Blood pressure
Target
• To reduce mean systolic blood pressure in the adult population by at least 5mm Hg by 2005 (baseline to be established by a new national survey).

HIV/AIDS
Target
• To reduce the percentage of injecting drug misusers who report sharing injecting equipment in the previous 4 weeks from 20 per cent in 1990 to no more than 10 per cent by 1997 and no more than 5 per cent by the year 2000.

Source: The Health of the Nation, CM 1986, 1992, p. 20.

Table 6.3 Health of the Nation: Risk factor targets

The role of legislation in influencing provision and priorities

This will be analysed by looking at the following legislation:

- statutory provision
- enabling legislation

Statutory provision

Statutory provision is legally required provision, laid down by Act of Parliament. Within these Acts, local authorities are often given duties and powers. A *duty* is something that a local authority must do, while a *power* is something they are able to do but do not have to. For example, it is the local authorities duty to provide Social services for disabled people, while they are empowered to provide leisure services, if they want to.

Enabling legislation

Enabling legislation covers services which can be provided at the discretion of the appropriate agency, using public funding.

We have already mentioned a number of Acts which have had major impacts on the health and care of individuals in this unit (e.g. 'Historical perspective' page 123) and other units (e.g. Children Act 1989, unit 2). Here we concentrate on the 1990 'NHS and Community Care' Act which, as previously mentioned, has had such a major impact on health care provision. As we have seen, it sought to decentralise the provision of health care and introduce more competition into the system by separating purchasers from providers (see page 124), creating an 'internal market' in health care. It is hoped that providers will become more cost conscious and that purchasers will be aware of 'best value' purchases of health care, thereby rewarding efficient providers with extra contracts. It is, of course, too early to fully evaluate the changes made.

Did You Know ?

Some of the concern for setting up internal markets' was to increase 'efficiency' and offset rapid cost increases. Between 1979 and 1992:

- real cost per GP consultation – up 86%
- real cost of drugs – up 55%
- real cost of dental services – up 30%

Care in the Community

However it is worth noting that patient care *outside* hospitals had already begun to increase. For example, the average stay in hospital for a patient has fallen from 11 days in 1979 to around 6 days in 1994. As well as establishing an internal market, the 1990 Act aimed to increase general 'care in the community', especially for the elderly, the mentally ill and handicapped, the physically disabled and children.

In fact it has long been recognised that these groups often have complex health and social problems which even specialist hospitals are not always well suited to deal with. Some piecemeal progress was made in the treatment of such patients outside hospitals in the 1970s and 1980s, but it was the 1990 Act which brought into law the main recommendations of the 'Griffiths report on Community Care' (Table 6.4).

Terms of Reference

- 'to review the way in which public funds are used to support community care policy and to advise . . . on the options for action that would improve the use of these funds as a contribution to more effective community care'.

Main Recommendations

- A clearer role for central government, including the creation of a Minister in the DHSS publicly identified as being responsible for community care.
- Social services departments identified as the lead agencies in community care. Their tasks: to identify needs, devise packages of care, and coordinate services. They should develop local plans for community care in consultation with health authorities, housing authorities, voluntary bodies and private providers of care.
- Where appropriate, specific care managers should be assigned to each case, to assess individuals' needs and to arrange packages of care.
- Social services departments should be given an enabling role. They should ensure that services are provided, within budgets, by private or public sectors according to where they can be provided most economically and efficiently.
- Social services departments' plans for community care should be reviewed and approved against national objectives, and alongside the plans of health authorities.
- A specific grant to local authorities for community care should be made available from central government, covering a significant proportion of the costs of an approved programme. This funding should be 'ring-fenced' in order to prevent it from being spent on other services.
- The perverse incentives which have led to the expansion of residential care should be removed. Social security payments should be limited to a basic level only, the balance paid by local authorities on the basis of individual care assessments.
- Collaboration at local level on training matters is necessary in order to prevent insularity of professions and promote mutual understanding of each profession's role.
- A need for a new multi-purpose auxiliary force of carers to be given limited training and to give practical help in the field of community care.

Table 6.4 Care in the Community: main recommentations of the Griffiths Report

Although the implementation of the 1990 Act was delayed for various reasons until 1993, funds have now been transferred from the social security budget to the local authorities in the form of a special transitional grant (STG). In the period 1993–94, the local authorities received over £1.5 billion in specially earmarked grants to help them cope with their new responsibilities. The local authorities must, if they are to receive these funds, agree with the health authorities on two main strategies. First, on the arrangements for placing of people in nursing homes, and second, on the procedures for discharging people from hospital in such a way that the new care assessment procedures are fulfilled.

Did You Know ?

Expenditure by the NHS is over £35 per week for an average family of 4.

Self Check ✓ **Element 2**

9. Local authorities have to provide certain essential services such as Housing and Education.
   True or False?

10. Local authorities have to provide other services such as libraries, noise control and recreational services to the people it serves.
    True or False?

11. Why do private companies give money to charities?
    A A way to reduce tax implications
    B A general ethos of 'doing good' or putting something back into society
    C A commercially sound thing to do because of Public Relations (PR), and marketing advantages that can be gained.
    D A whole range of reason including parts of the above three answers.

12. Why are increased funds (relative to inflation) required by the NHS year on year?
    A elderly population increasing
    B expectations of the population are increasing
    C population explosion
    D technology advances are expensive to provide on demand.

13. A resource is an item that can be used and has a worth.
    True or False?

14. (i) When '**empowered**' it is something that a local authority must do.
    (ii) A **duty** is something the local authority is able to do but does not have to.

    Are these statements True or False?

15. Look back at Fig. 6.3.
    What does it suggest?

16. Look back at Fig. 6.4.
    What does it suggest?

17. List five *areas* in which targets were set in the Health of the Nation Report.

18. List one main target for each area of concern.

19. List two ways in which *diet and nutrition* were targeted for improvement.

20. List two ways in which *smoking* was targeted for improvement.

6.3 Investigate ways in which services within health and social care operate

---

The services operating in health and social care

Here we look at

- Hospital and Community Health Services
- Social Work
- Early Education.

Hospital and Community Health Services

Hospital Health Services

All health authorities have at least one **district general hospital**. The main services offered by district general hospitals are:

accident and emergency (A&E)
x-ray facilities
maternity unit
medical wards (adults)
surgical wards (adults)
medical wards (children)
surgical wards (children)
out-patients clinics
rehabilitation services
–speech therapy
–physiotherapy
–occupational therapy etc.

Other hospitals include the following:

- **Day hospitals.** For minor operations; also provide occupational therapy and psychiatric treatment.
- **GP hospitals.** GP's treat their patients and do minor operations. Some may have control over a number of beds in larger hospitals.
- **Regional specialities.** Provided by regional units; plastic surgery, neuro-surgery, kidney treatment etc.
- **Cottage/community hospitals.** Many offer day surgery, maternity, and out-patient services.
- **Children's hospitals.** Better equipped to deal with children; have trained children's nurses who recognise the importance of parental contact and play.
- **Psychiatric hospital.** The aim now is to deal with psychiatric patients in the community. There are still, however, some psychiatric hospitals.

Community Health Services

Community health services can be viewed as:

> 'those front line services provided outside hospital, by community nurses, midwives, health visitors and other professions allying to medicine'.

Outside hospitals, includes:

School(s)
Clinics(s)
Health Centre(s)
Home(s)

Services include:

speech therapy
physiotherapy
dietetics
family planning
vaccinations and immunisations
health education
mothers and children's groups
health surveillance

Hospital services take up approximately 8 times more financial resources than the Community Health Services. Together they take up nearly three quarters of the total NHS expenditure (60% on average over the 1980s and early 1990s).

Social work

There is no one definition of **social work**. It is a term used in a broad sense. Social workers are involved in a broad area of work, including working in health education and with the police force (see Element 1).

The majority of social workers are employed by local authorities. Social work provision includes advice and counselling by social workers and practical facilities for people in need.

The broad area of work includes old age, handicap, mental illness, low income, family relationships, children, youth work and community work. Some duties of local authority's social services departments involve statutory responsibilities for children, including those children who have:

– got into trouble with the police,
– parents who are unable to provide adequate care.

The social work profession is made up of:

- field-workers, families and individuals in the community
- residential social workers
- day-care workers.

The *Barclay Report* (1982) saw residential social work as the 'Cinderella' service within social work. Workers suffer low pay and low status, and have a high incidence of demoralisation.

The *Seebohm Report* recommended that social workers in each geographical area become more *generic* (i.e. include all types of clients) rather than specialist.

Early Education

- **Family centres (Day nurseries)** These are provided by social services from approximately 1 year – 5 years (in some cases children from 6 months). Places are normally allocated on a priority basis e.g. single parents, special needs, deprived children, abused children and those with language difficulties.
  The service provides a stimulating, caring and warm setting to compensate for the limitations in the child's home.
  Many day nurseries are privately run for the under 5's. These have to be registered and inspected by the Social Services Department (SSD) of local authorities.
- **Nursery centres.** These are provided by local social services and local authority education departments; the main aim being to combine educational resources of the nursery class and the caring aspect of Day Nurseries. These must also be registered and inspected by SSD.
- **Play groups.** These are for under 5's; also included are parents and toddler groups where parents take their children once or twice a week to mix and play with other children. They vary in size and opening hours. The Social Services approve and register these groups. In some cases they may be given a small grant for material or allowed the use of premises.
- **Child minders.** They look after/care for pre-school children in their own home. They provide a flexible service. The child-minders are limited in the number of children they may look after at one time depending on the size of their house and facilities. They are free to charge their own fees. They are registered by the local authorities who make sure that the quality of care given is such that the health and safety standards are met. The social services keep a list of registered child minders that can be recommended.

The strategies for service delivery employed in health and social care

This will be explained by looking at 6 **strategies**, as follows:

- intervention
- remedial
- preventative
- therapeutic
- holistic
- multi-disciplinary

Intervention Strategy

An **intervention strategy** by a carer can be broken down into six separate categories:

1. **Prescriptive intervention** seeks to direct the behaviour of the client; e.g. give advice, be judgmental, critical or evaluative.
2. **Informative intervention** seeks to impart new knowledge and information to the client; e.g. instruct/inform, interpret.
3. **Confronting intervention** seeks to challenge any restrictive attitude, belief or behaviour of the client.
4. **Cathartic intervention** seeks to enable the client to experience painful emotion; e.g. release tensions by encouraging laughter / crying.
5. **Catalytic intervention** seeks to enable the client to learn and develop by self-direction and self discovery; e.g. be reflective, encourage self directed problem-solving.
6. **Supportive intervention** affirms the worth and value of a client; e.g. by approving, confirming, validating.

Remedial Strategy

This **remedial strategy** is where children with a learning difficulty are given help (often in their own existing school) by being provided with extra / special lessons or by being placed in a Special School. As a result of the 1981 Education Act and the admission of handicapped children to ordinary schools, it is important to understand the implications of a wide variety of disabling conditions on a child's ability to learn.

Preventative Strategy

A **preventative strategy** is aimed at individuals and families, enabling them to manage their lives more easily and avoid the occurrence of a breakdown or crisis.
Examples of preventative social work include:

    day care
    meals on wheels
    rotational care
    family centres
    warden services
    neighbourhood support groups
    volunteer work
    short stay care.

Therapeutic Strategy

This is the provision of 'palliative' care to terminally ill patients either in their own homes, hospitals, hospices, or hospice-type units within a hospital.

Part of the care is to help people to understand their illness and how their lives will need to be adapted as a result of the illness. An example of nurses who provide this care are Macmillan and Marie Curie Nurses (cancer relief). They provide domiciliary nursing services, e.g. nursing care for cancer patients in their own homes, day or night. The service is jointly funded by the foundation and the health authorities.

Many local charitable foundations have developed home care nursing teams outside the National Health Service, similar to the Macmillan Nursing services.

Holistic Strategy

This is a philosophy which looks at how the *parts* may work together as a *whole*, instead of looking at each part in isolation. A **holistic strategy** is important when dealing with a client.It will help the carer to see what makes a person behave in particular ways. The holistic approach recognises that all aspects of a person are significant and considers how these different aspects of the person can work together to help the whole person. A carer must not deal with one aspect in isolation. If they do, they will be left with an incomplete view of the client e.g. where a nurse refers to a client as 'the broken leg in bed 4'. The orthodox approach would be for the GP to give the client medication while the holistic approach would involve, perhaps in addition, some investigation into the client's lifestyle, recent changes relating to stress at work due to a new boss, etc. Dealing with these concerns may alleviate medical conditions in some cases.

Multi-disciplinary Strategy

This approach is one that looks at more than just one discipline within the health service. Sometimes *many disciplines* are combined to offer an effective solution to the client's problems. This approach should be completed in a 'seamless' way; e.g. the client should not be *aware* of the different departments involved and should see the health service as one system operating for the good of the client.

Self Check ✓ **Element 3**

21. Which service takes up the most of the NHS budget, is it?:
    A Community Health Services
    B Hospital Services
    C Voluntary Services
    D Management, Administration and Miscellaneous services

22. The majority of social workers are employed by local authorities.
    True or False?

23. The ———————— Report (1982) saw residential social work as the 'Cinderella service within social work'. Insert the missing word(s).
    A Health and Social Care
    B Barclays
    C National Health Service
    D Seebohm

24. It is the statutory responsibility of Social services to provide protection, fostering and adoption services for children in its area under 5 years of age.
    True or False?

25. Home care services provide which one of the following:
    A Supplementary care in the client's home
    B Day time nursery care in the client's home
    C Night time nursery care in the client's home
    D Complete care in the client's home

26. The following are examples of approaches in health care: holistic, preventative and intervention
    True or False?

Unit Test

Question 1
Statement (i)
The Department of Health is directly responsible for the organisation and finance of Regional Health Authorities (RHA's) in England.
Statement (ii)
The RHA's are responsible for the District Health Authorities (DHA's) which provide a range of services for people living in each district, by purchasing health care for its population.

Which option best describes the two statements:
A   Statement (i) True   Statement (ii) True
B   Statement (i) True   Statement (ii) False
C   Statement (i) False   Statement (ii) True
D   Statement (i) False   Statement (ii) False

Question 2
Self governing hospitals are run by:

A   Voluntary organisations
B   National Health Trusts
C   District Health Authorities
D   Local patients.

Question 3
The local authority is responsible for:

A   Charity based hospitals
B   Social Services Department
C   Voluntary services
D   Hospices for the terminally ill.

Question 4
Action on Smoking and Health (ASH) is an example of:

A   A statutory service
B   A voluntary service
C   A National Health Service
D   A community care service

Question 5
The main place to find information on the Health Services is:

A   Post Offices
B   Surgeries and clinics
C   Department of social security
D   Voluntary organisations

Question 6
Which one of the following is involved in the provision of primary health care?

A   Psychologists
B   Consultants
C   Occupational therapists
D   Health visitors

Question 7
GP Fund-Holders:

A   can buy services for their clients
B   can give financial assistance to their clients
C   must charge all clients for their treatment
D   receive their funding from private sources

Question 8
Decide whether each of these statements is True (T) or False (F)

(i) The term Welfare State refers to those services in the economy which are organised and provided by the government.
(ii) The National Health Service is no longer a part of the Welfare State

A   (i) T   (ii) T
B   (i) T   (ii) F
C   (i) F   (ii) T
D   (i) F   (ii) F

Question 9
The funding for Community Health Councils (CHC's) comes from:

A   Local Authorities
B   Voluntary contributions
C   Patients and donations
D   Health Authorities.

Question 10
Statement (i)
Special Health Authorities (SHA's) report directly to the Regional Health Authorities (RHA's).
Statement (ii)
District Health Authorities (DHA's) and FHSA's (Family Health Service Authorities) report directly to Regional Health Authorities (RHA's).

Which option best describes the two statements:
A   Statement (i) True   Statement (ii) True
B   Statement (i) True   Statement (ii) False
C   Statement (i) False   Statement (ii) True
D   Statement (i) False   Statement (ii) False

Question 11
The name given to the major programme of change in nurse education and training is:

A   Community Care Act
B   Care in the Community
C   Project 2000
D   Nursing Reform Act

Questions 12–15 share answer options A–D
Approaches used in the delivery of health and social care include:

A   Preventative approach
B   Therapeutic approach
C   Multi-disciplinary approach
D   Remedial approach

Which of these approaches are illustrated by the following examples?

Question 12
Providing palliative care to a terminally ill client.

Question 13
Providing special schooling for a child with learning difficulties.

Question 14
Providing an approach which is seen as seamless for the client although many health areas are involved.

Question 15
Providing vaccinations against certain diseases.

Question 16
There are several ways to be referred to the health care services. These include:

(i) GP referral
(ii) Self referral
(iii) Police referral
(iv) School referral

Choose from the following:
A   None of the above.
B   (i) and (ii) and (iv)
C   (i) and (ii)
D   All the above.

Question 17
Which two of the following describe the work of District Nurses?

(i) Head a team of nurses responsible for a district's health care.
(ii) Mainly provide home nursing care
(iii) Employed by Regional Health Authority
(iv) Are attached to GP practices

Is it:
A   (i) and (ii)
B   (ii) and (iii)
C   (i) and (iv)
D   (ii) and (iv)

Question 18
Aromatherapy is an example of:

A   Psychological therapy
B   Alternative medicine
C   Paranormal therapy
D   Conventional medicine

Question 19
Decide whether each of these statements is True (T) or False (F)
(i) Over the last ten years the amount of funds allocated to the NHS as a percentage of the total government budget has increased.
(ii) Approximately a third of the funding for the NHS comes from fees charged to patients.

Which option best describes the two statements?

A   (i) T   (ii) T
B   (i) T   (ii) F
C   (i) F   (ii) T
D   (i) F   (ii) F

Questions 20–23 share answer options A–D
Intervention strategies for service delivery in health and social care include:

A   Prescriptive intervention
B   Informative intervention
C   Cathartic intervention
D   Supportive intervention.

Which of these strategies are illustrated by the following examples?

Question 20
A recently bereaved widow is encouraged to release the anger she feels about her husband's premature death.

Question 21
An expectant mother is strongly advised to give up smoking.

Question 22
A patient recovering from major surgery is congratulated on the progress he is making.

Question 23
The wife of an alcoholic is given the address of a local self-help group.

Question 24
Holistic medicine

A   focuses on a patient's diet
B   believes in isolating the part of a patient's bodily system which requires treatment
C   looks at the way all aspects of a patient's life work together
D   is mainly concerned with encouraging physical exercise

Question 25
The function of a GP is to:

1. Diagnose and treat if possible.
2. Detect signs of illness.
3. Refer to other health specialists.
4. Carry out preventive health care such as immunisation.

How many of the above statements are true?
A   1 of the above
B   2 of the above
C   3 of the above
D   All of the above

Question 26
Privately run day nurseries:
A   are not officially approved or registered
B   are registered and inspected by the Social Services Department of local authorities
C   become part of the public sector when they receive approval from the Department of Education
D   cater specifically for children with special needs

Question 27
The role of local government includes the provision of which of the following:

(i)   Education services for children.
(ii) Electrical services for the elderly
(iii) Housing
(iv) Water services for disabled people.

A   (i) and (ii)
B   (i) and (iii)
C   (ii) and (iii)
D   (ii) and (iv)

Question 28
The organisation Shelter is an example of:

A   A government quango
B   A local authority service
C   A registered charity
D   A branch of the Department of Health.

Question 29
BUPA provides:

A   Free and independent medical advice
B   Private medical insurance cover
C   Help for those on low incomes
D   Lists of GPS in local areas.

Question 30
Insert the correct titles into the boxes labelled X, Y, and Z in Fig. 6.5.

A   X = RHA   Y = DHA   Z = SHA
B   X = SHA   Y = RHA   Z = DHA
C   X = SHA   Y = DHA   Z = RHA
D   X = DHA   Y = SHA   Z = RHA

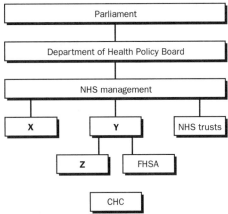

Figure 6.5

Answers to Self-check Questions

1. B. It was the Beveridge report on 'Social Insurance and Allied Services' which helped shape the 1946 Act setting up the National Health Service.

2. B. The District Health Authorities (DHA's) report to the Regional Health Authorities (RHA's).

3. A and B. Family Health Service Authorities (FHSA) manage the GP's (other than fundholders), dentists, opticians and pharmacists in their area. They are not purchasers. Hospital Trusts are providers not purchasers.

4. D. Hospital Trusts (rest are puchasers not providers).

5. False. The Community Health Comuls act as advisory and support bodies to District Health Authorities.

6. False

7. Primary-in the community; Secondary-via hospital staff; Tertiary-in institutions of long term care.

8. See page 130.

9. True-when part of their 'duties'.

10. False-not a duty. Being 'empowered' to provide such services does not mean that they have to provide them.

11. D. Other reasons can exist besides these first three.

12. A, B and D. The UK population is not exploding.

13. True.

14. Both statements are false. The reverse is true in each case.

15. The greater the rate of unemployment in a region, the more prescriptions are issued per person. In other words ill-health and unemployment seem to be related.

16. That an ageing population will need more to be spent on health care.

17. See Table 6.2 page 134.

18. See Table 6.2 page 134.

19. See Table 6.3 page 134.

20. See Table 6.3 page 134.

21. B. This has by far the largest budget.

22. True.

23. Barclays.

24. True.

25. A

26. True

Answers to Unit Test

Question	Answer	Question	Answer	Question	Answer	Question	Answer	Question	Answer	Question	Answer
1.	A	6.	D	11.	C	16.	D	21.	A	26.	B
2.	B	7.	A	12.	B	17.	D	22.	D	27.	B
3.	B	8.	B	13.	D	18.	B	23.	B	28.	C
4.	B	9.	D	14.	C	19.	B	24.	C	29.	B
5	B	10.	C	15.	A	20.	C	25.	D	30.	B

Unit Test Comments (selected questions)

Question 5
B. Some information might be obtained from the other three sources but B is the main source.

Question 6
D. The others are involved in secondary health care.

Question 15
A – because the aim is to prevent the contraction of disease.

Question 16
D. All of these methods of referral are possible.

Question 19
B. Only around 4% of NHS funding comes from fees. The remainder comes from general taxation (see page 10).

Question 20
C. Cathartic intervention encourages the release of emotions and anxieties.

Question 21
A. Prescriptive intervention involves giving advice and instructions.

Question 22
D. Supportive intervention involves giving sympathy, encouragement and emotional support.

Question 23
B. Informative intervention involves giving information to the client.

Question 24
C. Holistic medicine is based on viewing the client as a whole person.

Question 25
D. The work of a GP incorporates all of these functions.

Question 28
C. Shelter is a charity which helps the homeless.

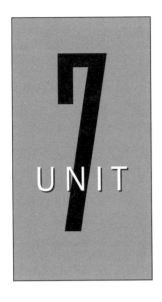

Care plans

Getting Started

This unit is made up of three Elements:

Element 1	Describe the development of care plans.
Element 2	Describe methods of assessing client need.
Element 3	Identify the purpose of monitoring and evaluation approaches within care plans.

In this unit we will be looking at what is involved in care planning (including assessment of the client's need), and in monitoring and evaluating those plans. We consider the development of care plans from the point of view of the client's personal needs, including gathering information about clients using primary and secondary sources of information. This Element will also discuss the rights of the client and how they can be protected during assessment. As we see below, this unit has much in common with a number of other units.

Cross-references:

Discrimination and its effects on individuals (Unit 1, Element 2)
Communication with individuals (Unit 2, Element 1)
Communication within groups (Unit 2, Element 2)
Client's rights in interpersonal situations (Unit 2, Element 3)
Development of individual identity (Unit 4, Element 1)
Threats to individual identity (Unit 4, Element 2)
Health Promotion (Unit 5, Elements 1, 2 and 3)
Structure of health and social care provision (Unit 6, Element 1)
Methods of deriving and using research information (Unit 8, Elements 1, 2 and 3)

Closed questions Questions which require a yes/no or specific answer.

Individual care A system where the carer performs all the tasks for a client.

Innate behaviour As for 'instinctive behaviour.

Instinctive behaviour Reflex types of behaviour.

Learned behaviour Conditioned types of behaviour.

Open ended interview No framework developed beforehand.

Open questions Questions which allow a client to express himself/herself.

Primary assessment Use of original information, e.g. obtained by face-to-face contact with client.

Secondary assessment Use of information on the client obtained second-hand from other sources.

Structured interview Setting of interview, questions to be asked, etc. carefully prepared beforehand.

Task oriented care A system where carers specialise in one task (or a limited range of tasks) for all clients.

Essential Principles

Relating care plans to personal needs

Before care plans are drawn up, it is important to remember that the client is a real person. It is vital that the care worker communicates with the client as part of the care that is provided. It is important to find out what the client is like as an individual as well as his/her physical needs. In other words to use the 'holistic' approach considered previously.

The two main types of care plans are:

- **Task oriented care** – This is when a care worker carries out *one task* (or form of care) for *all* clients. With this type of care each client could be cared for by many carers; the disadvantage is that the carers may not get to know the client in detail.

- **Individual care** – This is when one carer performs *all the tasks* and care for a client and can therefore get to know the client and develop a trusting relationship.

Types of personal need

It is also important to understand the "needs" of the individual. All individuals have basic needs. Maslow suggests that there are five categories of needs, arranged in a *hierarchy* from the basic (physical) needs to the higher needs involving self-esteem and creativity (see chart). However the higher needs cannot be met unless the basic needs have already been fulfilled.

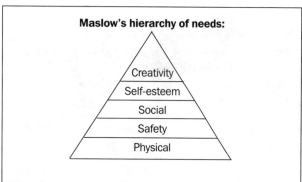

Maslow's hierarchy of needs:

Creativity
Self-esteem
Social
Safety
Physical

Physical needs. The need for food, drink, shelter, warmth and clothing.

Safety needs. These are needs for protection against danger and threats.

Social needs. The need to feel accepted; belonging to a family, peers, relationships with other groups, society, etc. The need to give and receive love and affection.

Self-esteem needs. The need to be respected, to receive recognition, to be productive. The need to have a stable evaluation of oneself.

Creativity needs. The need to develop as a person, to reach ones full potential (self actualisation).

A related but slightly different set of **personal needs** can be derived from Maslow's hierarchy of needs.

- physical needs
- emotional needs
- cognitive
- identity
- cultural

- **Physical needs:** (as above).
- **Emotional needs:** the need for love, self-worth, dignity, independence, choice, privacy. Even to experience 'negative' emotions such as loss, loneliness, separation, grief.
- **Cognitive needs:** intellectual needs which involve the need for communication, both verbal and non-verbal. Communication is important from birth onwards.
- **Identity needs:** a person develops a sense of identity from contact with the outside world, companionship in general and especially with ones own peer group.
- **Cultural needs:** related to the arts/spiritual aspects in general. May also involve participation in the beliefs and customs of a particular group to which a person belongs (Christian, Jewish, Muslim, etc).

An example of emotional, communicational and identity needs is when a baby smiles; people smile back and give the baby attention. The baby wants to feel warmth and affection, hence it develops *behaviour* which will encourage people to give that attention and affection.

As a result the child itself will develop attitudes about love and trust from its carers who themselves *give* affection and love.

Assessment of personal need

- **Assessing behaviour**
  Behaviour is the *observable* outcome of all the co-ordinating processes working within the body. Behaviour is a response from stimuli, either external or internal. Behaviour can be classed into 2 key categories:

  – instinctive (innate)
  – learned (conditioned)

  Instinctive behaviour – a person will withdraw his hand if he puts it on a hot oven ring. NB. Not all people do this – and an inability to respond in this way shows serious mental concerns or neurological problems.

  learned behaviour – children learn to play with other children. This can be by watching others at play.

- **Assessing physical condition**
  A health care worker need to assess the **physical condition** of the client. This will include:

  – appearance
  – strength
  – stamina
  – mobility
  – suppleness

Observation by the care worker or other health professionals (doctor's reports etc) clearly plays a part here.

- **Assess personal circumstances**
  Sometimes it is ease to identify **personal circumstances**, e.g. a diabetic who is dependent on insulin. A priority is then to satisfy the identified need, e.g. to give the insulin injection. Certain situations/conditions are not as easy to identify as others, e.g. it may be difficult, at least initially, to identify an incontinent person.

  Personal needs can change from day to day; e.g. a cold or flu could cause a person to be housebound so that they could not get to their rehabilitation centre or do their shopping. At other times changes are less obvious; e.g. a slow, gradual deterioration over a period of time until the situation has completely changed. This may be the case with rheumatoid arthritis which is a progressive condition. It is important that such individuals are *continually assessed* and that the changes are recognised and the care plan changed where appropriate.

  It is also important to *listen* to the client and not to make assumptions.

  Other personal details, which are required include age, family circumstances, personal history, and past events which may affect present care needs, such as bereavement of a partner. This may result in the client needing extra emotional or physical support.

Verbal reports
The client should be encouraged to express themselves verbally. This may not be as simple as it sounds. The carer needs to know the *framework* of the information required before discussion with the client; otherwise it can turn into just a general chat. The carer can be encouraged to discuss the following with the client to help him or her to open up:
– any reference to personal abilities
– autonomy – what can you do on your own?
– values – what do you believe in?
– identity – where are you in the world, and where are you going?
– intimacy – what are your close relationships?
– sexuality – what are your sexual needs?
– love, marriage, family – deeper commitments?
– career – where does work fit into your life?
– the wider community – neighbourhood, local and national activities?
– leisure – what do you do with your 'free' time?
– if the client has problems with speech, then get them to express themselves in writing.

Some of these may or may not be appropriate for every client, but it is a general framework. Good *notes* should be taken, highlighting key points from each section. If notes are taken while the conversation is on-going, make sure the client is made aware of *why* notes are being taken so as not to alienate the client. If this is thought to be the case, notes should be taken immediately afterwards. Other forms of note taking are by audio or video tape.

These forms of **verbal reports** are from the client directly. Other reports can be from any other carers involved with the client, such as relatives, neighbours, friends, work place colleagues, etc.

Care Plans
These can be divided into either macro or micro care plans.

- **Macro Care Plan**
This will identify the *overall* needs of the client. The macro care plan should also list the agencies that will be involved in providing the services. For example:

Client needs	– Surgical drying to left leg, daily
	– Improvement in hygiene levels throughout home
Action to be taken	– Nurse to dress and clean left leg, daily
	– Home help care to improve general hygiene
Provider	– District Nurse
	– Home help/carer

- **Micro Care Plan**
This describes the action plan of an *individual service provider*, e.g. a home carer.

Client needs	– daily hygiene (washing and drying of person
	– ensuring dressing has been completed by nurse and is intact.
Action taken	– assistance given to client in bathroom in relation to washing and drying
	– special assistance given to care/hygiene of left leg

Stages within the care plan
4 phases (or stages) will be considered.

- initial assessment
- repeated (second) assessment
- implementation
- monitoring and review

The stages in the care plan can be developed further and subdivided as shown below. A 'referral stage' can be introduced before the *initial assessment*. The *repeated assessment* can be broken down into 'devising a care plan' and 'setting objectives'. *Implementation* can remain as it is, but 'monitoring' and 'review and evaluation' can be separated.

This takes the four stages to a seven point plan as shown:

1. Referral
2. Initial assessment
3. Devising a care plan
4. Setting objectives
5. The care plan is implemented
6. Monitoring the care plan
7. Review and evaluation

We now consider these stages in more detail.

- **Referral and Initial Assessment**
Assessment of a client starts with the **initial referral**, which could have been by the client, friends, relatives or care worker(s). The care worker then obtains information *from the client* and from *secondary sources* such as: friends; relatives; the clients support network; health/medical records.

Ideally all the relevant information should be *brought together* to be able to give a holistic initial assessment. However, in reality there are two fundamental problems here,

(i) obtaining *ALL* the information
(ii) selecting what is *relevant*, as this will often change as developments occur.

Decisions have to be taken on the information available at the time, and maybe before detailed reports are prepared. In general the **initial assessment** needs to cover the following;

– self care – e.g. dressing, looking after one-self
– domestic skills – e.g. cooking, cleaning, taking medicine
– community skills – e.g. crossing road, using the telephone, public transport
– miscellaneous skills – e.g. budgeting with household money

This information will come from many sources;

- friends
- neighbours
- relatives
- workplace colleagues
- all other care workers involved – past and present

- **Devising a care plan**

It is from the initial assessment stage that clear **planning** now needs to take place. Planning takes place from the view: "What does this person need?" An *individual weekly care plan* can then be developed.

An example of this plan is shown in Fig 7.1.

Time	Mon	Tues	Wed	Thur	Fri	Sat	Sun
06.00–1000	R		R		R	R	
10.00–1400	CW	CW	CW	V	M	R	R
14.00–1800	CW	N	CW	CW	R	R	
18.00–0600	CH	RT	RT		RT	RT	CV

Key
CW = care worker
CV = church visitor
 N = community nurse
 V = volunteer visitor
 R = relative
RT = relative (telephone)
 M = meals on wheels

Figure 7.1

The plan needs to be:

- flexible
- continuous
- easy to understand, with roles clearly defined
- take the clients *degree of independence* into account – both as desired by the client and what can be realistically viewed as practical independence.

The plan has to be agreed by all parties.

The key factors affecting the **assessment** and **care plan** are:

- *physical impairments*; affects strength, stamina, mobility, co-ordination, suppleness, e.g. a person not able to walk up stairs.
- *sensory impairment*; e.g. reduction of hearing, seeing, smell, taste or touch.
- *mental impairment*, includes memory loss, loss of control, lack of communication skills and clear thought processes.
- *learning difficulties*; e.g. cannot read, write or count.
- *emotional impairment*; the lack of ability to receive and give kindness and affection.

Other factors to include might be:

- *Cultural factors* – this includes language, religious views and ritual beliefs.
- *Social factors* – where you work, spend your recreational time and with whom you live.
- *Environmental factors* – this can involve poor entrance facilities to a public building e.g. stairs, or excessive bad weather stopping a person's access to local shops, etc.
- *Housing* – if there is a housing need, then housing associations/providers need to be involved.
- *Transport* – are suitable transport facilities available?

- *Risk* – try to assess the risks involved. Involve the client here. Risks include – home risks – use of gas by people with debilitating illnesses, health risks – diabetes or epilepsy, etc.
- *Finance* – assessors need to consider the client's (and those of any people helping the client) ability to claim benefits for everything they are entitled to. Also whether the client can contribute to the cost of the care being given.

Each individual will need to be *reassessed* as part of the developing care plan. The frequency will depend upon the seriousness of the situation. It may range from hourly to monthly or every quarter or yearly. The assessment needs to review how the existing care plan is working (or not working), what improvements and changes have taken place, whether an increase or reduction in care is now necessary and why? The client *must* be involved at all times in this process. The plan needs to be flexible, but provide a continuous pattern of care.

- **Setting Objectives**

The main objective is that the care plan works and is reviewed as appropriate to continuously meet the client's changing needs. Around this main objective may be devised a *set of more specific* objectives which must be fulfilled if the care plan is to be effective; e.g. help at specific times with medical care, food needs, etc. These objectives need to be clarified to all concerned.

Before implementing the care programme, ways must be found of fulfilling these and other objectives, such as:

- Methods of monitoring ongoing progress.
- Making opportunities for receiving and giving feedback.
- Ways of maintaining the carer's commitment to the programme.

- **Implementation of the care plan**

This is when the plan is turned into reality; good planning, although time consuming, allows for good **implementation**. This includes

- good communication to client; e.g. the same message from all carers, not conflicting messages
- good communication between carers
- following the plan
- feedback on variance from the plan
- flexibility to change plan as required
- knowing when implementation is complete

- **Reviewing and monitoring the care plan**

The purpose of **monitoring** is to ensure that the provision continues to relate to the client's needs. Monitoring must involve regular evaluation of the impact of the care programme.

Clients rights with respect to assessment

Here we describe the *clients rights* with respect to assessment. In particular we consider

- independence
- identity maintenance
- choice and control
- confidentiality
- freedom from discrimination

First we should look at the *inequalities* that can occur between the client and the carer. The major problem is that the client may feel vulnerable and frightened due to having to cope with a new situation. Knowledge is power and the carer often has more knowledge, training and experience in relation to caring than the client. Additionally, the carer knows more about the client than the client knows about the carer. The client may feel dependent on the carer as the carer has the knowledge and expertise to deal with the situation, and has power over the access to resources.

• **Independence**
It is vital to know when to give help and when to encourage the client to be as *independent* as possible – independence can be defined as the ability to care for oneself.

It is important to always give encouragement and to appreciate the importance for many clients of feeling that they have achieved something for themselves. Generally, do *not* do everything for the client, but give help when required.

It is *not* the aim for the client to 'depend' on the health provision but for the client to move towards personal independence.

• **Identity maintenance**
The client has his or her own views and is an individual. This should not be forgotten. Therefore every care plan will need to be adjusted to the individual. For example, when the client is *resident* in a home, independence can be encouraged by allowing the client to:

– dress appropriately
– make own choices where appropriate
– have individual personal items, etc.

• **Choice and control**
The client must have **choices** and by allowing the client the right to make choices that suit his/her own needs, this gives the client **control** over his/her destiny.

The client has the right to know what his/her personal care plan looks like and be involved in the development of such a plan. The client has rights to what happens to them in relation to staying on their own (e.g. in their own home) or moving into a residential home.

• **Confidentiality**
It is important to respect the clients right to **confidentiality** at all times. At certain times this might be difficult especially if you think the information should be passed on to other team members. It is vital that you explain to the client *why* certain information should be passed on to other team members, so that the care plan might be adjusted in the interest of the client's well being. Difficult issues need to be discussed with the team leader.

• **Freedom from discrimination**
All clients should be treated equally, no matter what age, gender, sexual orientation, culture, religion, disability or ethnic background they come from. A carer must be aware that discrimination can take many forms, non-verbal, physical, verbal and by being judgemental etc. (see Unit 1).

Self Check ✓ **Element 1**

1. What are the two main types of Care Plan? Explain the difference between them.
2. What is the importance of Maslow's triangle?
3. What aspects are involved in the 'physical condition' of the client?

---

4. What are the fundamental phases or stages within a Care Plan?
5. A macro care plan lists all the agencies which are involved in providing the services for the client. True or False?
6. A micro care plan details the cost of the care provided. True or False?
7. The stages of a care plan consist of
   1 implementation
   2 repeated assessment
   3 initial assessment
   4 monitoring and review
   In what order would you carry these out.
   (A) 1, 4, 3, 2
   (B) 3, 2, 1, 4
   (C) 2, 3, 4, 1
   (D) 1, 3, 2, 4
8. Complete the missing stages in the seven point care plan.
   1 referral
   2 –
   3 devising a care plan
   4 –
   5 care plan implemented
   6 –
   7 review and evaluation
   Choose from:
   A setting objectives
   B initial assessment
   C monitoring the care plan
   A 2 = C   4 = A   6 = B
   B 2 = A   4 = B   6 = C
   C 2 = B   4 = A   6 = C

7.2 Methods of assessing client need

Some aspects relevant to this issue have already been considered in Element 1.

Primary methods involve face-to-face contact with the client. **Secondary** methods involve using the assessments of others.

Primary methods of assessment

Observation
Observation via a home visit etc. can be useful in gathering information on physical condition, individual behaviour and personal circumstances. For example, as regards *physical condition*, observation might indicate:

– marks on the face/legs/arms
– swellings
– redness and swollen areas
– appearance – dress sense, e.g. if the client has not been able to dress himself correctly
– lack of food/vitamins
– confidence level
– ability to take in information; e.g. request client to do something using their:
  – hearing
  – eye sight
  – memory

Clients that are not articulate, e.g. young children and babies, need especially careful observation. Clients can be asked to write or draw pictures where appropriate, or perform suitable tasks.

Verbal reports

Many clients, when given time, will be willing to explain their situations to a caring, listening person, especially if the client believes that benefits will follow from the discussion. Here are some "general rules' for use when the carer is receiving a **verbal report** from a client.

DO

1. listen – genuinely listen – to client.
2. good eye contact (without staring).
3. remain relaxed throughout session.
4. put the client at ease.
5 be well prepared.
6. also have an "open' posture.
7. make sure you understand what the client is saying? are you sure?
8. check understanding by asking questions.
9. take notes, where applicable.
10. encourage the client to be specific.

DO NOT

1. put words into the client's mouth.
2. interrupt the client, during mid-flow.
3. *pretend* to listen; your body actions will suggest whether or not you are *really* listening.
4. guess what the client is going to say.
5. ask meaningless questions.
6. rush the session.
7. appear nervous or unconfident.
8. take sides against the client.
9. impose your moral/religious views onto the client.
10. be vague.
11. build up false expectations.

Questioning

Asking *questions* may be part of the process of receiving a verbal report from a client or may be part of other interview approaches.

There are four *interview-types* in which questions can be asked

1. **Structured interview** – here all the questions are devised beforehand, and are strictly observed.
2. **Semi-structured interview** – as above, however some areas can be changed as the interview develops. Nevertheless the *framework* of the interview exists, and is kept to throughout the interview.
3. **Focused interview** – here a particular *focus* is agreed beforehand; however no questions are prepared in advance.
4. **Open ended interview** – here no questions or even framework is set before the interview. The conversation develops in its own way, not directed by the carer.

- **Types of question**
  Questions within the four types of interview can take different forms:

  – closed
  – open
  – probing

Closed questions. These give a response of yes or no or a direct answer. These are useful to obtain facts but not to develop arguments. For example:

> do you want '......' service? yes/no
> how old are you?
> how many times have you been in hospital?

Open questions These allow the client to express himself in his own way.

> "What is your view on ......?"
> "Why have you not eaten any food?"
> "What is the problem?"
> "How did it happen?"

Probing questions. These are an important tool of questioning. It is the technique of getting *specific* information from the client by asking additional or incidental questions on the topic (see Unit 8, Element 2).

Here are some examples of probing questions in the context of a woman, aged 26, complaining that her husband is physically abusive to her; she wonders whether she should get a divorce.

What is their marriage like outside the times of abuse?
What good points (if any) does their marriage have?
Are there other defects in their marriage?
What type of abuse? When does it occur? Is it in public/ private?
Is it after a specific event? (e.g. when he comes back from the pub, or comes home from work)
Does she react immediately to the abuse or some time later?
How long has it been going on?
How he (and she) feels about it, afterwards?
Has she discussed it with him? Results?
What previous 'solutions' have they tried?
Is he willing to seek help?

By this technique of probing, the carer can build up a detailed picture of the situation and the surrounding circumstances. It is important, however, not to allow the client to feel that they are being interrogated in a systematic way.

The questions would have to be asked in a way relevant to the clients and their needs. Likewise all this information may not all surface in one short meeting. It may be painful and embarrassing for the client and therefore time is required to obtain a complete picture. While questioning, therefore, be careful to *avoid* the following:

- patronising responses
- inaccurate empathy
- advice giving
- judgmental remarks
- over-use of probes (making the client feel grilled).
- closed, irrelevant or inappropriate questions.
- jargon responses
- condescending responses
- general, inappropriate comments

Secondary methods of assessment

This section describes how **secondary sources** can be used to obtain information about a client. It will approach the subject from the following four areas:

- relatives
- advocates
- support networks
- medical records

Relatives

Relatives can be a useful source of information. They may have lived with the client in the present or in the past and know individual details about the client. They can confirm information obtained directly from the client. They are also a useful support mechanism to be involved in the caring process.

Advocates

Information can also be obtained from **advocates**, e.g.:

- friends of the client – at school, club, work, in the neighbourhood
- neighbours
- work associated persons such as colleagues/boss/employees

Support networks

The carer may encourage the client to use a selection of the following examples of **support networks**:

Services for children and their families:

Health visitors
Children's home
Child minding
Day nurseries
Hospital
School
After school play schemes
Play groups
Toy library
NSPCC child time
Playgrounds
Gingerbread
One o'clock clubs
Teenage/children clubs
Cubs/scouts other youth groups for boys
Guides/brownies other youth groups for girls
Social workers
Other voluntary agencies

Services for elderly people:

Health visitors
Residential homes – long term
Respite care – short term
Sheltered housing
Day centre
Luncheon club
Home help
Pensions association
Age concern
Library services – mobile
Hospital

Services for people with, or recovering from, a mental illness:

Many of the above are available here plus:

Group homes
Community psychiatric nurse
Counselling
Adult education
Services for people with physical disabilities
Many of the above plus
Special equipment/adaptations
Occupational therapist
Care attendant
Welfare rights-mobility and attendance allowances
Physiotherapy
Laundry service

Services for those with a mental handicap:

– as above plus

Holidays
Sheltered employment
Adult training centres
Advisory services
Sports
Support groups
Home funding

These lists are not exclusive or complete but show a range of support networks available for different types of clients. These are useful for helping the client feel part of the community and encouraging participation with others.

Medical records

These are to be used to complete a view on the history and present medical condition of the client. **Medical records** can be used to confirm various points that the client has stated.

The medical records will also explain what medications have been given before, and the results. A carer can also find out information that may not be forthcoming directly from the client – e.g. incontinence – due to client embarrassment.

Clients rights with respect to assessment

These are described while looking at

- independence
- identity maintenance
- choice and control
- confidentiality

Independence (example – accommodation)

Clients have the right to their own **independence**. Clients who wish to stay in their own accommodation, as long as there is not a safety issue, have that right.

Identity maintenance

Clients rights to **identity maintenance** includes;

- privacy
- respect for dignity
- individuality
- right to take risks
- individual choice
- allowing client to achieve their own goals
- confidentially

Choice and control

It is important that the client is given the relevant information, so that they can make informed **choices** and thereby have **control** over their destiny. The information therefore needs to be presented to the client in a way that the client can understand, digest and then use as a basis for making informed decisions.

Confidentiality

The client needs to have the security of knowing that the assessment will be in **confidence**.

Principles of confidentiality for carers include:

- information should be used only for the purpose for which it was given.
- information about a client should normally not be shared without permission of the client involved, and even then only on a strict 'need to know' basis.
- all confidential information should be vigorously safeguarded.

Laws have been introduced to ensure that *computerised information* relating to a client is:

- obtained fairly
- kept up to date
- stored securely
- the client has a right to see and check the accuracy of the information.

- Recent acts include;

- Data Protection Act 1984
- Access to Personal Files Act 1987
- Access to Health Records Act 1990

Self Check ✓ **Element 2**

9. To obtain information from a client it is important to: 'listen genuinely, try to have eye contact and remain relaxed at all times'.
   True or False?

10. When trying to obtain information from the client it is important not to
    1 pretend to listen
    2 impose your views on the client
    3 rush the session
    4 give the client time to answer
    Choice
    A 1, 3, 4
    B 2, 3, 4
    C 1, 2, 3
    D 2, 1, 4

11. (i) A structured interview is when all the questions are devised beforehand, and are strictly observed.
    (ii) A semi-structured interview is similar to a

---

structured interview method, but the questions can be adapted or changed as the interview develops.
True or False?

12. Types of questions used are:
    1 closed
    2 open
    3 probing
    Match each of these to one of the answers below
    A used for 'teasing out' detailed information
    B the clients can express themselves
    C only one answer possible

13. In relation to care plans it is important not to give relevant information to the client, in case they interfere with the arrangements being made about their care.
    True or False?

14. Information needs to be presented to the client in a way that the client can understand.
    True or False?

15. Which of the following laws have been introduced to ensure that the client can be aware of computerised information relating to himself or herself?
    1 Data Protection Act 1984
    2 Access to Personal Files Act 1987
    3 Access to Health Records Act 1990
    4 Access to Personal Information Act 1992

16. All clients should be treated equally no matter what age, gender, sexual orientation, culture, religions, disability or ethnic background they come from.
    True or False?

7.3 Purpose of monitoring and evaluation in care plans

Monitoring progress in order to adapt care plans

This section looks at the purpose of monitoring progress in order to **adapt** care plans by looking at:

physical ability
cognitive ability
cultural influences
identity

Care plans have to be reviewed and monitored regularly. This process should be with the knowledge and agreement of the client in question.

The person who is responsible for assessment and implementation of care plans should also be responsible for the monitoring process. They should co-ordinate the monitoring process, bringing together all the people involved with the client's care, e.g. purchasing agents, service providers, managers who oversee the quality of their own services, clients themselves (contribute as well as being service users).

Physical ability

Over time **physical ability** changes. This can be a gradual process over years or an immediate concern after, say, an accident. Therefore regular monitoring and assessment is required.

Health authorities and social services can provide, as required, the following equipment at different stages of physical need.

– air ring cushions	– toilet aids
– bed cradles	– bath aids
– ripple mattress	– bath hoists
– continence aids	– over-bed tables
– commodes	– orthopaedic chairs
– sputum mugs	– dressing aids
– hoists	– special cutlery
– fracture boards	– kitchen aids
– walking aids	– stair lifts
– wheel chairs	– household aids
– voice amplifiers	– permanent hand rails
– voice amplifiers	– permanent hand rails
– feeding cups	– ramps
	– showers

This could be provided as part of a long term plan as agreed with the client.

Cognitive ability

Cognitive ability changes with time. A patient's condition could gradually deteriorate (e.g. senile dementia) and it may not be that obvious to begin with. It is important that regular monitoring takes place so that changes in the clients condition can be assessed and the care plan altered accordingly.

Cultural influences

There are many **cultural influences** which determine the expectations that individuals may have about care. When monitoring and evaluating care plans it is important to be *aware* of the cultural needs involved. For example in some cultures it is expected to cry and wail in response to emotional problems or to pain. This may not be understood by those from a different culture and may even be embarrassing to some.

Identity

If the clients circumstances change, for example the client becomes house-bound for a period of time, they could lose their sense of **identity**. It is important to adapt the care plan to meet such needs, for example arranging for the client to be taken to various groups which have previously been important to them in maintaining and developing their self-image.

Self Check ✓ **Element 3**

17. Cognitive ability does not change over a period of time. True or False?

18. A person who is responsible for assessment and implementation of care plans should not be responsible for the monitoring process of care plans. True or False?

19. It is important to review care plans
    - A every 3 years
    - B regularly
    - C not review
    - D only after 5 years

20. The delivery of service in the care plan should
    - A be kept a secret
    - B not be written into the care plan
    - C be written into the care plan
    - D be written down but kept by the person responsible for monitoring the care.

21. An 'informal carer' is:
    - A A carer who works in the private sector
    - B An unqualified carer
    - C A trainee carer
    - D An unpaid carer

Unit Test

Question 1
Task – orientated care means:

A   All tasks for a particular carer are performed by one carer.
B   Different carers focus on different tasks.
C   Clients are encouraged to carry out tasks for themselves.
D   Clients are shown how to carry out tasks.

Question 2
Individual care means:

A   A wide range of specialist carers are involved in the care of a single client.
B   All tasks for a particular client are performed by one carer.
C   The client is responsible for his/her own care.
D   Placing a hospital patient in a private room.

Question 3
Decide whether each of these statements is True (T) or False (F)
(i)   Care plans should be related to the personal needs of the client.
(ii) Care plans are confidential and should never be discussed with the client.

Which option best describes the two statements?

A   (i) T   (ii) T
B   (i) T   (ii) F
C   (i) F   (ii) T
D   (i) F   (ii) F

Question 4
In what order should individual care plans be developed?

(i)   Review and evaluation
(ii)   Devising a care plan for the client
(iii) Referral of client
(iv) Implementing a care plan
(v)   Monitoring and assessing the care plan

Is it
A   (iii), (ii), (iv), (v), (i)
B   (i), (ii), (iii), (iv), (v)
C   (ii), (iii), (v), (i), (iv)
D   (iii), (v), (ii), (iv), (i)

Question 5–8 share answer options A–D
Ways of assessing client need include:

A   Verbal reports
B   Observations
C   Using secondary sources
D   Consulting medical records

Which of these methods are illustrated by the following examples?

Question 5
In hospital, a patient's files are checked for details of previous medication.

Question 6
A client is interviewed and invited to discuss his/her needs.

Question 7
A district nurse on a home visit notices that a client is anxious and distressed.

Question 8
A doctor receives a letter from a man living in Australia expressing concern about his mother, who is one of the doctor's patients.

Question 9
Clients' rights with respect to assessment include which two of the following:

(i)   A written assessment report within 14 days
(ii)   Confidentiality
(iii) Identity maintenance
(iv) A written assessment report within 30 days

Is it?
A   (i) and (ii)
B   (ii) and (iii)
C   (iii) and (iv)
D   (i) and (iv)

Question 10
If information about a client is to be passed on to other members of the care team, it is important:

A   To protect the client by ensuring he does not find out
B   To explain to the client why you are doing this
C   To ask the client if he feels this would be an appropriate course of action
D   To ensure that other members of the care team do not let the client know that this has happened.

Question 11
Ways of obtaining information needed to make an assessment include how many of the following?

(i)   Observing the client's physical condition and general behaviour
(ii)   Taking into account the client's personal circumstances
(iii) Questioning the client
(iv) Obtaining reports from other sources

Is it?
A   (i), (ii), (iii), (iv)
B   (i), (ii), (iii)
C   (i), (iii), (iv)
D   (ii), (iii), (iv)

Question 12
How many of the following factors could affect a client's assessment?

(i)   The client's attitude towards being assessed
(ii)   Time restrictions
(iii) Not enough information about the client
(iv) The client's attitude towards the carer

Is it?
A   (i), (ii) and (iii)
B   (ii) and (iii)
C   (i), (iii) and (iv)
D   (i), (ii), (iii) and (iv)

Question 13
According to Maslow's hierarchy of needs, the first needs that have to be satisfied are:

A   Social
B   Physical
C   Safety
D   Self-esteem

Questions 14–17 share answer options A–D
Personal needs can be divided into the following five areas:

A Physical needs
B Emotional needs
C Cognitive needs
D Identity needs
E Cultural needs
Which of these needs are illustrated by the following examples?

Question 14
The need to develop a sense of oneself from contact with others

Question 15
The need for food and shelter

Question 16
The need for intellectual stimulation

Question 17
The need for support and sympathy from loved ones

Question 18
Decide whether each of these statements is True (T) or False (F)

(i)   Monitoring should take place throughout the implementation of a care plan.
(ii) Monitoring of a care plan should take place, but once the plan has been devised it should not be altered.

Which option best describes the two statements?

A (i) T   (ii) T
B (i) T   (ii) F
C (i) F   (ii) T
D (i) F   (ii) F

Question 19
Assessment of the physical condition of a client will include how many of the following:

(i)   Appearance
(ii) Morale
(iii) Mobility and suppleness
(iv) Strength and stamina

Is it

A (i), (ii) and (iii)
B (ii), (iii) and (iv)
C (i), (iii) and (iv)
D (i), (ii) and (iv)

Question 20
Assessment of a client's needs should take account of sensory impairment. Which one of the following is an example of sensory impairment?

A Senile Dementia
B Deafness
C Memory loss
D Inability to walk up stairs

Question 21–24 share answer options A–D
The following are four types of interview that might take place with a client:

A Structured interview
B Semi-structured interview
C Focused interview
D Open ended interview

Which of these types of interview describe the following?

Question 21
The conversation does not have a set framework and develops its own way.

Question 22
The questions are prepared beforehand and methodically worked through.

Question 23
The interview concentrates on a specific topic though questions are not prepared in advance.

Question 24
The interview has a definite framework though there is some flexibility within this.

Question 25
Which of the following best describes what is meant by a probing question?

A A question that is unnecessarily intrusive.
B A question that is asked as a preliminary to more searching questions.
C A question that seeks to elicit further information.
D A question asked at the very beginning of an interview to ascertain a client's state of mind.

Question 26
Which of the following is an example of a closed question?

A How did you get on with your parents?
B What is your address?
C Why did you decide to move?
D How are you feeling today?

Question 27
Decide whether each of these statements is True (T) or False (F)

(i) A care plan should involve the client's family.
(ii) A care plan should only involve the client.

Which option best describes the two statements.

A (i)   T   (ii)   T
B (i)   T   (ii)   F
C (i)   F   (ii)   T
D (i)   F   (ii)   F

Question 28
The Access to Health Records Act 1990:

A Grants access to a client's health records to all parties involved in the case of the client.
B Stipulates that health records can only be seen by the person who has compiled them.
C Grants clients access to their own health records.
D Restricts access to health records to qualified medical personnel.

Question 29
Which one of the following is an example of a cultural need?

A A client likes to keep his mind alert by tackling crossword puzzles.
B A hospital patient complains she is cold and asks for an extra blanket.
C A client is distressed and needs emotional support.
D A client wishes to fast on a particular day because it is a religious festival.

Question 30
Monitoring of a care plan serves which two of the following purposes?

(i)   The plan can be adapted to take account of the changing needs of the client.
(ii) It ensures that details of the care plan remain confidential and unknown to the client.
(iii) The client's feelings about the progress of the care plan can be ascertained.
(iv) It ensures that the care plan continues to be rigidly applied.

Is it?

A (i) and (ii)
B (i) and (iii)
C (ii) and (iii)
D (iii) and (iv)

Answers to Self-check Questions

1. Task Oriented Care – care worker carries out one task for all clients.
   Individual Care – carer performs all the tasks and care for one client.

2. Maslow develops five categories of need and the higher needs cannot be satisfied if the lower ones are not first met. See page 144.

3. Their general appearance, strength, stamina, mobility and suppleness etc.

4. This can be shown as four phases:
   1 – assessment of the client
   2.– planning their care
   3. – implementation of care plan
   4. – monitoring and reviewing the care plan.
   The four phases are sometimes broken down and shown as a 7-point plan (see page 145).

5. True. A macro care plan will also identify the overall needs of the client.

6. False. A micro care plan describes the action plan of an individual service provider, e.g. home help.

7. B. These stages can sometimes be further broken down into a 7-point plan.

8. C. It is important to the development of the care plan that it is carried out in the right order, to ensure good qualities of care for the client.

9. True. It is also important to remember that the carer must put the client at ease.

10. C. It is also important not to interrupt or put words into the client's mouth. The carer should also never take sides when dealing with clients.

11. True. It is important to use the correct method when trying to gather information about a client.

12. 1 = C, 2 = B, 3 = A
    It is important for you to know which types of questions you are using.

13. False. It is important to give the client the relevant information, so that they can make informed choices and thereby have control over their destiny.

14. True. The client can then digest the information and use it as a basis for making informed decisions.

15. 2, 3 and 4. The client also has a right to see and check the accuracy of the information.

16. True. A carer must be aware that discrimination can take many forms.

17. False. A client's condition could gradually deteriorate i.e. senile dementia.

18. False. They should co-ordinate the monitoring process and bring together all the people involved with the client's care.

19. B. This is important to make sure that appropriate care is given and that the care plan can be changed/updated regularly.

20. C. The care given by friends, relatives and neighbours should also be written into the care plan.

21. D. Someone qualified as a carer may still help a relative in an unpaid capacity (hence not B) – and be in this sense an informal carer.

Answers to Unit Test

Question	Answer	Question	Answer	Question	Answer	Question	Answer	Question	Answer	Question	Answer
1.	B	6.	A	11.	A	16.	C	21.	D	26.	B
2.	B	7.	B	12.	D	17.	B	22.	A	27.	B
3.	B	8.	C	13.	B	18.	B	23.	C	28.	C
4.	A	9.	B	14.	D	19.	C	24.	B	29.	D
5.	D	10.	B	15.	A	20.	B	25.	C	30.	B

Unit Test Comments (selected questions)

Question 3
B. Care plans are extremely confidential but it is a shared confidentiality between carers and clients.

Question 5
D. C is also correct here but D is preferable because it is a more precise answer.

Question 10
B. In some situations it may be appropriate to ask the client's opinion, but C implies that too much responsibility is placed upon the client – that too much of the burden of decision-making is transferred from the carer to the client.

Question 11
A. All of these actions can help when making an assessment.

Question 12
D. Again, all of these factors could come into play.

Question 18
B. A care plan should not be inflexible. One of the main purposes served by monitoring is that appropriate and necessary adjustment can be made.

Question 20
B. A and C are examples of mental impairment, and D is an example of physical impairment.

Question 26
B. A closed question invites a specific, limited response.

Question 27
B. (ii) would obviously be true if the client has no relatives, but generally it is important to enlist the co-operation of the client's family in care plans.

Question 30
B. (ii) is incorrect because the care plan should be made known to, and agreed with, the client. (iv) is incorrect because a care plan should be flexible and adjustments made when necessary.

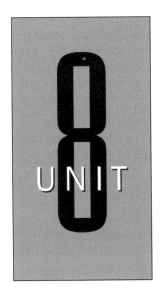

Research in health and social care

Getting Started

This unit is made up of three elements:

Element 1	Investigate types of research used in health and social care.
Element 2	Construct a structured research instrument to survey opinion.
Element 3	Investigate methods of interpreting information.

This unit investigates the types of research used in Health and Social Care. In Element 8.1 we introduce questionnaires, interviews and observation techniques and look at the advantages and disadvantages of each method. Element 8.2 looks at how you might construct a structured research instrument, such as a questionnaire, noting the importance of the types of questions and prompts to be used. In Element 8.3 we examine quantitative and qualitative research and how to present the information gathered in graph, table and text forms, including the basic statistical methods you might adopt in displaying and analysing your data.

The following elements contain material relevant to this unit.

Cross-References
Communication with individuals (Unit 2 Element 1)
Promote communication within groups (Unit 2 Element 2)
The Portfolio

Much of the work in this unit is relevant to the development of your **portfolio**. From time-to-time you will be referred to pages in the next (portfolio) chapter of the book.

Case Study A detailed study of one particular individual or small group.

Controlled observation The deliberate setting up of a situation in which certain behaviour patterns can be observed.

Correlation The presence (or absence) of a relationship between two or more variables.

Covert observation Where researcher hides his /her identity and purpose from the subject being observed.

Cross sectional Usually the study of a person or group at a particular point in time.

Longitudinal Usually the study of a person or group through time.

Mean The simple average of everyday understanding.

Median The observation which is half-way in the distribution.

Mode The observation which occurs most often.

Naturalistic observation Observation in a natural setting e.g. home.

Overt observation Where researcher declares their intentions of observing behaviour before hand.

Participant observation Where the researcher himself/herself joins a group that is to be studied. Can be overt or covert.

Primary data Data you have obtained yourself.

Random sample One in which each person or item has an equal chance of selection.

Secondary data Data others have collected.

Standard deviation A measure of the spread or dispersion of a variable around its average.

8.1   Investigate types of research used in health and social care.

In this element we will investigate the ways in which research and sampling methods are relevant to health and social care, outlining the main advantages and disadvantages of each technique.

Sources of data

Data is a set of facts or figures. There are two types of data: primary data and secondary data.

Primary data   This is information that *you* obtain first-hand by carrying out your own investigations. Primary data would include, for example, the results of experiments you have set up and of questionnaires you have devised and distributed.

Secondary data   This is information collected by others or from books, newspaper and similar sources. Examples of secondary data might be information from the ten-year Population Census, from Social Trends or the Monthly Digest of Statistics, from a particular newspaper report, and so on.

Primary data

Advantages	Disadvantages
– The researcher can get the exact information required. – The information will be up to date.	– The researcher may collect more information than is required. You must be clear about what you want to achieve. A common error is to collect all the information related to the subject in question, only to find that far too much information has been collected, causing confusion. – The researcher may need to learn new skills to obtain the information needed. These skills may include survey design skills, computer inputting skills and analytical skills. – It can be time consuming and costly, both in manpower and other resources required.

Secondary data

Advantages	Disadvantages
– The information is readily available; for example from reference libraries. – It is a good starting point; this information can then be modified if required. – A wide range of information is available – including newspapers, periodicals, magazines, reference material from libraries and books.	– The information was compiled *without* your particular need in mind; i.e. it is other people's information. – Only certain information is available. – The information may be out of date. – Statistics are not always correct; problems of interpreting figures. – The information is available to everyone. – The information may conflict with other published material.

Due to the advantages and disadvantages of the above data sources many organisations and researchers use a *combination* of primary and secondary data. Often the starting point will be secondary data with specific primary data being sought to meet the needs of the project in question.

We look at sources of *primary data* in the next section. You will find a comprehensive list of sources of *secondary data* in the Portfolio chapter (pages. 180–188)

Data Collection

Collecting primary data

The most common methods of assembling **primary data** include the following:

- **Experiments**. Before deciding to carry out an experiment, consider whether there are any practical difficulties which may prevent a properly controlled experiment taking place. (In the example of the nursery experiment mentioned earlier, for instance, could you be sure that others would not speak to or distract the children as they were carrying out the tasks?) Another potential disadvantage of experiments is that in creating a controlled situation you are also creating an artificial environment, in which the circumstances of the experiment do not correspond to those of 'real life'. (See also page 158).

- **Observation**. This usually involves systematically observing the behaviour of a group or individual. If you take part in the activities that are being observed (you may for example be studying a group to which you belong) this is known as *participant observation*. If you do not take part (e.g. you observe a group but are not a member of it) *non-participant observation* takes place. Both these methods can be time-consuming, but if the assignment is based upon your work-placement or your school or college this may be less of a problem. Another drawback is that people may behave differently if they realise they are being observed. If you are observing them without their knowledge, ethical objections may arise (see next section, 'Ethical considerations'). Another form of observation is *self-recording*, which in effect involves asking the subjects of the research to observe themselves. If you are investigating teenage smoking habits, for example, you may ask a group of friends to make a note, each time they smoke a cigarette, of the time of day, where they are and who they are with. If you are considering using this research method you must again think about practicalities. Are you sure your subjects will keep an accurate record? They may not intend to give you misleading information, but pressures of time and other distractions may prevent them maintaining a complete record of their actions.

- **Surveys**. You might decide to carry out a survey among a group of people, in order to ascertain their needs or opinions, or to gain factual information from them. The two principal forms of survey are:
  (a) *Interviews* If a large number of interviews need to be conducted, this can again be time-consuming. If you re seeking similar information from each interviewee, it is important that similar questions are asked at each interview. One of the keys to

successful interviewing is careful preparation, and this will be discussed more fully on page 187.

(b) *Questionnaires* These are a way of avoiding the need to carry out a long series of face-to-face interviews (unless a questionnaire is used as the basis for the interviews), but there is a danger of a patchy response, especially if the questionnaires are sent through the post. Great care must be taken in framing the questions for the questionnaire (see page 160).

- **Case Studies**. A case study is an in-depth investigation of a specific situation – often of an individual client. Rather than focusing on one aspect of the situation, a case study aims to give a more comprehensive picture by looking at several different aspects and considering how they inter-relate. In a study of an individual client, for example, the client's medical history, family situation, financial circumstances and living conditions might all be considered. Correspondingly, a variety of research methods is likely to be used – interviews, observations, self-recording. You need to be sure that your subject is willing to co-operate, and that your research will not be intrusive. You also need to consider what your case study is intended to achieve. Usually the hope is that a close investigation of one person's experiences will enable helpful general conclusions to be drawn, which will throw light on the experiences of others who are in a similar situation.

Collecting secondary data

A detailed outline of the methods you might use in collecting secondary data, and the sources available, is presented in the Portfolio Chapter (pages 180–188).

Comparison of data collection techniques

In this section we need to understand the main advantages and disadvantages of different data collection techniques. We therefore look in more detail at some of the techniques previously mentioned.

INTERVIEWS AND QUESTIONNAIRES

Structured Interviews (Standardised Interviews)
Consist of a list of fixed questions.
Everyone interviewed is asked the same questions, in the same way, and in the same order.

Advantages	**Disadvantages**
– They are easily repeated.	– The information is limited, and non specific.
– The structure of interviews can be agreed in advance by all concerned.	– The respondent is not prompted by the interviewer; because of this the person being interviewed may be unable to develop an answer and therefore feel inhibited.
– It is easy to verify the results	

Unstructured Interviews (Personal)
Consist of an informal, relaxed discussion. Many topics can be discussed. The interviewer can probe and gain more information. The questions are not imposed on the respondent.

Advantages	**Disadvantages**
– They are more likely to reveal what the respondents actually think and feel.	– It is difficult to verify information.
– The interviewer can examine more complex issues, such as those involving personal views and feelings.	– It is time consuming, therefore expensive.
– It is possible to compare different ideas.	– The interview is hard to duplicate, therefore reliability of results may be in question.
	– Interview bias may be present which can influence the respondent's answer; respondents give the answers they think they ought too.
	– The interviewer needs lots of training and experience to perform unstructured interviews.
	– The respondent can be influenced by the interviewers age, appearance, accent, gender, race and class.

Questionnaires
Questionnaires are a list of questions which can be in many forms (see pages 160–161).

Advantages	**Disadvantages**
– They are relatively easily constructed.	– The number of possible answers is often limited, and therefore they cannot deal easily with complex issues.
– They are easy to analyse.	– Information may be interpreted in different ways.
– The samples are usually large, and relatively cheap to obtain compared to other methods.	– People may give the wrong information, either deliberately or by mistake.
– They can be conducted by face-to-face contact, post or telephone.	– The respondents may wish to present themselves as socially acceptable and therefore give answers which are expected.
	– With postal questionnaires, as high as 95% are not returned, so the views of non-respondents are unknown.

OBSERVATIONS

Observations fall into three categories: Naturalistic – Controlled – Participant. This approach involves observing behaviour and recording it, but making no attempt to control it. Observations are good for describing what happens, but not why it happens. Methods of recording observations include written notes, tape recordings, video-recordings and photographs.

Observations can be **overt**, when the researchers declare their intentions beforehand, or **covert**:, when the researchers hide their identity and purpose from the subject being observed.

Naturalistic observations

These occur in a natural setting, such as at school, home, work, or a hospital. An example could be observing the interaction between a mother and child during feeding time, or a nurse while at work. This would usually be carried out in a non-participatory way, e.g. when the researcher simply looks on and tries to be unobtrusive.

Advantages	Disadvantages
– Individuals are studied in a real-life setting.	– The researcher may not observe accurately.
– The researcher can study complete behaviour.	– People may act differently if they know that they are being observed.
– The researcher can study one aspect of behaviour in detail; for example babies at play.	– It can take a long time to complete a study because the researcher has to wait for behaviour to occur; as a result it can be expensive to carry out.
– Less artificial than other methods of research.	

Controlled observation

Controlled observation is the deliberate setting up of a situation in which certain behaviour can be observed, which may not be possible to do using naturalistic observation. Example: leaving a child alone with toys and waiting for the behaviour to occur (perhaps recording with the use of hidden cameras, or two way mirrors.) The persons or groups that are being observed may not be aware of the fact; this would be an example of covert observation.

Advantages	Disadvantages
Researchers can decide before-hand what they want to study. The observed are usually not aware that they are being watched; as a result they tend to act normally.	The researcher might have to wait a long time for the required behaviour to occur. The set-up costs may be high.

Participant observation

The researcher joins a (often) small group that is to be studied. The group is not aware that they are being observed. The researcher could join a doctors' practice as one of the receptionists to observe the length of time that doctors spend with male and females patients, perhaps to find out if it is the same for both sexes. This is also referred to as **participatory observation.**

Advantages	Disadvantages
The researchers can gain real insight into what is happening, as they become one of the group. Those observed tend to act naturally, being unaware of the presence of the observer.	– It is costly and time consuming; (could spend years on one study.)
	– The researcher could become too involved.
	– There can be problems with interpreting the information.
	– There can be the problem of bias with the researcher. For example, if the researcher gets too involved, the researcher might sympathise with the group.

Observation is a subjective method of research. Findings depend on the observations and interpretations of the researcher. It has a limited usefulness for generalisation to a large population. It is not easy, and sometimes impossible, to repeat the study.

Other techniques used in data collection and research are: case studies, experiments, longitudinal and cross sectional studies. We now look at each of these in turn.

CASE STUDIES AND EXPERIMENTS

Case study

This is a detailed study of one individual or a small group. For example the study of one child's social and emotional behaviour, physical development, abilities, home background and medical history. The main methods of obtaining information is by interviews and by examining case histories, such as medical records and school records.

Advantages	Disadvantages
The researcher can get a lot of detailed information about the behaviour and development of one individual, or a small group.	The sample is small, usually 1 person or a small group; as a result it is not easy to generalise. If children are involved, parents may not give accurate and reliable information about the child being studied.

Experiment

An experiment is a method in which the investigator manipulates one variable to see what effect it may have on another variable. The investigation usually takes place in a laboratory or other controlled situation. Information is gathered by treating the subjects in some way or giving them some tasks to perform.

Advantages	Disadvantages
– The researcher can establish a cause and effect relationship by manipulating one variable (the Independent Variable) to see what effect it has on another variable (the Dependent Variable).	– It is an artificial situation; not like real life.
– It can be repeated fairly easily under the same conditions.	– Children (and adults) may behave differently because they know they are being studied (the Hawthorne effect). The researcher may be biased and conduct the experiment so that it is likely to support his or her views.

LONGITUDINAL AND CROSS-SECTIONAL STUDIES

When studying children the researcher is often interested in looking at the development of behaviour over a period of years. For example, changes in the play behaviour of children from 1 year to 5 years. This can be done in one of two ways:

Longitudinal Study
In this approach the same group of individuals are studied at different ages *over a period of time* – often many years.

Advantages
- The same group is studied all the time, so the profile of development is clearer and more reliable.
- Generalisations from sample to population are more reliable.

Disadvantages
- It can take a long time to complete – often years.
- Loss of subjects – they may move and not leave a forwarding address, fall ill, or notes are lost.
- It can be expensive.
- Circumstances of subjects may change over the years (e.g. parents may divorce) which effects the normal course of development.

Cross-Sectional Study
In this approach, subjects in different age groups are studied *at the same time* to give some idea of the course of development over a period of years.

Advantages
It does not take as long as a longitudinal study. There is little danger of loss of subjects.

Disadvantages
The picture of development may not be as good as in the longitudinal study because subjects in the different age groups may not be comparable.

Sampling Methods

In this section we identify four different types of sampling methods: (a) **Random**, (b) **Quota**, (c) **Stratified** and (d) **Opportunity** sampling methods.

If your research involves a survey of some kind, it may be necessary to select a sample from the total population of potential subjects. In statistics, a 'population' is the total number of people in a particular group. If you were investigating client needs at a local health centre, for example, the population would be all the clients who use the health centre. If your survey population is small it may be possible to interview each member of it, or to ask each one to complete a questionnaire. If the population is large, however, this becomes impossible and sampling has to take place.

Imagine for instance that you wish to assess your fellow students' knowledge of preventive health services (cancer screening, immunisation etc.). If the study was confined to your own class, you could probably include every student in the survey. If you wanted to investigate the entire student population of your school or college, it would be more sensible to use a sample. To select the sample you could use one of two common methods:

Random sample
Here every person has an equal chance of being selected. You could simply pick names out of a hat, but random sampling is usually approached more systematically than this, as care must be taken to ensure that the sample is truly representative. Suppose for example that for your preventive health services survey you decided to distribute questionnaires to 1 in 20 of the college student population. You might simply stand outside the college gates on Monday morning and hand out questionnaires to every twentieth person entering the college. If you later discovered that several classes did not attend college on Mondays (because of work placements, for example) your sample would not be representative. In any case, some students would inevitably be absent for other reasons (e.g. ill health) so simply stopping 1 in 20 of those coming into college would not ensure that your questionnaires reached 1 in 20 of the student population. A better approach might be to approach the college office and ask for access to a computer print-out of enroled students; you could then select every twentieth name from this list.

Quota sample
Here the sample is selected according to certain specific criteria. If the survey population has a wide age-range, for example, the sample might comprise five individuals aged between 20 and 30, five aged between 30 and 40, and so on. In the case of the preventive health services survey, you might decide to select four students from each department of the college.

Pilot study
Conducting a few 'mini-surveys' as a pilot study will help you to check the accuracy of your sampling method. If the samples are truly representative, the results of each survey should be similar.

In your final report you should explain clearly how many people were involved in the study, and how they were selected. If a pilot study took place this should also be described.

Stratified (layer) sample
This is used to give the representation to the various 'layers' or sub-groups, within the population. The sample is chosen so that if, say, 30% of the *population* is composed of women under 40 years, then 30% of the *sample* will be women under 40 years. In this way the sample then reflects the attributes among the population, e.g. the proportion of law, middle and high income earners. The particular individuals selected for the sample *within* each strata (layer) may be selected randomly.

Opportunity sample
This is where researchers are faced with an (often unexpected) opportunity of studying a particular individual or group, perhaps suffering from an unusual disease or being in unusual circumstances. This is a convenient, but not necessarily representative, means of devising a sample.

Self Check ✓ Element 1

1. Explain the difference between primary and secondary data sources.

2. Identify four ways of collecting primary data.

3. List 3 advantages and 3 disadvantages of each of the following
   (a) Unstructured interviews
   (b) Questionnaire
   (c) Naturalistic observation.

4. What is a target population?

5. What is a sample?

6. Why study samples of people?

7. Explain what is meant by:
   (a) Random Sample
   (b) Quota Sample.

8. What must the researcher be sure of before generalisation can be made of their results to the wider population?

9. Do you think that hospital clients could be representative of the wider society? Discuss.

10. Distinguish between cross-sectional and longitudinal studies.

8.2 Structured research

This element is designed to help you construct a structured research instrument to survey opinion.

Defining the research problem

It is vital that you know what you want to find out and the different types of information that will be required. Therefore the research problem needs to be clearly defined.

In research work a **hypothesis** is often used. This is a statement at the beginning of the research which proposes a tentative idea about the relationship between two variables or conditions. The hypothesis to be tested is called the **null hypothesis**. The **alternative hypothesis** is the hypothesis against which you test the null hypothesis. For example:

Null hypothesis: women between 40 and 50 years are most at risk from breast cancer.
Alternative hypothesis: there is no age factor affecting the risk of women contracting breast cancer.

Having stated your hypothesis you must identify the *sources of information* needed to test your hypothesis. As we have seen, should you require *primary data* then you must select between the following methods of acquiring such data, bearing in mind the advantages/disadvantages already outlined for each.

- experiment
- observation
- survey
- questionnaires
- interviews
- case studies

Types of questions and responses

In all these methods you may be involved in asking *questions* of respondents. You need to be aware of the different types of questions and responses you might use or encounter.

Open and closed questions

There are two main types of questions: open and closed. In an **open question** the respondent's answer is not restricted. An example of an open question is 'Why do you think a balanced diet is important?' The respondent is free to reply as he or she wishes. **Closed questions**, which invite a more limited reply, take various forms. They are much easier than open questions to analyse afterwards. Although most questions in a questionnaire should be closed, it is a good idea to have at least one question inviting more general comment at the end of the questionnaire. Open-ended answers may be hard to analyse, but they do produce accurate and often interesting information.

Types of closed question

There are six major forms of closed question:

1. **Tick one box.** Respondents in a questionnaire are asked questions and invited to answer by placing a tick against one of several answers on the form.
   Example
   I feel that the media coverage of National No Smoking Day was:

Biased in favour	☐
Neutral	☐
Biased against	☐

2. **Rating scales.** Here some dimension of feeling, opinion or attitude is expressed as two extremes, with a number of intermediate points also available.
   Example
   How would you rate access to leisure facilities for the disabled in your area?

Very good	☐
Good	☐
Average	☐
Bad	☐
Very bad	☐

3. **Checklists of descriptive words or phrases.** The respondent is asked to tick all of those which apply to him or her.
   Example
   What did you like about this assignment? (Tick as many boxes as you wish.)

More freedom than usual	☐
Being able to work on my own	☐
Being able to work at home	☐
Discussing my work with my tutor	☐

4. **Yes/No.** Choosing a single 'Yes' or 'No' answer to a question.
   Example
   Did you find talking about your feelings helpful?

Yes	☐
No	☐

5. **Ranking.** Here several items (usually not more than about six or eight) are numbered by the respondent in order of importance.

Example

The following have been said to be advantages and benefits of assignment work. Put them in order of importance by placing 1 alongside the statement you consider most important, 2 alongside the next most important and so on.

Improves analytical skills	☐
Makes work more interesting	☐
Helps you to work as part of a team	☐
Gives understanding of practical problems	☐
Helps you to become more independent	☐
Helps you to look at issues in greater depth	☐

6. **Semantic differential**. Like 2 above but with a *bi-polar* scale often used for each response, such as:

fair – unfair;
good – bad;
strong – weak;
active – passive;
fast – slow

Often used for measuring attitudes or opinions.

Advantages/disadvantages of question types:

Open Questions

Advantages	**Disadvantages**
– Allow self expression	– Difficult to analyse
– Allow for answers that the researcher has not considered	– Time consuming Numerous areas covered
– The respondent can develop a point being made	

Closed Questions

Advantages	**Disadvantages**
– It is simple to analyse the results either manually or by a computer. There is no personal choice allowed by the respondent.	– Difficult to analyse
	– Time consuming
– As computers can be used to analyse the returned data, a large sample can be used *without* a delay occurring at the analysis stage.	– 'Leading' questions have to be used as the respondents cannot add their own comments.
– These types of question are easy for respondents to complete. Little effort is required to tick one box from a choice of two boxes.	– There is less chance of new and unexpected information being obtained from the questions asked.
– They enable people who cannot speak to communicate, i.e. make choices; e.g. a geriatric patient in a nursing home who cannot speak can shake or nod their head to answer.	

Question development

– It is important that the wording of the questions are clear, unambiguous and non threatening.
– It is important that the questions are understood; it is a good idea to try the questions out first by carrying out a *pilot* (a small scale survey) to see that the answers are along the lines expected.

Some factors to consider when preparing a questionnaire:
– The question must be kept simple
– They must be written in language that the respondent can understand.
– The questions should produce the types of answer that are expected.
– The questions asked should not be too personal
– Irrelevant questions should not be asked
– It is important that the right amount of questions are asked, not too many or too few. Refer back to the original purpose of the questionnaire. Do you really need to know the answers to some of the questions you have asked?
– Leading or suggestive questions should not be asked; e.g. Don't you agree that female doctors are more understanding than male doctors?
– Questions must not be ambiguous or confusing; e.g. Do you feel better or worse after your appointment with the consultant?

Tick One
☐ yes
☐ no
☐ maybe
☐ don't know

Question order and layout

The first few questions are normally of an easy nature to 'warm up' the respondent. For example; initial questions should consist of questions like:

Name and Address (if appropriate)
Male or female (please tick box)
Age (if necessary) This could be the exact date or indicated by a range of scales.
Marital status.

More personal questions such as:

Have you been tested for the HIV virus?
How much do you earn?
How often do you have sex?

would need to be asked later on during the questionnaire, if they were to be used at all. The exact wording would have to be thoroughly investigated *before* the questionnaire is used. It is important to consider:

- the topics which are going to be included in the questionnaire
- the questions which will be asked
- the number of questions which are going to be asked
- the number of questions which will be of the open and closed type
- which questions will include *follow-up* questions; e.g. If you answered Yes, now go to question 3; if you answered No, go to question 4.
- how useful the questions will be in providing information which can be analysed easily

Also remember the following:

- The questions should have a logical order.
- The printing, spacing, typing, can all affect how a question is interpreted. Have any of the questions got diagrams, pictures or charts associated with them? These all need to be positioned correctly on the page.

What happens after the questionnaire has been completed? This also has to be clear. Does the respondent post it back to a specific address? Has the postage been paid? Has his been explained? Is there a covering letter required? Is the questionnaire put into a box in the waiting room of the doctors, or given to the receptionist Has the issue of confidentially been covered? Has the respondent been identified by the questionnaire, or is the respondent anonymous? What affect may this have on the results obtained?

A structured questionnaire can lead a respondent down various avenues by the use of the technique of **funnelling**. For example: 'if you answered yes, go to Q2, if no go to Q3'. This can continue at questions 2 and 3 to funnel respondents further down the structured questionnaire.

You can find more applications and discussion of survey techniques, including questionnaires, in the Portfolio chapter which follows.

Self Check ✓ **Element 2**

11. What is a hypothesis?

12. What is a Null hypothesis?

13. Explain the difference between open and closed questions.

14. Describe, with examples, 4 different types of closed question.

15. List 3 advantage and 3 disadvantages of
    (a) open questions
    (b) closed questions

16. Write down your own example for each of the following types of closed question
    (a) Rating scales
    (b) Checklists
    (c) Ranking
    (d) Semantic differential

17. Identify some principles which may help you decide on the types of questions to use in a questionnaire.

18. What is 'funnelling'

19. The following question is an example of a closed question.

When did you give up smoking?   tick one box
up to 6 months ago   ☐
up to a year ago   ☐
1–4 years ago   ☐
over 4 years ago   ☐

However, what more *specific types* of information about smokers and non-smokers might be missed by this closed-question?

8.3 Investigating methods of Interpreting information

This Element looks at various types of research, the presentation of data and the use of various statistical methods in analysing and interpreting data.

Types of research

- **Quantitative research** involves the use of numbers in the search which are usually obtained by counting or measuring some aspect of behaviour. This type of quantitative research is useful for giving insights into amounts and frequency of use, but it has limitations. For example a structured interview or questionnaire which is investigating drug taking in teenagers might concentrate the questions around how often and how much they take the substance while ignoring the *circumstances* in which it is taken, such as at parties or because of a lack of job, boredom or poverty. Failure to understand and *reasons* behind why young people take drugs, may limit the uses which can be made of the research

- **Qualitative research** is research which cannot easily be quantified, i.e. converted into a number format. Examples include:

  - case studies
  - informal interviews
  - diaries
  - introspective reports

Respondents explain how they have experienced an event or their feelings about the event. This type of information is useful for understanding the meaning people give to their actions.

Reliability and validity of data
Reliability refers to the extent to which a method of data collection gives a consistent and reproducible result when used by other researchers at another time. The use of *standardised* questions in a social survey investigation may help reliability. So too would a tightly controlled *experimental* investigation (see page 191).

Validity refers to whether a test measures that what it is supposed to measure. Does an intelligence test accurately measure intelligence?

The reliability and the validity of data are different. High reliability indicates nothing about validity.

Sources of error

Potential **sources of error** arise from the collection methods, analysis methods and the interpretation of data. These include:

- leading questions
- non-response
- misuse of statistics
- sampling errors.

Leading questions

Leading questions are ones which are so phrased that they almost invite a particular response. This includes, for example, questions which being 'Do you agree that...?' Such a question tends to suggest that the respondent should answer 'Yes'.

Interviewers who are not trained can interact with the respondent and thereby alter the respondents replies. This can be a form of leading the respondent.

A subtle form of leading can also cause the respondent to want to please the interviewer; and this encourages the respondent to reply with the answer that they believe the interviewer wants to hear. This is a form of distortion and therefore causes errors.

Non-response

The *type* of research method used will affect the number of respondents, and the number of non-respondents. Postal questionnaires typically get less than a 5% response rate. Telephone questionnaires can get higher results if administered carefully.

Response rates to personal surveys depend on the *setting* of the respondents. If you are trying to get patients views as they leave a busy hospital you most likely will be less successful than in a warm doctors surgery when respondents have to wait for the doctor anyway.

Likewise certain *types of people* are more inclined to complete a questionnaire than other people. A person who does not speak or write clear English may be less inclined to participate, than someone familiar with the language.

A danger with a high *non-response rate* is that when you analyse the data of those who *have* responded, you may get a biased or misleading result. For example, if those who wish to *avoid* a certain outcome respond more readily to a questionnaire, then your results may over estimate the opposition to a particular course of action; or vice versa.

Misuse of statistics

In the later parts of this Unit (pages 164–170) and in the following chapter on the Portfolio you will find many examples of the use and misuse of statistical information; for example changing the *scale* of an axis to show a line rising more or less steeply, depending on the effect desired; changing the *values* at which the labelling of the axis begin; selecting only statistical data which supports a *particular viewpoint*; and so on.

Be especially careful when using statistical information provided by sources which have a vested interest in a particular issue.

Sampling errors

If a sample is being used, then by definition an error is being introduced as the complete population is not being used. If **random sampling** is used, i.e. each respondent has an equal chance of being chosen to become part of the sample, then errors are calculable. However, unless every possible respondent has an equal chance of inclusion then the sample is **non-random**. For example, if you are completing a questionnaire at a few hospitals in your local area, then respondents further afield will not have the opportunity to be included in the sample. This will increase the probability of error if you try to *generalise* your result to all hospitals. It may be that patients from higher income groups are admitted to that hospital, so that a survey of attitudes is not representative of typical patients.

Presentation of data

Data which is untreated is called **raw data**. In research our aim is to treat the raw data so that if becomes more meaningful, e.g. revealing patterns and trends. Here we look at how we can use various types of table, graph and chart to present information and data.

The ability to construct and interpret statistical diagrams is also a requirement of the Core Skills Unit 'Application of Number'. It is important however to choose the right form of presentation. You should consider carefully the advantages and disadvantages of the alternative available to you and decide which method of presentation is the most appropriate for the findings you have to present.

Note that a spreadsheet programme (see page 170) makes it possible to use a computer to present numerical information in many of the forms discussed here (line graphs, bar and pie charts and so on). Using a computer in this way would help you to satisfy the requirements of the Information Technology Core Skills unit.

Tables

Tables are the most straightforward method of presentation. An advantage of them is that the results of the research can be easily seen. However, they can be visually less effective than other forms of presentation and harder to interpret, especially if a lot of information has to be shown – patterns may not emerge clearly from rows of figures. For this reason it is sometimes appropriate to present the information *initially* in the form of a table and then in another form (a line graph or bar chart, for example) so that trends or patterns in the findings become more apparent.

If you use a table try not to include more information than is necessary but make sure that the columns are clearly labelled. Below is a table resulting from a survey of teenage drinking habits. Forty teenagers aged 16–19 (ten from each of the possible ages) were asked whether they exceeded the recommended maximum sensible amount of 21 alcohol units per week.

Alcohol units per week	16	17	18	19
0–21 units	8	6	5	6
22 units and above	2	4	5	4

Of course a pre-requisite to presenting a table may be to organise your *raw data* into **groups**. This is considered in more detail on page 168.

Line graphs

Line graphs are one way of showing changes and trends more clearly. They can be used to indicate the relationship between two variables. In the case of the teenage drinking survey, for example, you want to establish if there is any significant relationship between the ages of teenagers and the amount that they drink. A line graph will help you to see if your findings suggest there is such a relationship.

The first stage in constructing a line graph is to sort your data into two groups of figures. One of these groups will be plotted on horizontal axis (known as the 'x' axis) and the other on the vertical axis)known as the 'y' axis). It is usual to place the dependent variable on the 'y' axis and the independent variable on the 'x' axis. You may recall that the terms 'dependent and independent variable' were defined on page 158. Essentially, the dependent variable is something that is determined by, or depends upon, another variable. In the case of the teenage drinking survey, the dependent variable is the amount of alcohol consumed because its value depends upon the age of the teenagers concerned. The opposite is clearly not true – the age of the teenagers does not in any way depend upon the amount that they drink. The age of the teenagers is therefore the independent variable and is plotted along the horizontal axis.

We now have a problem. The vertical axis needs to be used to plot the amount that the teenagers in the survey drink. However, our findings do not present us with this information in a simple way. The graph would be easier to construct if we had a single figure for each of the four ages, telling us the average amount of alcohol consumed by a teenager of that age. Instead we have two sets of figures – the numbers in each age group who consumed more than the recommended maximum sensible amount and the number who consumed less. For the purposes of our graph we only need one set of figures. We could construct a graph showing how many of the teenagers in each age group have sensible drinking habits, but we are more likely to be interested in how many do not. The figures to use for the graph are therefore those that refer to the number in each group whose alcohol consumption exceeds 21 units a week.

The next step is to construct a scale for each axis. The point at which the axes cross on a graph is known as the origin and variables usually have a value of zero at this point. However, our horizontal axis is only to be used for plotting the ages of 16–19. The ages between zero and 16 do not concern us so if they were plotted on the horizontal axis the result would be a lot of wasted space. We could therefore begin the horizontal axis at 16 and measure out three equal units taking the age up to 19.

In constructing a scale for the vertical axis we might convert the figures into percentages – this is easily done as 10 subjects were used, so a percentage can be calculated by multiplying each figure by 10. (Thus 2 = 20% and so on.) We can therefore construct a ten unit scale, starting at zero and ending at 100%. This is a useful conversion of the figures because it will enable us to show clearly the percentage of each age group which exceeded the sensible drinking limit.

The resulting line graph is shown in Fig 8.1.

Note how the pattern of alcohol consumption is now seen clearly – it increases markedly between the ages of 16 and 18 but then tapers off between 18 and 19 (though a worrying 40% of those surveyed still exceeded the recommended maximum sensible consumption). Note also that the axes are labelled so that it is clear what they are measuring.

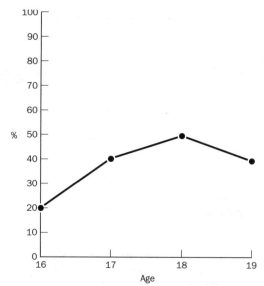

Figure 8.1 Line graph showing percentage of survey teenagers aged 16-19 whose alcohol consumption exceeded 21 units per week.

Line graphs can also be useful for making *comparisons* between sets of figures. Imagine for example that the survey referred to above only involved male teenagers, and that another, similarly constructed survey was carried out among female teenagers. The two sets of results could be plotted on the same graph, as in Fig. 8.2.

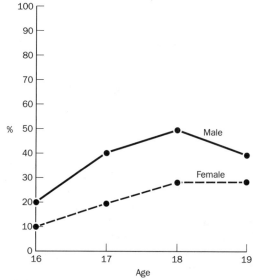

Figure 8.2 Line graph showing percentage of male and female teenagers (aged 16-19) surveyed whose alcohol consumption exceeded 21 units per week.

Note how the two lines are clearly labelled 'Male' and 'Female'. To distinguish them further you might draw each line in a different colour. This graph shows that as with male teenagers excessive drinking among the female teenagers surveyed increased between the ages of 16 and 18, and that the increase was then halted. It also shows that for every age group fewer females drank excessively than males.

As these examples illustrate, line graphs are often used for indicating trends over time. They are commonly used for instance in recording the changes in an infant or young child's height and weight as he or she grows older (these are known as percentile charts). In such graphs time is always the independent variable and is plotted along the horizontal axis. The example below records the progress made over a 10-week period by a client trying to give up smoking. The horizontal axis refers to the time period (in weeks) and the vertical axis to the number of cigarettes smoked (the client was asked to total up the number smoked at the end of each week).

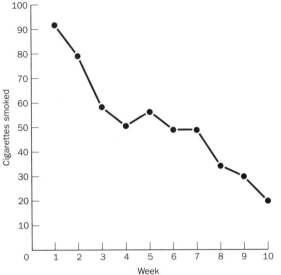

Figure 8.3 Line graph showing progress made over a 10-week period by client who was attempting to give up smoking.

The graph shows how the client gradually reduced the number of cigarettes he smoked over the 10-week period, though his progress was interrupted in the middle weeks. This example also illustrates how it is often possible to make *predictions* from line graphs. If the graph shows a clear trend then, providing there is no change in circumstances, the trend is likely to continue – in this case, by week 12 or 13 the client is likely to be smoking even fewer cigarettes, and may even have stopped altogether.

Bar Charts

A **bar chart** consists of a set of bars of equal width, separated by spaces of equal size. Each bar indicates the size of a particular category. The bar chart below shows how the findings of the survey of drinking habits among male teenagers could be represented:

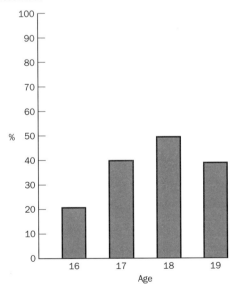

Figure 8.4 Bar chart showing percentage of surveyed male teenagers (aged 16-19) whose alcohol consumption exceeded 21 units per week.

Note that as with line graphs the bar chart has a brief explanation beneath it and the axes are clearly labelled.

Multiple bar chart
Multiple bar charts can be used if there is more than one set of figures for each category. In the case of the above chart, for example, we could incorporate the figures for female teenagers by changing it into a multiple bar chart:

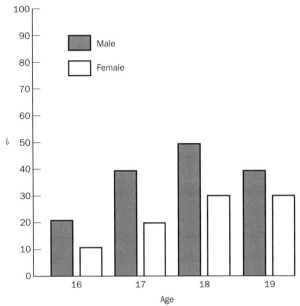

Figure 8.5 Multiple bar chart showing percentages of male and female teenagers (aged 16-19) surveyed whose alcohol consumption exceeded 21 units per week.

Note how a different type of shading has been used for male and female and that a 'Key' has been included to explain this. If the chart is drawn by hand an alternative is to use a different colouring for the different subdivisions of each category.

Component bar chart
An alternative to the multiple bar chart is the *stacked* or **component bar chart**. Here the different components of each category are 'stacked' on top of each other. The teenage drinking survey for example, found that out of 20 16 year olds questioned, three (or 15%) exceeded the maximum recommended limit for alcohol consumption. Of these, one (= 5%) was female, while the other two (= 10%) were male. If we carry out similar calculations for the other age groups the component bar chart below can be produced:

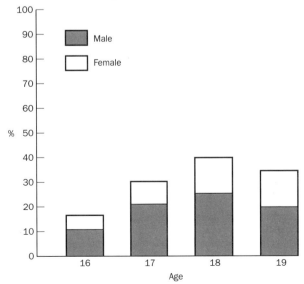

Figure 8.6 Component chart showing percentages of surveyed teenagers (aged 16-19) whose alcohol consumption exceeded 21 units per week.

Component bar charts are useful for showing how a category is made up of different subdivisions, but they should be avoided if more than two or three subdivisions are involved as the resulting chart is often hard to understand. Another disadvantage is that comparisons between the component parts of different categories can be difficult – in the above example it is easy enough to compare the overall totals for each age group and the totals for males, but the differences in the totals for females are less easy to spot.

Bar charts are an appropriate method of presentation when you have many different sets of figures and are not seeking to identify a trend (line graphs are usually more effective for this purpose). Your aim rather may be to show differences between categories. The bar chart below, for example, based on a survey undertaken in 1993, shows the percentage of National Health Service patients in each region of the country who had been waiting over 12 months for treatment. The way the information is presented makes it relatively easy to make comparisons between different regions. Another point of interest about this bar chart is that the information is shown horizontally rather than vertically. Either style of presentation can be used, but computer packages tend to favour verticle bar charts. (Using a computer to present graphical information will help you to fulfil the criteria for the Information Technology Core Skills Unit.) Finally, note that the *source* of the information used in the bar chart below is given – if you have not compiled the information yourself, you should always do this.

Percentage of National Health Service patients waiting over 12 months: by region, 1993[1]

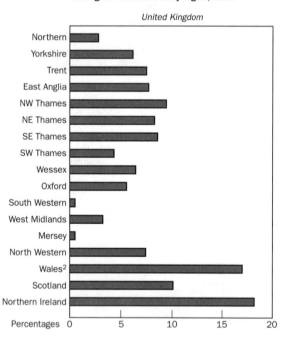

United Kingdom

[1] At 31st March
[2] Only non-urgent cases waiting over 12 months

Source: Department of Health; Welsh Office; Scottish Health Service, Common Services Agency; Department of Health and Social Services, Northern Ireland

Figure 8.7

Histograms

Visually, **histograms** are similar to bar charts except the bars adjoin each other rather than having spaces between them. They are often used to present continuous data rather than data that has been divided into categories. Histograms help you see where most of the data in a table can be found. For example, in

Fig. 8.8 we can see that in a class of 20 pupils, the largest number of pupils (6) is in the class interval 135–139 cm.

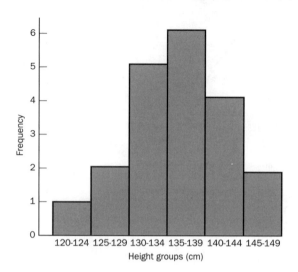

Figure 8.8   Histogram of pupil heights (cm)

The *areas* of the rectangles are important in a histogram. The *heights* of the rectangles are equal to the class frequency (i.e. number of observations in the class interval). However if the *base* of any rectangle is different from any other (say double) then you must adjust the height in proportion (i.e. halve the height). This is because the areas of the rectangles represent the class frequencies.

Pie Charts

A **pie chart** is a circle divided into segments. The circle represents a whole number, and each segment represents a share or proportion of that number. Imagine for instance that you interviewed 20 working mothers with children under five and asked them how their children were cared for while they were at work. Their responses were as follows:

School/nursery school	5
Unpaid family or friends	7
Paid childminder/nanny	5
Local authority scheme	2
Workplace facility	1
	20 TOTAL

The first step in constructing a pie chart is to calculate each category's share of the total. We can do this by converting each number into a percentage (see page 168). This gives the following:

School/nursery school	5	25%
Unpaid family or friends	7	35%
Paid childminder/nanny	5	25%
Local authority scheme	2	10%
Workplace facility	1	5%
	20	100% TOTAL

A pie chart is a circle of 360°. Each of the five survey categories needs to occupy an area of the circle corresponding to its percentage of the total. Thus the segment which indicates the 'school/nursery school' category will have an angle which is 25% of 360°.

$$360 \times \frac{25}{100} = 90°$$

If we perform a similar calculation for all five categories we arrive at the following:

School/nursery school	90°
Unpaid family or friends	126°
Paid childminder/nanny	90°
Local authority scheme	36°
Workplace facility	18°

To draw the first of these segments we find the mid-point of the circle and draw a radius. Using a protractor we then mark off an angle of 90° and draw another radius so that the angle between the two radii is 90°. The procedure is then repeated for the other segments to produce the pie chart below:

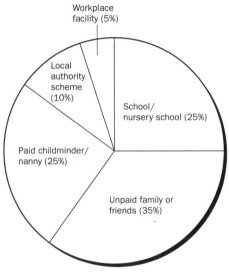

Figure 8.9

A pie chart can be a useful means of showing the relative importance of different components of a total figure. The segments can be further distinguished from each other by giving each segment a different shading (see example below). However, it is sometimes difficult to see when one segment is larger than another. For this reason, percentages (or the original figures before conversion to percentages) should also appear on the pie chart, either within the segments or immediately outside. Note also in the above

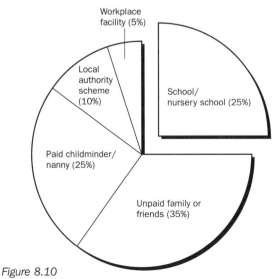

Figure 8.10

example that the category to which each segment refers is clearly labelled.

Another disadvantage of pie charts is that too many divisions can make the chart difficult to interpret – about 6–8 segments is usually considered the maximum that a pie chart should contain. They can also be difficult to calculate and to draw, though computer packages can be used to construct pie charts. A computer also make it possible to focus attention on one or more segments by 'exploding' them, as in the example presented (Fig. 8.10).

Pictogram

This is a chart shown in picture format. It is used for it's eye catching quality and it is easy to understand. However it is at the expense of accuracy; you would need to go back to the raw data to get accurate information. In Fig. 8.11, the 1993 figure is clearly over 5,000, but it is not clear if it is 5,200 or 5,300 etc.

The pictogram could be developed by using different figures for men and for women for each of the three years shown.

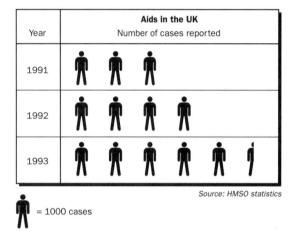

Figure 8.11 Pictogram of annual number of confirmed cases of Aids in the UK.

Correlation and the scattergram

Correlation is an indication of how closely two different factors might be related. You may wish to test for example whether there is a relation between the ages of adults and the number of visits they make to their GP in the course of a year. To do this you could select 10 people of different ages and ask them how many times they had visited their doctor in the past 12 months. The findings could then be presented in the form of a *scattergram*, which is a form of diagram used to compare two sets of figures. In the scattergram (p.168), the vertical axis represents the number of visits to the doctor and the horizontal axis the ages of the adults involved. The dots represent each person's score on the two variables.

In this case (Fig 8.12a)) there is a *positive correlation*, which means that those who score highly on one variable tend also to score highly on the other. In other words, the survey found that as the ages of the adults increased, so too did their visits to the doctor.

Imagine though that an opposite pattern emerged – that the older adults made fewer visits to the doctor. This would mean a *negative correlation*, which occurs when people who score highly on one variable tend to have a low score on the other. The resulting scattergram would look something like that in Fig. 8.12b).

If there is not a strong relationship between the two variables (neither a positive nor a negative correlation) this would again be evident from the scattergram in Fig. 8.12c).

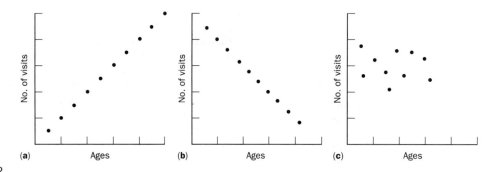

Figure 8.12

Note how the dots are more widely scattered and do not form a clear pattern as in the previous two scattergrams.

Scattergrams are useful because they can give a quick visual impression of the relationship between two variables. However, you should remember that a strong correlation between two variables does not necessarily mean that the relationship between them is one of cause and effect – an increase in one variable is not necessarily the reason for the increase or decrease in the other. The correlation may be the result of other factors or of coincidence.

Text

Reports are examples of narrative **text**. Most reports these days have a summary of a page or so which highlight the key points. Busy managers have not got the time to read in-depth, detailed reports, although they need to be reassured that the research has been completed in a logical and detailed fashion. If the reader wants to know the in-depth information, it should be available in the appendices, clearly labelled. In the next chapter (Portfolio) you will find more information on how to write both short and longer reports, together with some actual examples.

Basic Statistics

Here we consider some basic statistical terms and methods widely used in analysing data.

Grouping data

Data needs to be **grouped** and classified before it can be analysed. This means sorting the bits of information you have obtained into logical groupings. If a small range of figures or responses is involved this is usually straightforward. If for instance you asked a ward of hospital patients to grade the quality of information they had received on admission to hospital on a scale of 1 (inadequate) to 4 (excellent), you would only need to sort the responses into these four categories. Here the groupings suggest themselves, but if a large range of figures is involved you need to reduce them to a smaller number of groupings.

Imagine for instance that in a survey 100 adults were asked to fill in a questionnaire) instead of 10. Their responses would be easier to analyse if you put them into groups according to age. Usually you need around 5–10 groupings. Fewer than this may mean you are generalising too much and obscuring the details of your findings; more than this and the purpose of grouping the data (which is to make it more manageable by summarising it) begins to be lost. You also need to ensure that each grouping covers a similar range. In this case you might use the following groupings:

18 and under 30 years
30 and under 40 years
40 and under 50 years
50 and under 60 years
60 and under 70 years
70 and under 80 years
80 years and above

In deciding the groupings care needs to be taken to ensure that every figure (in this case, every age) is accounted for and that no figure belongs to more than one group. Thus a groupings such as the following would be incorrect:

18–30 years
30–40 years
40–50 years
    etc.

This is incorrect because people who were 30, 40 or 50 years old could be placed in two different groups.

Fractions, decimals and percentages

Fractions, decimals and percentages are all ways of expressing parts or divisions of a whole.

Fractions are calculated by dividing the number that refers to the part by the number that refers to the whole. Thus if a survey found that one out of four patients in a hospital ward was dissatisfied with the meals served in the hospital, we can express this as a fraction: $^1/_4$. If the number referring to the part and the number referring to the whole have a *common denominator* – that is, a number by which both can be divided – we divide the two numbers by the common denominator. Thus if instead of one out of four patients our findings involved three out of twelve patients, we would first express this in fraction form as $^3/_{12}$. As 4 is the common denominator of 3 and 12 we divide both numbers by 3 and arrive again at $^1/_4$. The fraction is the same in both cases because the *proportion* of patients expressing dissatisfaction (that is, the part or division of the whole) is the same in both instances.

Fractions can be a useful way of simplifying your findings or of making a trend or pattern in the findings more obvious. If you conducted a survey in a school, for example, and found that 37 out of 72 questioned considered the sex education they had received to be inadequate, you might observe in your discussion of the findings that 'around half of the pupils interviewed felt that the sex education they had received had been inadequate'.

A **decimal** is a fraction with a denominator of 10, or of some power of 10 such as 100, 1,000 and so on. A decimal is calculated by dividing the upper part of a fraction by the lower part, adding noughts to the upper number as required. Before the first nought is added a decimal point is inserted in your answer and for each additional nought the point is moved one place further to the left. Thus $^1/_4$ can be converted to a decimal as follows:

$$\frac{1}{4} = \frac{1.0}{4} = \frac{1.00}{4} = 0.25$$

$$0.25 \times 100 = 25\%$$

Again these calculations can easily be performed on a calculator. In the first of the above examples the stages in the calculation are:

$$1 \div 4 \times 100 = 25$$

Percentages are useful in analysing the responses to questions in a questionnaire. If for example survey found that seven our of thirty two expectant mothers questioned at an ante-natal clinic smoked during pregnancy, this could be expressed as a percentage. The part (7) is divided by the whole (32) and the resulting fraction multiplied by 100:

$$\frac{7}{32} \times 100 = 21.875\%$$

It is the usual practice to express such percentages to the nearest whole number, or to one decimal place. This is done by rounding figures of 5 or more up, and figures that are less than 5 down. The above percentage therefore becomes:

22% to the nearest whole number
21.9% to one decimal place.

Percentages can also be used to express the response rate to a questionnaire. If you distribute 100 questionnaires and 83 are returned, the response rate would be 83%. A further use of percentages is to make your findings easier to comprehend. Imagine, for example, that you have found out from your local authority that the most recent estimate of the population of the borough in which you live is 115,073. These are distributed among the following types of property:

52,203 – owner-occupied properties
37,411 – council-owned properties
21,879 – private rented accommodation
3,580 – other accommodation/unaccounted for.

These figures might be easier to grasp if they were expressed as percentages:

45% – owner-occupied properties
33% – council-owned properties
19% – private rented accommodation
3% – other accommodation/unaccounted for.

You should be careful to ensure however that any percentages you use do not give a misleading impression. This is especially a danger with a small study using only a limited number of subjects. Suppose for instance that you were investigating the amount of information given to hospital patients about their treatment and interviewed four patients who had recently had operations, three of whom were dissatisfied with the information they had received. As the number of patients interviewed was so small, it would be misleading to report 'The survey found the 75% of patients were dissatisfied with the amount of information they had received before their operations'. It would be better simply to say 'Four patients who had recently had operations were interviewed, and of these three expressed dissatisfaction with the amount of information they had received before their operations'.

Averages (Mean, Median, Mode)

When you have a group of figures or scores it is often useful to have one figure which indicates the overall tendency. In everyday language this is known as an *average*, but in statistics there are different kinds of average, including *mean, median* and *mode*.

- **Mean**

The most commonly used is the **mean**, which is the simple arithmetic average. It is calculated by adding up all the scores and dividing the total by the number of scores. Imagine for example, that you asked 10 teenage smokers to record how many cigarettes they smoke on a particular day and the reported total were as follows:

5, 15, 12, 40, 10, 10, 4, 9, 5, 10

The mean is calculated by adding these scores up and dividing by the number of scores:

$$120 \div 10 = 12$$

An advantage of the mean is that it takes into account all the individual scores. A disadvantage is that extreme scores can influence the mean so that the mean actually gives a misleading impression. In the above example, there is one extreme score – 40 – and this makes the mean greater than it would otherwise be. If the score of 40 were omitted, the mean of the other scores would be 9 (to the nearest whole number). If a report on these findings stated 'On average the teenagers in the survey smoked 12 cigarettes a day' this would be quite misleading as in fact only three of the teenagers smoked 12 or more cigarettes.

- **Median**

The **median** is the middle score of a group of scores. It is found by placing the scores in numerical order and identifying the number that is in the middle. Thus if eleven scores were arranged in numerical order the median would be the sixth score because this would have five scores to the left of it and five scores to the right. If there is an even number of scores the median is the arithmetic average (the mean) of the two middle numbers. To return to the above example, if we place the scores in numerical order we have the following:

4, 5, 5, 9, 10, 10, 10, 12, 15, 40

As there is an even number of scores there is not a single middle number but two (10 and 10). The mean of these two numbers is 10, which is therefore the median. (If the middle numbers were 10 and 12, the median would be 11; if they were 10 and 11, the median would be 10.5.)

An advantage of the median is that it is less influenced than the mean by extreme scores and is therefore more representative than the mean when there are extreme scores. In the example of the smoking survey, 10 cigarettes per day is a more representative average score than 12 cigarettes per day. A disadvantage however is that it is mathematically less precise than the mean and does not give a true arithmetic average.

- **Mode**

The **mode** is simply the number that occurs most frequently in any given set of scores. Thus if we take the original set of scores in the smoking survey –

5, 15, 12, 40, 10, 10, 4, 9, 5, 10

– the mode is 10, because this score occurs three times, which is more frequently than any of the other scores. An advantage of the mode is that it is usually easy to find. However, difficulties arise if the same rate of frequency is shared by more than one number. It is also a crude measure of the average score, especially if there is not a great difference in the frequencies of the scores (in the above example, 5 occurs almost as frequently as 10).

If you mention an average in an assignment, always explain whether it is a mean, median or mode. If the average seems in any way unrepresentative or misleading (if it has been distorted by an extreme score, for example) point this out also.

Range and Standard Deviation

As well as finding an *average* we are often interested in how the data is *dispersed* around that average. The range and standard deviation are ways of indicating how scores are distributed within a set of figures. They are useful because they can show if the scores are close together or far apart.

- **Range**

  The **range** is the difference between the highest and the lowest scores. In the smoking survey the highest score was 40 and the lowest 5, so the range was 35:

  $$40 - 5 = 35$$

  A disadvantage of the range is that it only uses the extreme scores so can give a misleading impression if one number is markedly higher or lower than the rest. In the smoking survey, the range becomes very different if we omit 40 from the list of scores. The lowest number is still 5 but the highest is 15, so the range drops to 10. The original range (35) was misleading because it implied that the scores were more highly scattered than they in fact are.

- **Standard deviation**

  The number of items in the range is called the **frequency count**. A more satisfactory measure of distribution is the **standard deviation**. This is a measure of the spread of scores around the mean value. If the scores are grouped closely around the mean value, the standard deviation is small. If the scores are widely distributed, the standard deviation is large. The distribution curves below (Fig. 8.13) represent large and small standard deviations:

  The small standard deviation curve indicates that most of the scores are close together; the large standard deviation curve indicates that they are spread quite widely.

Although a knowledge of range is a GNVQ requirement, a knowledge of standard deviation is not. However, you may wish to make use of the concept of standard deviation in your assignments. You should be able to find a more detailed explanation of standard deviation in any book on statistics, or your teacher may be able to help.

Probability

If a distribution of a variable is *normal*, i.e. perfectly symmetrical about mean (see Fig. 8.14), then a number of important points follow.

(a) Mean, median and mode will be the *same value*
(b) We can work out exact *probabilities* of a particular observation being a certain number of standard deviations away from the mean.

Spreadsheets

Many of the calculations we have been discussing in this statistics section can be performed on a computer using a **spreadsheet** program. A spreadsheet is a program for handling numerical information. On screen it appears as a grid of boxes or 'cells', each of which can contain a number or a formula to act upon the contents of other cells. For example, a very simple calculation would be to add the numbers in two cells together; another would be to express one number as a percentage of another, or as a percentage of the total of all the numbers on the spreadsheet. Not only can a spreadsheet perform a large range of calculations, it can also present numerical information that has been entered, and the results of calculations that have been carried out, as charts and graphs.

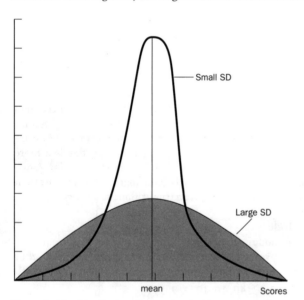

Figure 8.13 Distribution curves showing large and small standard deviations

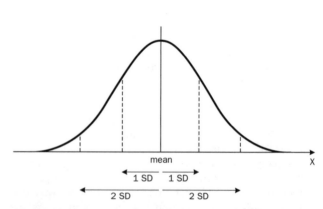

68.26% of distribution lies within ± 1 standard deviation (SD) of mean

95.45% of distribution lies within ± 2 standard deviations (SD) of mean

Figure 8.14 Probability and the normal distribution.

Self Check ✓ Element 3

20. Identify two *types* of research and distinguish between them.

21. Must a *reliable* test be a *valid* test?

22. Give 3 examples of your own of *leading* questions

23. List 4 potential sources of error involving data collection and interpretation.

24. List 3 reasons for a low *response* rate in a survey of G.P. patients opinions by questionnaires sent by mail.

25. The age of children in a nursery are as follows: 6, 7, 7, 6, 5, 8, 4, 3,
    (a) Find the mean age
    (b) Find the median age
    (c) Find the range
    (d) FInd the frequency count

26. Given a range of salaries of hospital staff as follows.
    (£000 per annum):
    8, 8, 10, 10, 10, 15, 15, 16, 20, 45

    calculate the:
        mean
        mode
        median
        range

27. If the directors' salary above was £75000 instead of £45000, how would this change the above calculations?

28. What is the difference between the mean and the standard deviation?

29. What do you understand by the phrase 'positive' correlation between two variables?

30. Draw a diagram showing *negative correlation* between two variables.

Unit Test

Question 1
Primary data is:

A   Data obtained at the beginning of a research project.
B   Data that the researcher obtains through his/her own investigations.
C   The data that is of greatest importance in a research project.
D   Data that has not been analysed.

Question 2
Secondary data is:

A   Data that may be unreliable.
B   Data that is surplus to a researcher's requirements.
C   Information that has been collected by others.
D   Data that is of relatively minor importance.

Question 3
You are undertaking a piece of research. Which one of the following might be an example of the primary data that you collect?

A   The results of a questionnaire that you devise and distribute.
B   The books that you consult at the beginning of the research.
C   Details of the most important relevant research already carried out by others.
D   An Action Plan showing how you intend to allocate time during the research project.

Question 4
You are undertaking a piece of research. Which one of the following might be an example of the secondary data that you collect?

A   Eyewitness accounts of a road accident obtained by interview.
B   The findings of a survey that you carry out.
C   The results of interviews that you conduct.
D   Information obtained from Department of Health statistics.

Question 5
As part of an investigation into group behaviour you observe the fellow members of your school or college class during a lesson. This kind of research is known as which one of the following?

A   Non-participant observation
B   Survey
C   Participant observation
D   Self-recording

Question 6
Decide whether each of these statements is True (T) or False (F).
(i) A disadvantage of postal questionnaires is that the response might be patchy.
(ii) An advantage of experiments is that they can be repeated under similar conditions.

Which option best describes the two statements?

A   (i)   T   (ii)   T
B   (i)   T   (ii)   F
C   (i)   F   (ii)   T
D   (i)   F   (ii)   F

Question 7
A case study is:

A   A classic, widely quoted piece of research.
B   Research into a specific medical problem.
C   The detailed study of one individual or small group.
D   Research carried out by a group of people.

Questions 8-11 share answer options A-D
Data collection techniques include the following:

A   Structured interviews
B   Unstructured interviews
C   Naturalistic observations
D   Controlled observation

Which of these techniques are illustrated by the following examples?

Question 8
An informal, relaxed conversation with a hospital patient.

Question 9
The behaviour of the patient during the course of a day is watched and recorded.

Question 10
A list of questions is prepared and then the patient is asked them.

Question 11
The patient is moved to another ward for the day and her behaviour watched and recorded.

Question 12
Decide whether each of these statements is True (T) or False (F)
(i) An open question can be answered equally effectively by a 'Yes' or 'No'.
(ii) A closed question invites a specific, limited response.

Which option best describes the two statements?

A   (i)   T   (ii)   T
B   (i)   T   (ii)   F
C   (i)   F   (ii)   T
D   (i)   F   (ii)   F

Question 13
Which one of the following is an example of a closed question?

A   How old are you?
B   What is your attitude towards smoking?
C   Why do you believe health education to be important?
D   What are your views on abortion?

Question 14
Which one of the following is an example of an open question?

A   What is your address?
B   Have you visited this day centre before?
C   Do you agree or disagree with a smoking ban on public transport?
D   What causes teenagers to take drugs?

Question 15-18 share answer options A-D
Listed below are four types of sampling method.

A   Random sample

B   Quota sample
C   Stratified sample
D   Opportunity sample

Which of these techniques are illustrated by the following examples?

Question 15
For a survey of attitudes among the over-60s, a researcher interviews five people aged 60-64 , five aged 65-69, five aged 70-74 and five aged 75-79.

Question 16
A school of 800 pupils has 360 (45%) who are male and 440 (55%) who are female. A researcher decides that 45% of her sample of pupils from the school will therefore be male and 55% female.

Question 17
A doctor investigating a rare tropical disease finds that a patient recently admitted to his hospital is suffering from the disease and he therefore has a chance to carry out some useful research.

Question 18
For a survey of public opinion a group of researchers stand outside a supermarket and interview every tenth person to enter the shop.

Question 19
In a questionnaire, a ranking form of question is which of the following?

A   The respondent is invited to tick one box from a choice of several boxes.
B   The question employs a rating scale.
C   The respondent is invited to tick more than one box from a choice of several boxes.
D   The respondent numbers several items in order of importance.

Question 20
Decide whether each of these statements is True (T) or False (F).
 (i) The responses to open questions can be difficult to analyse.
(ii) Closed questions are usually harder than open questions for the respondant to complete.

Which option best describes the two statements?

A   (i)   T   (ii)   T
B   (i)   T   (ii)   F
C   (i)   F   (ii)   T
D   (i)   F   (ii)   F

Question 21
Which of the following is an example of a leading question?

A   Would you agree that racial discrimination is wrong?
B   Do you support or oppose capital punishment?
C   Are you aged 21 or over?
D   How much do you weigh?

Question 22
A high non-response rate:

A   Reduces the size of your sample but does not invalidate your findings.
B   Is always caused by apathy.
C   Means that your research may produce biased or misleading results.
D   Is usual with all questionnaires.

Question 23
Line graphs:
A   Cannot be used to record trends over time.
B   Show the relationship between two variables.
C   Are visually less effective than tables.
D   Are also known as bar charts.

Question 24
A histogram:
A   Comprises adjoining bar shapes.
B   Is a circle divided into segments.
C   Is a chart shown in picture format.
D   Is a form of table.

Question 25
Correlation:

A   Means drawing up the two axes for a line graph.
B   Is an indication of how closely two different factors might be related.
C   Means checking the validity of research findings.
D   Always shows a positive relationship between two variables.

Questions 26-28 share answer options A-C
Three kinds of statistical averages are:

A   Mean
B   Median
C   Mode
Consider the following sets of numbers:
2, 2, 2, 3, 5, 8, 11, 14, 16

Identify each of the numbers below as the Mean (A), Median (B) or Mode (C) for the above set of numbers.

Question 26
5

Question 27
2

Question 28
7

Question 29
The range of a set of scores is:

A   The number of different scores recorded.
B   The total number of scores recorded.
C   The difference between the highest and lowest scores.
D   The highest score recorded.

Question 30
The median is:
A   The middle score of a group of scores.
B   The most frequently occurring number in a group of scores.
C   The difference between the highest and lowest scores.
D   The arithmetic average of a group of scores.

Question 31
Decide whether each of these statements is True (T) or False (F).
 (i) A positive correlation exists between smoking and lung cancer.
(ii) A negative correlation exists between stress and heart disease.

Which option best describes the two statements?

A (i) T (ii) T
B (i) T (ii) F
C (i) F (ii) T
D (i) F (ii) F

Question 32

A scattergram:

A Is based on a random sample.
B Can only be constructed from a large range of scores.
C Always depicts a negative correlation.
D Is a set of dots representing the relationship between two variables.

Question 33

A positive correlation:

A May be the result of coincidence.
B Always proves that a cause and effect relationship exists.
C Proves a hypothesis to be correct.
D Means that a piece of research will have beneficial results.

Question 34, 35 and 36

From the Diagrams the following can be stated:

A No correlation exists.
B Negative correlation exists.
C Positive correlation exists.
D Cannot determine from information available.

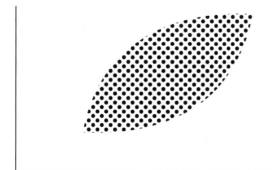

Figure 8.15

Question 34 refers to Fig. 8.15

Choose from the above list:

A B C D

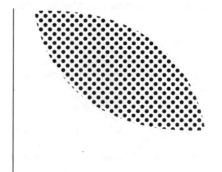

Figure 8.16

Question 35 refers to Fig. 8.16

Choose from the above list:
A B C D

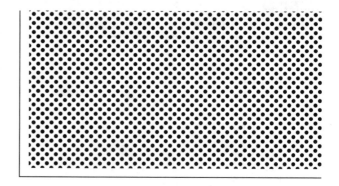

Figure 8.17

Question 36 refers to Fig. 8.17

Choose from the above list:
A B C D

Answers to Self-check Questions

1. Primary – you collect; Secondary – others collect; etc.

2. Experiments; observation; surveys; case studies

3. See pages 157–158.

4. The complete population involved in the experiment, test or under observation.

5. A part of the total population.

6. It saves money, time and effort and the results represent (statistically) the total population.

7. See page 159.

8. That the sample is accurate and represents the wider population and the minimum of errors have been introduced.

9. Have *particular* needs and experiences, may not therefore be fully representative; also depends on type of hospital (private/public) and catchment area (high/low income) etc. as to whether representative of the wider society.

10. At a particular point in time; over time; etc.

11. A theory or assumption about something.

12. The hypothesis to be tested.

13. Open – respondent's answer not restricted; closed – only limited types of response possible.

14. See page 160.

15. See page 161.

16. Many examples possible: see page 160.

17. See page 161.

18. A technique for guiding respondents as to the questions they answer in a structured questionnaire.

19. Possible types of information missed by such an open question might include:

- Cigar and pipe smokers are not separated out.
- No differentiation made between male and female smokers or non smokers.
- The age of smokers is not determined.
- The age of smokers that have given up is unknown.
- The number of times a smoker has given up smoking is not recorded.
- The *reasons* why the smokers gave up are unknown.
- Why some smokers have *not* given up smoking is unknown etc.

20. Quantitative involves number format while qualitative does not.

21. No. *Reliable* tests give consistent results which can be reproduced. *Valid* tests measure what they are supposed to measure. A reliable test could be quite *invalid*.

22. Many possible answers here.

23. Use of leading questions; high non-response rate; misuse of statistics; sampling errors.

24. Various possibilities: e.g., complex questions; another item of 'junk' mail to respondents; time when questionnaire sent out (e.g. Xmas when much other mail); incorrect addresses; etc.

25. mean = [46/8] = 5.75 yrs; median = 6 yrs; range = 5 yrs; frequency count = 8 items of data.

26. Number in the sample = 10

mean = 157/10 = 15.7 = £15,700

mode = 10 (i.e. 3 values) = £10,000

median = (10 + 15) /2 = 12.5 = £12,500

range = 45 – 8 = 37 = £37,000

27. Number in the sample is still 10

mean = £18,700   i.e. 187k / 10

mode = £10,000   i.e. same as before.

median = £12,500   i.e. same as before.

range = £67,000   i.e. £75k – £8k

28. Mean is a measure of average; standard deviation is a measure of the distribution (dispersion) of data around that average; etc.

29. The two variables move in the same direction; e.g. as X rises, so does Y and as X falls so does Y.

30. See pages 167,168.

Answers to Unit Test

Question	Answer	Question	Answer	Question	Answer	Question	Answer	Question	Answer
1.	B	9.	C	17.	D	25.	B	33.	A
2.	C	10.	A	18.	A	26.	B	34.	C
3.	A	11.	D	19.	D	27.	C	35.	B
4.	D	12.	C	20.	B	28.	A	36.	A
5.	C	13.	A	21.	A	29.	C		
6.	A	14.	D	22.	C	30.	A		
7.	C	15.	B	23.	B	31.	B		
8.	B	16.	C	24.	A	32.	D		

Unit Test Comments (selected questions)

Question 3
A. B and C are both examples of secondary data.

Question 4
D. A, B and C are examples of primary data.

Question 11
D. This is controlled observation because the situation has been set up by the researcher.

Question 13
A. A closed question invites a specific limited response.

Question 14
D. A, B and C are examples of closed questions.

Question 20
B. (ii) is false because closed questions are usually easier to answer than open questions.

Question 21
A. This is a leading question because it encourages the respondent to say 'yes'.

Question 23
B. Line graphs can be used to record trends over time and usually they are visually more effective than tables.

Question 26
B. 5 is the middle score in the group.

Question 27
C. 2 is the number that occurs most frequently.

Question 28

A.   7 is the arithmetic average of the scores.

Question 31

B.   (ii) is false because a positive correlation exists between stress and heart disease.

Question 33

A.   B is incorrect because while a positive correlation may suggest that a cause and effect relationship exists, it does not 'always prove' this.

Question 34

C.   Both variables move upwards (and downwards) together.

Question 35

B.   As one variable increases, the other variable decreases.

Question 36

A.   This is a random scatter of points. There is no correlation here.

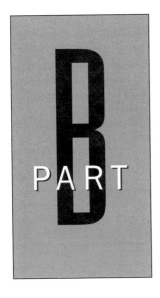

The Portfolio

This final section of the book is devoted to the **portfolio of evidence** that you will compile in order to achieve your GNVQ. Most of the section examines closely the various skills that might be involved in putting together a portfolio. To illustrate these skills, some examples of student work are included and their merits and shortcomings assessed. From time to time you will be referred to topics and pages in Unit 8 which has already covered some of the key skills required in researching and presenting the portfolio. We begin however with some general information on the content and presentation of the portfolio, and on grading criteria and the 'core skills'.

What is a portfolio?

A **portfolio** collects together all of the *evidence* you are submitting to show that you have fulfilled the GNVQ standards, including the criteria for the Mandatory, Optional and Core Skills units and, where applicable, the grading criteria for a Merit or Distinction. As it will represent two years' work and will probably contain many different types of evidence (see below), it is unlikely that it will be a simple folder. More typically, the evidence will be presented in a box file.

What will a portfolio contain?

The portfolio is likely to contain a *variety* of evidence. Listed below are some of the most common forms of evidence:

- Assignments
- Reports
- Projects
- Essays
- Case Studies
- Letters
- Memos
- Artefacts produced by the student
- Care plans
- Work experience logs
- Peer group assessments
- Self assessments
- Reports or assessments of simulation/role play exercises
- Photographs
- Audio and video recordings
- Internal tests

During the course you may also be assessed by observation or oral questioning. The portfolio would contain evidence of the assessments carried out and, where appropriate, of your own planning and evaluation of the activities. Some evidence from sources other than the GNVQ course may also be used. This might include for instance evidence of prior achievement (e.g. GCSE certificates) and references from employers if you work part-time.

1 Presentation and record-keeping

As the portfolio will contain a large amount of material, it is essential that it is *well organised*. An Assessor or Verifier should be able to see clearly how the evidence within the portfolio relates to the GNVQ units and to the grading criteria for a Merit or Distinction.

The task of organising the portfolio is made easier by **accurate record-keeping**. The examining bodies supply standardised **forms** which are filled in for each assignment, explaining which Unit criteria the assignment has met. There are additional forms for Action Plans, assessments and self-evaluations, as well as summary forms on which you indicate that all the necessary criteria have been met and where in the portfolio the evidence can be found. Alternatively, your school or college may have designed their own forms for these purposes.

Some of the forms in most common use are listed below:

- **A portfolio front or cover sheet**, stating your name, the name of your school or college, and the name of the qualification (Advanced GNVQ in Health and Social Care).

- **A contents sheet**, listing the assignments, assessments and other forms of evidence included in the portfolio. Each piece of evidence might be given a code number, to facilitate cross-referencing.

- **A summary record sheet**, indicating the units that have been completed.

- **An element record sheet** for each unit element, confirming that the performance criteria for that element have been met and indicating what form the evidence takes.

- **A cover sheet for each activity (including assignments) undertaken**, listing such details as the date of completion, the task that was set and the performance criteria covered.

- **An activity assessment sheet**, on which assessments made by assessors and internal and external verifiers are recorded. (See Figure 1).

- **An Action Plan sheet** for each activity where it is appropriate to have one.

- **An Evaluation sheet** (again for activities where this is appropriate).

- **A grading information sheet** for appropriate activities, explaining how you have shown in the activity the skills necessary for a Merit or Distinction.

- **A grading record sheet,** used to keep a record of the Merit or Distinction grading themes you have covered.

Do not worry if you find all this paperwork hard to come to terms with at first. Once you have completed a few assignments and become familiar with the procedures it should all begin to make more sense. It is important however to try to ensure that the appropriate sheets and forms are correctly filled in as your course progresses. This will save you a lot of headaches when the time comes to hand in your completed portfolio. If there is anything you are unsure about you should not hesitate to ask your teacher.

GNVQ		TUTOR:	
LEVEL			
YEAR		STUDENT:	

ASSIGNMENT TITLE

UNIT	ELEMENT	ASPECT OF RANGE	TUTOR COMMENTS

THEMES	CRITERIA	MERIT	DISTINCTION	ASSESSOR COMMENT
PLANNING	1	M	D	
MONITORING	2	M	D	
SOURCES	3	M	D	
VALIDITY	4	M	D	
EVALUATING	5	M	D	
JUSTIFYING	6	M	D	

CORE UNIT	CORE ELEMENT	ASPECT OF RANGE	TUTOR COMMENTS

SIGNATURES
TUTOR:

STUDENT:

Figure 1 Assignment Assessment Sheet

2 Grading criteria

If you satisfy the performance criteria for all of the required units you will achieve a GNVQ. For a Merit or Distinction you need to show that you have satisfied the additional **grading criteria** for these two levels of achievement. A more detailed breakdown of these criteria will be given shortly, but essentially they require you to take increased responsibility for planning, monitoring, carrying out and evaluating the activities you undertake. For a Merit or Distinction to be awarded it is not necessary for every piece of evidence submitted to meet these criteria. Rather, the portfolio must contain 'consistent' evidence that the criteria have been met, which means at least one third of the total evidence contained in the portfolio must satisfy the Merit or Distinction requirements. In practice this usually means that much of the evidence is produced in the later stages of the course, when students are better equipped to work independently.

The criteria for a Merit or Distinction are divided into three **themes,** each with two criteria. We shall now look at each of these in turn and consider what they entail.

Theme 1: Planning

This relates to the planning and monitoring of activities and assignments. The two criteria under this heading are:

(a) **Drawing up plans of action.** For a *Merit* you need to draw up action plans (perhaps with the help of a teacher) for series of discrete (that is, separate or isolated) tasks. You also arrange the tasks in order of priority. For a *Distinction* you *independently* draw up action plans for complex (that is, inter-related) activities. You again need to arrange the tasks in order of priority.

(b) **Monitoring courses of action.** For a *Merit* you independently monitor the progress of your activities and recognise when intended courses of action need to be modified. Revisions to plans are made with guidance from teachers. For a *Distinction* the significant difference is that revisions to plans are made independently.

Theme 2: Information-seeking and information-handling

This theme is concerned with locating sources of information and checking the validity of information that you obtain. The two criteria are:

(a) **Identify and use sources to obtain relevant information.** For a *Merit* you independently access and collect relevant information for series of separate, self-contained tasks. You identify the main sources of information independently and receive guidance on other sources from teachers. For a *Distinction* the information is acquired for series of inter-related activities. You independently identify and use a range of sources of information, and justify the selection of these sources.

(b) **Establishing the validity of information.** For a *Merit* you independently identify information which needs to be checked for validity and use methods which have been shown to you to carry out these checks. For a *Distinction* the important difference is that you independently select and apply appropriate methods to check validity.

Theme 3: Evaluation

This involves retrospective (looking-back) self-assessment. At the end of an assignment or other activity, you look back over it and review such things as the degree of success achieved, the decisions that you made and alternative courses of action that you might have taken. The two criteria are:

(a) **Evaluating outcomes and alternatives.** For a *Merit* you judge the success of activities undertaken by measuring their outcomes against your original targets and criteria for success. You also identify alternative criteria that could be applied in order to judge the success of the activities. For a *Distinction* you go one stage further and apply a range of alternative criteria to judge the measure of success achieved.

(b) **Justifying particular approaches to tasks/activities.** For a *Merit* you justify the approaches that you used and indicate that alternative approaches were identified and considered. For a *Distinction* your justification is based on a detailed consideration of the advantages and disadvantages of the approaches employed. You also identify alternative approaches that might have been adopted and ways in which your own approaches could have been improved.

In the remainder of this chapter we shall make frequent reference to these grading themes and criteria, explaining at appropriate points ways in which they might be fulfilled. You will find that many of the sections that follow are relevant to the various grading themes: for example, 'Choosing a research method' (page 190) is relevant to Theme 1: *Planning*; 'Sources of information' (page 180) is relevant to Theme 2: *Information-seeking and information-handling*; and 'Evaluating reports and projects' (page 197) is relevant to Theme 3: *Evaluation*.

In the portfolio some of the evidence for these grading criteria may be on **standardised forms** – there are forms for Action Plans, for example, which would help you to achieve the Planning criteria. In other instances the evidence would be an integral part of the assignment itself – in a research project you might for instance assess the validity of your findings, thereby meeting certain of the criteria for Information-seeking and information-handling. Occasionally, however, you may need to add an explanatory page or two to an assignment indicating how particular grading criteria have been met. You might for example add a justification of the sources of information that you consulted. The important thing is that the portfolio should contain *clear evidence* that the criteria have been met. For this reason some kind of grading information sheet and/or grading record sheet (see page 178 above) is helpful.

3 Core skills

To achieve a GNVQ, the evidence in your portfolio will need to show that in addition to the mandatory and optional units you have also completed the three **Core Skills** units:

- Communication
- Application of Number
- Information Technology

The specifications for these units are common to all Advanced GNVQs. The intention is that the Core skills should be *integrated* into the work undertaken for each GNVQ course. What this means is that while all of the work you undertake will be relevant to the specific field of Health and Social Care, some of this work will also give you the opportunity to demonstrate the three Core Skills. In this way you will build up the evidence to show that you have completed the Core Skills units. Some assignments are likely to include tasks which specifically relate to the Core Skills units. As part of a report on a health centre, for example, you might be asked to calculate the floor area of each of the main offices, which would help you to satisfy the performance criteria for the Application of Number Core Skills unit. Other assignments or activities will enable you to satisfy performance criteria for *both* the mandatory or optional units *and* the Core Skills units. To take three examples:

- You might make a presentation to your group on teenage substance abuse and lead a discussion following the presentation. This would help you to satisfy performance criteria 5.3.1 in the Health Promotion unit ('main risks to health associated with substance abuse are investigated') and also contribute to the completion of Element 3.1 in the Communication Core Skills Unit ('Take part in discussion with a range of people on a range of matters').

- You might undertake a survey of dietary habits among a group of fellow students. This could help you to satisfy performance criteria 3.3.5 in the Physical Aspects of Health unit ('factors that affect choice of diet are explained') as well as Element 3.1 in the Application of Number Core Skills unit ('Gather and process data').

- You might design and produce with the aid of a computer a leaflet intended to warn children of the dangers of smoking. This would relate to both Element 5.2 in the Health Promotion unit ('Present health promotion advice to others') and to Element 2.3 in the Information Technology Core Skills unit ('Select and use formats for presenting complex information').

The emphasis is thus on *practical* and *relevant* applications of the Core Skills.

It is important to note that the Core Skills do not have to be assessed on every occasion they are demonstrated. Communication skills, for example, are likely to play a part in most of the activities and assignments you undertake, but formal assessment of these skills does not need to take place every time. There do however need to be sufficient assessments during the course for you to demonstrate that you have completed the full range in all three Core Skills. As with the mandatory and optional units, a record of these assessments is included in the portfolio together with the relevant evidence of achievement.

A brief outline of what is contained within the three Core Skills units is given below.

Communication
This has four key themes:

- Taking part in discussions;
- Preparing written materials (e.g. reports, letters, memos) that conform to rules of grammar, spelling and punctuation and are effectively organised and expressed;
- Using images (e.g. sketches, diagrams, charts) to illustrate points made in writing and discussions;
- Reading and responding to written material and images.

Application of Number
This has three key themes:

- Gathering and processing data (e.g. carrying out surveys; design and use of questionnaires and observation sheets; organisation of data);
- Representing and tackling problems (e.g. use of fractions, decimals, percentages; calculation of perimeters, areas and volumes);
- Interpreting and presenting data (e.g. identifying trends; drawing conclusions from data; constructing and interpreting statistical diagrams).

Information Technology
This has five key themes:

- Storing and inputting information (e.g. entering textual, graphical and numerical information; using new and existing storage systems);
- Editing and organising information (e.g. moving and copying information in and between files; use of tabulation and indents);
- Presenting information (e.g. use of format options to display effectively complex textual, graphical and numerical information);
- Evaluating procedures and features of applications (e.g. facilities offered by applications to save time, reduce costs, increase efficiency and improve accuracy in a work setting);
- Dealing with errors and faults (e.g. correct identification of errors and faults and taking appropriate action to identify them; awareness of health and safety requirements).

In the remaining sections of the book we shall occasionally suggest where activities undertaken to produce different kinds of evidence for the portfolio might give you an opportunity to *demonstrate* the Core Skills. You will find that certain sections of this and the previous chapter are especially relevant to particular Core Skills: for example, 'Other Writing Skills' (p.207) is relevant to Communication, 'Analysing Data' (p.162) to Application of Number and 'Ways of Presenting Information' (p.170) to Information Technology.

Make use of opportunities to demonstrate Core Skills. The important points to remember are that opportunities to demonstrate the Core Skills should arise naturally out of your work, and that you should make use of these opportunities when they do arise.

We shall now examine a wide range of the skills involved in putting together a portfolio. We look first at sources of information and how this information can be put to effective use.

4 Sources of information

In this section we shall discuss the various **sources of information** available to you when you begin an assignment. You will of course have from your school or college your own lecture notes, handouts and so on and you should make full use of these. It is likely however that you will need to locate some information independently, and the grading criteria for a Merit or Distinction do in fact encourage this. We shall therefore be considering in detail how you might approach an information search for an assignment. Among the sources we shall consider are libraries, books, newspapers, periodicals, television and radio broadcasts, and specialist information services. The kind of information you will require and where you might expect to find it will of course depend on the exact assignment you have been set. The aim of this section is to give you some hints on where to look, and advice on how to extract relevant information from the sources that you consult. The emphasis will be on information which might be useful to a student of Health and Social Care. The section ends with a list of addresses and telephone numbers of organisations you might decide to consult.

Information-seeking and information-handling are important skills and are included in the criteria for a Merit or Distinction. You need to show that you can identify appropriate sources of information and make effective use of them. You also need for a Merit or Distinction to recognise any information which needs checking for validity, and to carry out such checks.

Libraries

Libraries are of course one of the most important sources of information and for many assignments it is to libraries that you will turn first in your search for information. We shall now consider the uses that can be made of libraries under the following four headings:

- Types of library;
- Finding what you want;
- Reference material;
- Use of databases.

Types of library

(a) **School / College libraries.** You should make full use of your own school or college library. If the GNVQ course in Health and Social Care is being taught at the institution, it may well have a stock of books specifically intended for students on the course. If you are starting at a new school or college, pay an early visit to the library. It will prove extremely useful to find out as early as possible in your course such information as the following:

- What is the general layout of the library? (Where is the reference section? Where are magazines and periodicals kept? Are there quiet areas for private study?)
- Where on the shelves are the books most likely to be of interest to you? Where for example are the books on Medicine, Psychology and Sociology? Does there seem to be a good range? If you visit the library early in the year you may be able to borrow especially useful books before other students get to them! Don't forget to familiarise yourself with the reference section as well.
- Find out where the library's cataloguing system is located and how to use it. Are there any card indexes, printed catalogues or microfiches? Or is the cataloguing information stored on computer? (For more on this see 'Finding what you want' below.)
- Find out the magazines and periodicals that are stocked. Are there any that might be of particular relevance to you – the British Medical Journal, for

instance? Are back numbers of periodicals stored in the library?

- Ask if there are any special collections of books or other materials (e.g. project packs) relevant to your course. Often these are stored behind the library counter.
- Join the library as soon as you can. Find out the borrowing arrangements – how many books can you take out, and for how long?
- What are the opening hours? You may be able to use the library for private study in the evenings.
- Are there photocopying facilities?
- Find out how to order books. If the library does not have a book you want they may be willing to buy it for you (ask how long this usually takes). Alternatively, there is probably an inter-library loan system which means that if another school or college library in the area has the book they can get it for you. If the book you want is out on loan to another student you should be able to reserve it.
- Don't be afraid to ask the library staff about any of these points.

(b) **Public libraries.** Most of the above applies to public libraries as well. Familiarise yourself with the libraries in your area (there are probably several that you are eligible to use) and with the books, magazines, reference materials and so on that they contain. They are usually bigger than school or college libraries and may well stock a wider range of books and periodicals. The reference sections of public libraries are especially useful for information about the local community (annual health reports, for example) and for official records and statistics (see 'Reference material' below).

(c) **Libraries at universities and other colleges.** These may have a wider range of academic books than your own school or college library. They are unlikely to allow you to borrow books but if you telephone first you may be able to visit such libraries to carry out research. It may also be possible to photocopy any especially useful material you find there.

(d) **Medical libraries.** There is likely to be a medical library at your local District General Hospital, especially if it is a teaching hospital. Many are closed to the public but if you contact the library and explain why you wish to visit it you may well be able to use the library for reference purposes. (In the United States, a patient who used a medical library in California correctly diagnosed her own illness as lead poisoning after unsuccessful consultation with twenty two physicians!)

(e) **Patient information libraries.** Some parts of the country now have patient information libraries. Your local health centre, hospital or health authority should be able to tell you if there is one in your area.

Finding what you want

In order to find what you want in a library you need to know how the library's stock of books is classified and arranged. The **classification system** used by the majority of libraries is the **Dewey Decimal System**. This numbers books according to the following main categories:

    0 – General Works
  100 – Philosophy

200 – Religion
300 – Society
400 – Languages
500 – Science
600 – Technology
700 – Arts
800 – Literature
900 – History

Within each of these main categories there is a progressive breaking down into smaller divisions and sub-sections. Thus a division of Technology is Medicine, which has the number 610. This in turn has smaller division such as Human Physiology (611) and Surgery (617). These divisions are then further sub-divided, so that Diseases (616) for instance includes Diseases of the cardiovascular system (616.1) and Diseases of the digestive system (616.3).

The books in most libraries are arranged on the shelves in numerical order, using the above system. Locating the book or books that you need is relatively straightforward provided you know one of two things:

Either the classification number of the subject you are interested in;

Or if you are searching for a specific book and know the title and author, the classification number of that particular book.

In both cases the relevant number can be found by consulting the library indexes and catalogues. These are of four main kinds:

1. **Subject index.** Here subjects are arranged in alphabetical order and the classification number for each subject is given. For any one assignment you may need to look up several different subjects. For an assignment on the relationship between living conditions and illness, for example, you might look up such subjects as 'poverty', 'housing', 'health' and 'disease'. If you cannot find the subject you are interested in listed in the subject index try to think of a word with a similar or closely related meaning. Thus for an assignment on smoking you might not find 'cigarettes' listed but might have better luck with 'tobacco'.

   After consulting the subject index you may find when you go to the shelves that there are a very large number of books on the subject, and you are not sure where to start. You could try to narrow your search by deciding which particular aspect of the subject you are interested in and then returning to the subject index to see if it is listed. Alternatively, it might be fruitful to spend some time glancing along the titles on the shelves, taking out any books that look as if they might be of use and skimming the contents or index pages to check what they cover.

2. **Classified catalogue.** This lists the books in the library in numerical order. Thus if you know the classification number of the subject you are interested in you can check which books the library has on that subject. This catalogue includes books which are not on the shelves because they are out on loan, and often also lists books which can be found in other libraries within the same borough, county or town.

3. **Author index.** This lists authors' names alphabetically, and gives the titles of books by each author together with their classification number. If you are searching for a particular book and know the author's name, this is the index to use.

4. **Title index.** Here books are listed alphabetically. For each title the index identifies the author and the classification number.

These indexes and catalogues come in various forms. Often they are on microfiche – that is, sheets of acetate which are placed on a viewer for scanning. It is also common for the information to be stored on computer. These two methods of storing and presenting information have generally replaced printed catalogues and card indexes, though these can still be found in some libraries.

Reference material

The **reference section** of any library contains encyclopaedias and other reference books which cannot be taken out on loan. The great advantage of a reference section is that the books and other material contained within it should always be available for consultation. When you go to a reference section to carry out research for an assignment, take with you a list of key subject areas your assignment covers, and about which you are hoping to gain information. Always make a careful note of the source of any information that you find as this will need to be included in your assignment (see 'References to books' on page 184) and Bibliographies (page 186). Listed below are some of the main types of reference material that might prove of use to you.

(a) **Encyclopaedias.** These will not cover individual subjects in as much depth as complete books on those subjects but are handy for quick reference if you want a brief summary of a subject. They are also useful if you are looking for specific items of information (if you wanted to discover when the World Health Organisation was founded, for example, most encyclopaedias would be able to tell you). Some encyclopaedias are divided into several volumes, with a separate index volume which you should usually consult first – this will tell you if different aspects of a subject are dealt with under separate headings. Two multi-volume encyclopaedias found in many libraries are:

The Encyclopaedia Britannica
Chambers Encyclopaedia

(b) **Official statistics.** These are an extremely useful source of both national and local information on health and social issues. They provide helpful background information for many assignments, and can often be quoted in the assignment itself. If you were tackling an assignment on diet, for instance, the Ministry of Agriculture, Fisheries and Food publish statistics for fruit, vegetables, meat, fish and other food stuffs, estimating how much the average person consumes and recording how dietary patterns have changed over the years.

All government departments produce volumes of statistics, which are published by Her Majesty's Stationery Office (HMSO). Thus the Department of Health produces a volume entitled *Health and Personal Social Services Statistics for England*. As a tremendous range of official statistics is available, it might be sensible to begin by consulting one of two general guides to government statistics:

• *Government Statistics – A Brief Guide to Sources.* This contains headings for different subject areas and lists under each heading the publications available.

- *Central Statistical Office – Guide To Official Statistics.* A more detailed guide, this covers all official statistics, which are again grouped under general headings (such as 'National Health Service: General Statistics' and 'Hospital Services'). The Guide indicates where the relevant statistics are to be found.

Some of the main sets of statistics from different government departments are collected together in two invaluable publications, both published annually:

- *Social Trends.* This includes national statistics on population, income, expenditure, health, housing and other matters. The section on health, for example, includes statistics on such diverse subjects as cot deaths, Aids, smoking, immunisation and hospital waiting times.
- *Regional Trends.* This covers a similar range of information, but the information is given on a regional rather than a national basis. It can be very useful if your assignment involves a local study.

Another helpful source of local information are the *Annual Public Health Reports* produced by local health authorities. These give detailed information about the state of health of local residents and also explain the policies and future plans of the health authority.

If you are interested in obtaining information on world health, *World Health Statistics*, is an annual publication of the World Health Organisation.

(c) **Bibliographies and Indexes.** These are specialist publications which give comprehensive lists of books and articles related to particular subjects. The library indexes and catalogues referred to earlier (p.10) only include books that can be found in the library, but these publications aim to list all relevant books in print as well as including details of articles in journals, which the ordinary library indexes do not. Some also include an abstract (or summary of contents) for each item listed.

(d) **Directories.** Directories of national organisations can indicate whom you might contact for further information about a particular topic. Such directories include:

- Directory of British Associations (CBD Research)
- The Health Directory (Bedford Square Press)
- Voluntary Agencies (National Council for Voluntary Organisations)

Your public library might also have separate directories of local organisations.

(e) **Handbooks, guides and manuals.** A wide range of these is published, some annually, by a variety of organisations. Many can be found in public libraries. *The Disability Rights Handbook*, for example, is published annually by Disability Alliance and gives a comprehensive guide to rights, benefits and services for all people with disabilities and their carers. Another example is the *National Aids Manual*, which covers all aspects of HIV and Aids, including transmission, prevention and treatment.

(f) **Newspapers, journals and magazines.** Libraries usually carry a large stock of these, and often keep back issues of some publications. There are also indexes to help

you locate articles on a particular subject. For more advice on making use of this source of information, see the separate section on page 184.

(g) **Information technology.** An increasing amount of information can now be accessed by computer. For example, most libraries can key into the information systems of other libraries and organisations and produce a printed list of the literature available on a specific subject. There are a growing number of databases listing sources of information for different subject areas (the Department of Health Database, which covers a range of health care subjects, is but one example). Many libraries now make use of CDROM, which stands for Compact Disc Read Only Memory. These are discs which are capable of storing massive amounts of information and which can be read on a computer screen. Many indexes listing sources of information – in some cases providing abstracts (summaries) of books and articles – are available. An example of a CDROM index is CINAHL (Cumulative Index of Nursing and Allied Health Literature). Increasingly, complete books (such as encyclopaedias and dictionaries) and back issues of newspapers and journals are being transferred to compact disc, making quick access to information even easier.

Making use of books

It can be very daunting in the early stages of an assignment to be faced by a pile of books, all of which appear to be of relevance to your topic. Reading all of the books from cover to cover would not only consume an enormous amount of time, it would also almost certainly be a *waste* of your time. Books are only of use to the student if your reading of them is *selective*. Time can also be wasted by reading a book but not 'taking in' its content, so that within a day or two (or even sooner!) you have to all intents and purposes forgotten what the author had to say. Reading therefore has to be *effective* as well as selective.

Before any detailed reading of a book takes place, you need first to establish which parts of it are likely to be relevant to your needs. You should scan the contents and index pages, looking for relevant subjects, terms and topic headings. It is also worth scanning individual chapters, looking at introductory paragraphs, sub-headings within the chapters, opening sentences of paragraphs (which often tell you what the paragraph is about) and concluding paragraphs (which sometimes summarise the contents of the chapter).

Assuming you have selected what you are to read, you now need to make sure that when you do read you do so effectively. Your task is to extract from what you read information that will be of use to you and to ensure that you retain this information. One method that can be used if the book is your own is to mark the text as you read through it. You might draw lines in the margin alongside significant parts of the text, underline the relevant parts or use a highlighter pen. Bear in mind though that if you are likely to need the book again for further assignments marking it too much or too often can cause confusion. Whichever method of marking the text you use your aim is the same: extracting from it what is important. This might include terms, definitions, significant facts and important points or stages in an argument. As you read the book, you might also write occasional thoughts and comments in the margin. You might for instance note down which part of the assignment a particular section of the text will be relevant to, links or contrasts with other material you have read, examples to illustrate points made in the text, and any questions that come to mind.

An alternative to marking the text (though the two methods can also be combined) is to take notes. This is necessary if the book has been borrowed, but is in any case a valuable and productive study skill. Compiling a proper set of notes forces you to think – about what the author means, about the structure of his or her argument and about which parts of the text are relevant to your needs. The notes should be clear, concise and well organised. Do not simply write line after line of continuous prose – make use of headings, numbered points, indentation and underlining. Use abbreviations and write in note form rather than in complete sentences. (Remember though that the notes need to be sufficiently clear for you to understand them later on.) The advice given above about marking the text applies equally to note-taking: only include that which is relevant and important. Generally, you should not copy direct from the text, though you will need to copy down factual information such as dates and statistics and may transcribe a few passages word-for-word so that you can later quote them. For most of the notes however you should try to use your own words. This helps you to check that you have understood the author's argument and will save some time later on, when in writing your assignment you will need to use your own words in any case.

Finally, when you have finished with a book always check to make sure that you have noted down the author, title and other details necessary for inclusion in your bibliography. (See 'Bibliographies', page 186)

References to books

As indicated above, the great majority of an assignment should be in your own words. If an assignment consists of lengthy quotations from other people's work with very little of your own argument in between you will get very little credit. Even worse is copying from books and presenting the work as if it were your own. Assignments written in this way usually do not read well because of the jarring differences of style between the parts that the student did write and the parts that were taken from other sources. You would again receive little credit for work of this kind. Using your own words will be rewarded because you will be showing the teacher marking the assignment that you have understood what you have read and incorporated it into your own argument.

If in the course of an assignment you include a paraphrase of what an author has written (that is, you express his or her argument in your own words) it is customary to mention the author's surname and the date of the publication to which reference is being made. The following examples illustrate how this can be done:

> Seedhouse (1986) equated good health with having the necessary resources to live one's life to the full.

OR

> Another view of good health is that it means having the necessary resources to live one's life to the full.
> (Seedhouse, 1986).

Fuller details of the book (author, title, publisher and date of publication) would then be included in a bibliography (see 'Bibliographies' on page 186).

Occasionally, however, you may wish to quote an author's actual words. Quotations might be appropriate:

- where the precise language used is especially significant (as might be the case with a definition, for example);
- to illustrate a point of view;
- to support a point that you have made;
- when you intend to challenge or question what is in the quotation.

Quotations should usually be clearly separated from the rest of the text. This can be done by indenting the whole of the quotation. It should begin on a new line and when the quotation is complete you should again give the author's name and the date of the publication, before returning to your own argument on a new line. The following example illustrates these points:

> Another view of health is expressed by Seedhouse:
>> "A person's optimum state of health is equivalent to the state of the set of conditions which fulfil or enable a person to work to fulfil his or her realistic chosen and biological potentials." (Seedhouse, 1986).
> This is very different from the definitions of health discussed earlier.

Again the book would be given a more detailed listing in the bibliography.

Newspapers, journals and magazines

Health and social care issues are of great public interest and are covered extensively in the press. Reading newspapers helps to keep you up to date with current information and new developments. It may also help you to think of interesting ideas for assignments and may provide you with material that you can draw upon when completing assignments. Government reports and changes of policy, the findings of surveys and campaigns by pressure groups are all reported in newspapers. You should consider keeping a file of newspaper cuttings for reference purposes. The 'quality' or broadsheet newspapers carry regular health sections (you may find the Guardian on Fridays and the Independent on Tuesdays of particular use) and stories and features relevant to health and social care also occur frequently in the popular press. Local newspapers often contain useful information on the area in which you live. Care should be taken with newspaper articles however. You should consider whether the article is biased or sensationalised. (See 'Checking the validity of printed sources' on page 186).

In addition to newspapers there are a number of more specialist publications, ranging from popular magazines to more serious journals and periodicals. The former category includes 'Here's Health' (monthly) and 'Which Way to Health?' (published bimonthly by the Consumers' Association). Publications targeted at health and social care professionals include the 'British Medical Journal', 'Lancet' and 'Nursing Times' (all weekly). These and other relevant publications are stocked by most public libraries, who may well have a supply of back issues also.

Other sources of printed information

More information is available in the form of leaflets, brochures and booklets. You will probably find a range of such literature at your local library, Citizens Advice Bureau,

Community care 'failing to improve lot of carers'

David Brindle
Social Services Correspondent

MORE than one in four people caring for an elderly or disabled relative or friend has not heard of the community care system introduced a year ago, a survey shows today.

Almost three in four carers say there has been no assessment of the needs of the person they look after. Fewer than one in seven thinks community care has brought any improvement.

The survey was carried out for the Carers' National Association among 426 carers in touch with some form of voluntary group.

The association fears that other "hidden" carers would know even less about community care and have had even worse experience.

Twenty-seven per cent of those surveyed said they had not heard of the community care system, by which local authority social services departments have assumed responsibility for assessing the needs of elderly and disabled people and arranging services for them.

Seventy-four per cent said ther had been no assessment since April of last year of the needs of the person they cared for, 79 per cent thought the changes had made no difference to them, 8 per cent believed services had got worse and only 13 per cent thought it had become easier for carers' needs to be recognised.

Norman Warner, former Kent social services director and author of the survey report, said the findings showed the need for better information for carers, for more encouragement of take-up of assessments and for possibility giving carers a statutory right to assessment of their own needs.

"The jury is definitely still out on whether the community care changes will improve the lot of carers.

"On the evidence of this preliminary study, carers are distincly underwhelmed," said Mr Warner, now a senior fellow at Kent University.

The association of Directors of Social Services said it was "entirely unrealistic" to expect that all 5 million carers would have experienced assessments in the first year.

Denise Platt, ADSS president, said " Ensuring carers' needs are addressed is a key priority of our community care programmes, and we have received additional money for this year, and next, to help with our respite care schemes."

A separate report today warns that the assessment system is rationing places for elderly people in care homes. Some people who wish to enter a home are being turned down, says the report from Counsel and Care, a voluntary group working with the elderly.

Jef Smith, the group's general manager, said "The effect for many of the older people who will now be assessed as not needing places in homes is actually to narrow their choice relative to those who entered homes before 1993."

Community Care: Just a Fairy Tale?; CNA, 20-25 Glasshouse Yard, London EC1A 4JS; price £12.50. More Power to Our Elders, Counsel and Care, 16 Bonny Street, London NW1 9PG; price £5.

DOCTORS TOLD TO OFFER WOMEN MORE CHOICES ON HOW THEY GIVE BIRTH

Mother knows best in new baby Charter

WOMEN are to be given more freedom of choice than ever before when they have babies.

A new Childbirth Charter is to be launched next month by junior Health Minister Baroness Cumberlege.

And it will enshrine in the Patient's Charter a woman's right to choose how and where she has her baby – and who looks after her.

The charter follows a pioneering Health Department report last year, which said maternity services were not giving women what they wanted.

The report was bitterly opposed by some obstetricians who said a move to more midwife-only care and home births would put babies at risk. But Ministers have given it full backing and have told health authorities that they have five years to introduce services which respond more to women's needs. Most authorities will draw up initial plans this year.

Leaflets and videos released nationally this spring will spell out the options for women.

And the Health Department plans training programmes for doctors so that they can give objective advice. The shake-up means more women will be able to have their babies at home or be cared for throughout pregnancy by a midwife they know. Every woman will also have the right to ask for a specialist to manage her case.

Officials say it will free specialists to deal more thoroughly with really needy cases.

Baroness Cumberlege said last night that the changes would take time, but she urged women to grasp the opportunity to make their needs known.

Explore

'It is essential that there is more choice and we are looking at ways that we can help women to be better informed,' she said.

'We also feel that the professionals find it extremely difficult to give unbiased information because theit training has worked against it. We feel they need some help here, so we would like to explore ways of improving training.

'This is a wonderful moment for women actually to sat what they want because the professionals are getting more receptive.

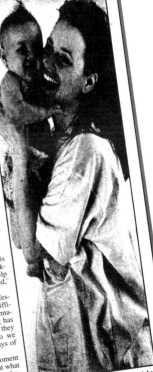

CHOICE: Mothers will be given new rights

Figure 2   Newspapers can be a valuable source of up-to-date information

health centre and hospital. However, if you are seeking information on a specific topic you may well need to approach a specialist organisation. Names, addresses and telephone numbers of some organisations relevant to health and social care are listed on page 188. Many of these supply information leaflets and booklets free of charge.

If the organisation that you wish to approach has an office near you, you may be able to call in person to collect the information, though you should telephone first. Alternatively, you could write requesting information (see 'Letters', page 212) or telephone and ask if information can be sent to you. With all these approaches you need to explain clearly the kind of information that is required and why it is needed. Keep copies of all correspondence as these could be included in an appendix to your assignment. Remember also that some organisations can take time to send out material so any requests for information should be made at the beginning of the research stage of the assignment (when you draw up an Action Plan – see page 205 – this should be one of the first tasks listed). Any literature received and used in the completion of the assignment should of course be listed in your bibliography.

Bear in mind that literature produced by such organisations may be promoting a special interest and may in some cases have a commercial purpose. You need to be objective in your use of this kind of information – an organisation may have been very helpful to you, but that does not mean you have to agree unquestioningly with everything they tell you! (For more on this see 'Checking the validity of printed sources' that follows.)

Bibliographies

Any printed sources of information that you have made use of should be listed in a bibliography at the end of the assignment. The names of authors and of organisations whose literature you obtained should be set out in alphabetical order. With books it is customary to list details in the following order:

1. Name or names of author(s) (surname first, followed by initials);
2. Title of book;
3. Publisher;
4. Year of publication.

Below is an example:

Seedhouse, D. Health: The Foundations for Achievement. John Wiley and Sons, 1986.

For journal, magazine and newspaper articles the usual form of listing is:

1. Name or names of author(s);
2. Title of article;
3. Title of journal/magazine;
4. Volume and/or issue number of journal/magazine, or date of newspaper;
5. Inclusive page numbers of the article.

For example:

Lowry, S. Housing and health: health and homelessness. British Medical Journal, 300, 32–34.

An accurately compiled and presented bibliography provides important evidence of efficient information-seeking.

Checking the validity of printed sources

As was explained earlier (page 179), to achieve a Merit or Distinction you need to show evidence of checking and establishing the validity of information obtained for an assignment. With printed sources of information (books, articles, leaflets and so on) the following points should be borne in mind:

- How up to date is the information? For example, if the research on which the information is based was carried out 10 years ago, are you aware of any changes in circumstances during the intervening period which might mean that different findings would result if the same piece of research were carried out now? Is more recent information on the topic available so that comparisons can be made?

- If the information was research-based, what methods of research were used? Do you think that different methods might have produced different results? If a sample was used, how big was it and was it representative?

- Can the information be double-checked in any way? If more than one source of information is available to you, it might be possible to make cross-checks between them.

- Is the information being used to support an argument or a particular point of view? For example, does it have a political purpose? If so, it might be possible for you to find a book or article which expresses an opposing viewpoint, so that you can weigh up the opposing arguments and arrive at balanced conclusions.

- If the literature has been obtained from an organisation, is it promoting a special interest? For instance, there is a pressure group in favour of smoking as well as one against it, and both use sets of statistics to support their case. Can you be sure the information you have obtained is not biased in any way?

- Does the literature have a commercial purpose? That is, is its ultimate objective to generate business of some kind so that the organisation which has produced the literature makes a profit? Again this may make the information biased and checks with other sources of information should be made if possible.

- If you have found the information in a newspaper or magazine, can you find the original source of the article? For example, newspapers often summarise the findings of reports and surveys. The newspapers's account can be checked if you are able to obtain the report or survey on which the article is based.

- Newspaper articles should also be checked for bias and sensationalism. Stories may be slanted towards a particular political viewpoint or dramatised in order to arouse the interest of the readers. What are the actual facts on which the article is based?

- If the information is in the form of research data check how this has been presented. Does the method of presentation distort the findings in any way? Imagine for example that in a particular area the number of children placed on the At Risk register has increased from 90 to 100 over a 3 year period. Both the line graphs in Fig 3 present this same piece of information:

Note how the different *scale* used for the vertical axis in Graph A makes the rise seem far more dramatic than it does in Graph B.

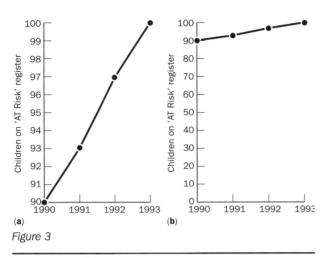

Figure 3

Obtaining information by telephone

We shall now consider other sources of information, beginning with information that might be obtained over the **telephone**. This is an especially useful method if the person or organisation you wish to speak to is too far away for you to visit, or if you are seeking brief factual information (if you have more probing questions to ask you may find their response is less forthcoming than if you speak to them in person). It can also be an appropriate method if you have been unable to obtain literature from an organisation, or if you have obtained literature but it leaves some questions unanswered.

Before making the telephone call you should prepare your questions in advance. Decide exactly what it is that you need to know – there is nothing worse than putting the phone down and realising you forgot to ask a crucial question. Make sure you have a pen with you to note down answers. When you make the call be courteous and explain clearly the information that you require and why it is needed. Before finishing the call check that you have the name of the person you have been speaking to – this will be needed for the 'Acknowledgements' section of your assignment (see p.188) and will also be helpful if you need to call the organisation again. At the end of the call thank the person for his or her assistance.

Checking validity

Some of the points made in the previous section about checking the validity of information apply also to information obtained over the telephone. You should be careful about accepting information solely on a word of mouth basis. You might find that another telephone call to a similar or related organisation will enable you to check what you have been told. Bear in mind the position of the person who gave you the information – if he was a spokesperson for an organisation he would naturally seek to portray that organisation in a flattering light and this may have influenced what he said to you.

Interviews

An alternative to asking questions over the telephone is to arrange a **personal interview** with the person concerned. This is generally preferable as it usually results in a fuller and more co-operative response.

The initial approach may be by letter or telephone (you should certainly not turn up unannounced!). Explain clearly why you want the interview and the kind of information you need. Be flexible and accommodating about the date and time of the interview. When the interview has been set, write a letter of thanks confirming such details as the date, time and who you are to see.

Prepare for the interview by drawing up a *list of questions*. Think carefully about what you need to know. Although some of the questions may only require brief, factual answers, you should also include open questions which allow for a freer, more extended response from the interviewee. Decide whether you are going to take notes during the interview or use a tape recorder – if the latter, you should ask the consent of the interviewee beforehand.

During the interview, try to adopt a relaxed manner and try also to help the person you are interviewing feel at ease. Although you should make sure that no important questions are omitted, be prepared to depart from your set list of questions in order to explore issues in greater depth or if your interviewee makes an unexpected remark. At the end of the interview remember to thank the person concerned for his or her co-operation.

Afterwards, you should make a fuller set of notes while the interview is still fresh in your mind. If you leave it too long, the notes you made at the interview itself may not make much sense to you. Make sure you have a record of the date and venue of the interview, and of the name and position of the person interviewed – these details can be included in your assignment later.

Checking validity

Finally, the points made in the previous section about checking the validity of information obtained by telephone apply equally to personal interviews.

Visits

Visiting an organisation gives you an opportunity to learn first-hand abnut how the organisation works. Before paying such a visit always make a formal request some time in advance, either by telephone or in writing, explaining clearly the purpose of the visit. Again you should prepare for the visit by deciding before you go what it is that you need to know. If people are working and you are allowed to observe them, be unobtrusive and do not ask them questions when they are busy. Make notes during the visit and write up a fuller version when the visit is over.

Television and radio programmes

Like newspapers and magazines, **television and radio programmes** are a useful source of topical information. Television documentary series such as 'Horizon' and 'Everyman' frequently feature health and social care topics, and other items of interest regularly appear in news programmes. On radio there are series such as the magazine programme 'Medicine Now' and 'Does He Take Sugar?', which features items for and about disabled people (both programmes are on Radio 4). You might be able to record television and radio programmes so that you can watch or listen to them at your own pace and extract relevant information.

Make a note of any programmes that you use for inclusion in your bibliography.

Health promotion services

Your local health authority will have a **health promotion department**, responsible for promoting good health within the community. You can obtain through them a wide range of health education literature, including leaflets and information booklets on health topics and from voluntary groups. They will also provide information on such matters as community health projects and local self-help groups.

Acknowledgements

As mentioned previously, printed information sources along with any television and radio programmes used in preparation of the assignment should be listed in a **bibliography**. Other assistance received from individuals and organisations can be mentioned in a separate '**Acknowledgements**' section. Usually the entries are listed alphabetically, with a brief explanation where appropriate of the nature of the help given, as in the following example:

> I should like to thank the following for the help and information they provided: Mersey Regional Health Authority (Health Promotion Department); Clive Ryan, who showed me around the Cranridge Day Centre and agreed to be interviewed about the Centre's work; the Royal National Institute for the Blind; Sue Smith of the Disablement Information and Advice Line.

Useful addresses and telephone numbers

Action on Smoking and Health (ASH), 5/11 Mortimer Street, London W1N 7RH (Tel. 0171-637-9843)

Age Concern, Astral House, 1268 London Road, London SW16 4EJ (Tel. 0181-679-8000)

British Homoeopathic Association, 27a Devonshire Street, London W1N 1RJ (Tel. 0171-935-2163)

British Sports Association of the Disabled, 34 Osnaburgh Street, London NW1 3ND (Tel. 0171-383-7277)

Cancer Information Service, 121-3 Charterhouse Street, London EC1M 6AA (Tel. 0171-608-1661/0800-181199)

Carers National Association, 29 Chilworth Mews, London W3 3RG (Tel. 0171-724-7776)

Cruse-Bereavement Care, Cruse House, 126 Sheen Road, Richmond, Surrey TW9 1UR (Tel. 0181-940-4818/9407)

DIAL UK (Information and advice for the disabled), Victoria Buildings, 117 High Street, Clay Cross, Chesterfield S45 9DZ (Tel. 01246-250055)

Disabled Living Foundation (Information on aids and equipment for the disabled), 380-4 Harrow Road, London W9 2HU (Tel. 0171-289-6111)

Family Planning Information Service, 27-35 Mortimer Street, London W1N 7RJ (Tel. 0171-636-7866)

Friends of the Earth, 26-8 Underwood Street, London N1 7JQ (Tel. 0171-490-1555)

Hospice Information Service, 51-9 Lawrie Park Road, Sydenham, London SE26 6DZ (Tel. 0181-778-9252 Ext 262)

Institute for Complementary Medicine, 21 Portland Place, London W1N 3AF (Tel. 0171-636-9543)

MENCAP (Royal Society for Mentally Handicapped Children and Adults), 117-123 Golden Lane, London EC1Y 0RT (Tel. 0171-454-0454)

Midwives' Information and Resource Services, Institute of Child Health, Bristol BS2 8BJ (Tel. 01272-251791)

MIND (National Association for Mental Health), 22 Harley Street, London W1N 2ED (Tel. 0171-637-0741)

National Association for Patient Participation, 13 Manor Drive, Surbiton, Surrey KT5 8NE (Tel. 0181-399-4122)

National Association for the Welfare of Children in Hospital, Argyle House, 29-31 Euston Road, London NW1 2SD (Tel. 0171-833-2041)

National Autistic Society, 276 Willesden Lane, London NW2 5RB (Tel. 0181-451-1114)

National Childbirth Trust, Alexandra House, Oldham Terrace, Acton, London W3 6NH (Tel. 0181-992-8637)

National Self-Help Support Centre, 26 Bedford Square, London WC1B 3HU (Tel. 0171-636-4066)

Pregnancy Advisory Service, 11-13 Charlotte Street, London W1P 1HD (Tel. 0171-637-8962)

Royal Association for Disability and Rehabilitation, 25 Mortimer Street, London W1N 8AB (Tel. 0171-637-5400)

Royal National Institute for the Blind, 224 Great Portland Street, London W1N 6AA (Tel. 0171-388-1266)

Royal National Institute for the Deaf, 105 Gower Street, London WC1E 6AH (Tel. 0171-387-8044)

SKILL: National Bureau for Students with Disabilities, 336 Brixton Road, London SW9 7AA (Tel. 0171-274-0565)

Terrence Higgins Trust (Information on HIV and Aids), 52-4 Gray's Inn Road, London WC1X 8LT (Tel. 0171-242-1010)

Women's Health and Reproductive Rights Information Centre, 52-4 Featherstone Street, London EC1Y 8RT (Tel. 0171-251-6332)

5 Reports and projects

Many of your assignments will take the form of reports and projects. We now look at the skills involved in producing these.

5.1 Short reports

Reports can vary considerably in length, and also in scope. Long reports (which we shall examine in the next section) frequently require extensive investigation and research, and may for example be written in order to test a hypothesis or to arrive at recommendations for future action. **Short reports**, which we shall consider first, may arise from a more limited investigation or may be an account of an event (e.g. an accident). Sometimes the writing of a short report simply entails the completion of a standard printed form (accident report forms, for example, are common in many organisations). All reports, regardless of length, involve the structured presentation of information on a specified subject, for a specified purpose. In presenting this information use is often made of headings, sub-headings, numbered sections and indentation.

Many short reports adhere to the following standard structure:

1. Introduction
2. Main body (The heading 'Findings' is often appropriate here)
3. Conclusion

In the *Introduction* the purpose and scope of the report should be clearly stated. The situation that has given rise to the report can also be mentioned here. The *Main body* contains all the important facts, information and findings. Material should be arranged in a logical order and use made of paragraphs and sub-headings as appropriate. The *Conclusion* is a brief summing-up and in a short report may incorporate recommendations for action (in a larger report 'Recommendations' would be a separate heading – see next section).

Imagine for example that you have been asked to visit your local health centre and then write a short factual report of about 250 words, describing the organisation of the centre and outlining the services that it provides. (A limited task such as this might well form part of a larger assignment examining the health services available in a particular area.) An example of the kind of report you might produce is given below.

Report on Kenslow Medical Centre

Introduction

The Kenslow Medical Centre was visited on 12 January 1994. Interviews were conducted with Dr Roy Fraser and Mrs Clare Andrew (a Centre receptionist). Information was obtained on the services offered by the Centre and on staff, opening hours and the areas that are served by the Centre.

Findings

Staff
The Medical Centre has 26 members of staff. These include:
- 3 Doctors
- 13 Practice Staff (6 receptionists; 3 practice nurses; 2 secretaries; 1 practice manager; 1 assistant practice manager)
- 10 Attached Staff (7 district nurses; 2 health visitors; 1 midwife)

Services Available
In addition to normal medical services, the Centre offers the following: contraceptive advice; immunisation; maternity care; women's screening clinic (e.g. cervical smears, breast examination); medical examinations required for insurance purposes or by prospective employers; minor surgical procedures (e.g. cyst removal, skin biopsy); health promotion and disease surveillance clinics (e.g. heart disease prevention, foreign travel service, asthma control).

Opening Hours
The Centre is open from 8 am to 6.30 pm Monday to Friday and from 8 am to 11.30 am on Saturday. On Sunday the Centre is closed. The doctors also make home visits and there is an emergency telephone number for urgent advice or treatment outside surgery hours.

Areas Covered By The Centre
The Centre covers Kenslow, Little Shoreham, Waltham Green, Friarby and Midhurst.

Conclusion

The visit was an informative one and gave an interesting insight into the organisation of a medical centre and the functions that such a centre has. The Centre staff were very helpful and indicated that they would be happy to assist in any future research projects.

This is an effective short report. The Introduction provides relevant background information in a concise manner and clearly outlines the scope of the report. The main Findings section organises the information obtained from the visit in a logical way and makes appropriate use of sub-headings.

5.2 Long reports/research projects

Projects and **long reports** usually involve more extensive research than short reports. They are also much more detailed and have a different format. We shall now consider the various stages involved in producing a research project or a long report, looking first at the choice of a topic and a title.

Choosing a topic and a title

Of course you may already have been given a title by your teacher, in which case you can skip both this and the next section. However, it is quite possible that at some stage in your course you will be given the opportunity to suggest and devise assignments. GNVQs are intended to promote active learning, and to encourage and reward independence and initiative. In particular, devising your own project will help you to display the planning skills required for a Merit or Distinction.

When you decide upon a topic and a title, bear in mind the following points:

- Make sure you will be able to obtain information on the topic you choose. Earlier we looked at sources of information (page 180) and shortly we shall look at other kinds of research you might carry out. You might find that information is more readily available if you base your assignment on the local community. If you have a work placement you might choose a topic where you will be able to make use of the research possibilities available to you there.

- Avoid broad topics which may prove unmanageable, or which you will only be able to cover in a sketchy, superficial way. Instead, choose a specific, clearly defined topic which will enable you to undertake research which is both original and thorough. For example, if you wanted to investigate facilities for the disabled, it would make more sense to concentrate on one area rather than to seek to carry out a nationwide study. It might also be sensible to focus on one type of facility – e.g. leisure facilities (cinemas, theatres, restaurants, sports facilities etc.).

- Remember that the best projects are analytical rather than descriptive. Projects which do no more than gather together information in the form of leaflets, magazine articles and so on will get little credit. You therefore need to give yourself a title which will require you to investigate, analyse and arrive at conclusions. This might be helped by devising a title which poses a question: 'How adequate are leisure facilities for the disabled in Midwick?' might well produce a more analytical project than 'Leisure facilities for the disabled in Midwick'. (Alternatively, the project could test a hypothesis – see the next section, 'Formulating a hypothesis'.)

- Be realistic. Will you be able to carry out the research required? Will it involve a lot of travelling around, and will you be able to afford this? Are you sure the people you may wish to speak to will be prepared to spare you the time? Have *you* the time to carry out the research, analyse your results and write up your final report? Bear in mind the deadline for the assignment – are you sure you will be able to meet it?

- All of the above questions can be more easily answered if you draw up an *Action Plan* before embarking on the assignment. Here you work out the stages involved in completing the assignment, and allocate time to them. An Action Plan helps you to test the feasibility of the project: thinking through each stage in advance should enable you to spot if any aspect of the project is impractical. Action Plans also help you to satisfy the criteria for a Merit or Distinction. They are discussed more fully opposite.

- Remember to consult your teacher. It is worth checking that your topic and title are appropriate before setting to work in earnest.

Formulating a hypothesis

You might decide that your research will test a **hypothesis**, ie a theory or assumption.

> **Hypothesis**
> A theory or assumption which seeks to explain a particular situation or occurrence.

Often the most effective way to test a hypothesis is by carrying out an *experiment*. This means that a controlled situation is set up by the experimenter, who then observes what takes place. Suppose for example that your work placement is in a nursery and that you have noticed that children who are given a task to perform (building a house with toy bricks, for example) tend to retain an interest in the activity and persevere longer if they are praised for their efforts and given other verbal encouragement. You could decide to investigate this further by formulating a hypothesis and then testing it. Your hypothesis might be:

> 'Children who are given five set tasks to perform and who are given verbal encouragement as they undertake these tasks will retain an interest in the tasks for a longer period than children who do not receive such encouragement.'

Note that the hypothesis is specific (the reference to 'five set tasks') rather than general (it does not state that children who are encouraged will show greater interest and perseverance in any situation). This is because although you may have a general theory about children's behaviour (that encouragement increases motivation) you will only be able to test the theory in these specific circumstances. When you formulate a hypothesis, remember to ensure that you will be able to test it and discover how far it is correct.

Choosing a research method

Having decided upon a title or formulated a hypothesis, you now need to decide *how* you will undertake your research. The data that you collect is likely to be of two kinds:

Primary data. This is information that you obtain first-hand by carrying out your own investigations. Primary data would include for example the results of experiments you have set up and of questionnaires you have devised and distributed. For more on how to collect primary data, see Unit 8 (pages 156–160).

Secondary data. This is information collected by others or from books, newspapers and similar sources. For more on how to obtain and use secondary data, see the earlier section on 'Sources of Information' (page 180).

Ethical Considerations

When you devise and carry out research you must be careful to protect the rights and interests of your subjects. Usually you would explain your intentions and ask the subjects for their consent. This means telling them the purpose of the study, what they will be required to do and who is likely to be shown the results of the research. You should also explain whether they will be identified by name in the study. (This is usually unnecessary – pseudonyms can be used, or if several subjects are involved each can be allocated a number.)

You may however wish to observe subjects without them knowing, so that you can observe their natural behaviour. You should only carry out research without informing your subjects if you are certain that they will not experience any pain or distress and that you are not intruding upon their privacy. Ethical considerations are especially important where vulnerable groups are concerned – children, the elderly or those who are ill. You must always be careful to ensure that subjects drawn from such groups retain their dignity, and that their rights are never threatened. If you have any doubts about the ethics of your research you should consult your teacher.

Action Plans

Assuming you now have a title for the assignment and know the research approach you are going to adopt, you should now draw up a *plan* for the preparation and completion of the assignment. These are known as **Action Plans** and they are necessary and helpful for all but the briefest of assignments. In an Action Plan you decide the various activities that need to be undertaken and set a timetable for their completion. An Action Plan ensures that you adopt a structured approach to the assignment and that you allocate an appropriate period of time for each activity. It will also help you to see at an early stage if any aspects of your research strategy are unrealistic. For example, if you have a month to complete an assignment and intend using postal questionnaires, you will need to allocate time for devising the questionnaires, getting them photocopied or printed, sending them out, waiting for them to be returned, chasing up those that are not returned, analysing the results and writing up the final report – when you have done this you may well decide that given the time available another research method would be more practical!

Some of the tasks that might be involved in completing an assignment are listed below. In an Action Plan you would show how much time you expected to spend on each, and when you intended to begin and complete each task. For a Merit or Distinction you would also *prioritise* the tasks. This means deciding which are the most important and the order in which they need to be completed.

- Sending for information (leaflets, brochures etc.)
- Collecting secondary data (information from books, other printed sources etc.)
- Carrying out research into secondary data
- Requesting permission to carry out research
- Preparation for interviews
- Conducting interviews
- Preparation for visits
- Visits to obtain information
- Devising a questionnaire
- Testing the questionnaire
- Circulating the questionnaire
- Collecting the completed questionnaires
- Conducting an experiment
- Conducting an observation
- Collecting together results of research
- Analysing results of research
- Planning final report
- Writing first draft
- Writing final draft
- Writing evaluation.

Remember to allow for unforeseen delays. Especially with major assignments it is advisable to set a completion date that is at least a week earlier than the date given to you by your teacher. You should also be prepared to *revise* your Action Plan when necessary. For example, if a visit to a particular institution cannot take place until a date later than you originally intended, it would be sensible to try to bring something else forward (you might for instance re-schedule an interview date). Monitoring your plan of action and making appropriate revisions are again skills which can help you to achieve a Merit or Distinction.

Your school or college may well provide you with printed forms on which to fill in your Actions Plans, or your teacher may suggest an appropriate format. If not, you will need to decide on a layout. One approach is to have separate columns for each of the following:

Task/ Activity	Time Allocation	Date for Completion	Resources	Monitoring	Comments/ Revisions

For a specimen Action Plan using this format, see Specimen Assignment B on page 205.

Diaries / Logs

During the completion of the assignment you should keep a **diary** or **log**. Here you keep a record of the progress you are making, including problems you encounter, decisions made about alterations to your approach and general thoughts about how the project is developing. A diary is useful because it enables you to explain and justify *revisions* to your plan of action or research method. It should also prove very useful

when you reach the final stage of the assignment, the Evaluation.

Pilot Studies

A **pilot study** tests a method of research to make sure it is reliable. It is a 'trial run' of the research intended to show up flaws and weaknesses which you can then correct before carrying out the research proper. It is especially appropriate if your research method involves an experiment or a questionnaire. Imagine for example that you intend distributing a questionnaire to 30 subjects. Before doing this you could test the questionnaire on a smaller sample of 8 or 10 people. It may then become apparent to you that certain questions are ambiguous, difficult to understand or incomplete. Suppose for instance that your questionnaire included the following question:

How did you find out about the playgroup?

Word of mouth (friends, neighbours, relatives)	☐
Telephone directory (e.g. Yellow Pages)	☐
Local Press	☐
Other publicity (e.g. posters)	☐

If when you carry out the pilot study four out of the ten people taking part do not tick any of the boxes, you should re-think the question. Is there another important source of information about the playgroup that you have omitted? Or perhaps you could add to the list of possible answers 'Other (please specify)'.

A trial run of an experiment may reveal practical problems (e.g. the room in which you intended to carry out the experiment may be too noisy), difficulties in measuring results or a need to clarify the instructions you give to those taking part.

You can include a report on the pilot study in the final version of the assignment, explaining any changes it causes in your approach. You can also assess the value of the pilot study in the Evaluation. As a pilot study helps you to monitor, revise and evaluate your project it gives you another opportunity to fulfil some of the criteria for a Merit or Distinction.

We shall now consider how you would actually carry out your research, looking in turn at each of the research methods referred to in Unit 8.

Carrying out research: Experiments

For the newcomer to the **experiment**, the method and the language used may at first seem complex. In fact, the essence of the experimental method is simple – it is the study of cause and effect. Experiments deliberately manipulate one variable – the *independent variable* – to see if it has any effect on another variable – the *dependent variable*.

To take an example: suppose that you are interested in the effect of exercise on the heartbeat. An experiment could be devised where the independent variable would be the number of minutes of exercise taken, and the dependent variable a measure of the heartbeat. The independent variable is therefore a condition selected by the experimenter, while the dependent variable is the variable which is observed and measured. The dependent variable is so named because its value *depends* on the value of the independent variable.

Another important aspect of the experimental method is *control*. Suppose for example you were interested in the effect of positive feedback on memory. Your hypothesis is that giving verbal encouragement (positive feedback) to people as they attempt to remember something makes them more likely to remember it successfully. The independent variable would be encouraging feedback and the dependant variable might be a score on a memory test. In a typical experiment you would select two groups – the experimental group and the *control group*. The experimental group would take the memory test and be given feedback (in the form of verbal encouragement) as they did so. The control group would take the same test but receive no such feedback.

We might suppose that any difference in the performance of the two groups would be due to the independent variable (feedback). However, there are several other things which might affect the result. By chance the people (or, to use the correct term, *subjects*) in the experimental group might have higher IQs or better memories. There may be differences in levels of education between the two groups. Problems like these are known as *confounding variables*, because they are factors which can confound or mislead the experimental findings.

The experimenter could overcome such problems by attempting to *match* the two groups. This could be done by giving subjects a preliminary memory test and assigning them to the control and experimental groups in such a way that any individual differences in memory 'span' were equalised in the two groups. Other individual differences (such as age) could also be equalised between the two groups. If the two groups are alike in other respects, with the independent variable the only difference between them, we can be fairly confident that the difference (if any) in memory scores is due to feedback.

As well as individual differences, we must also control *extraneous variables* between the groups. An example of an extraneous variable would be noise levels in the room in which subjects were tested, or the time of testing. If we tested the experimental group in the morning in a light, quiet, airy room and the control group in the late afternoon in a small, stuffy room, with noisy roadworks taking place outside, the different results of the two groups may be due not to the independent variable but to these extraneous variables. An experimenter must therefore ensure that subjects are tested in similar environments.

The *design* of an experiment is also important. The two basic experimental designs are:

- Independent Subjects Design
- Repeated Measures Design

Each of these designs uses subjects in a different way. With the **Independent Subjects Design** a group of subjects is obtained for the experiment and individuals are allocated randomly to either the experimental condition or the control condition. (This might be done, for example, by tossing a coin or by picking names out of a hat.) With the **Repeated Measures Design** subjects perform under *both* conditions, experimental and control.

Below is an example of the allocation of subjects to conditions, in an Independent Subject Design and in a Repeated Measures Design. In the table S1, S2 and so on refer to individual subjects.

Independent Subjects Design		Repeated Measures Design	
Condition A	Condition B	Condition A	Condition B
S1	S2	S1	S1
S3	S4	S2	S2
S5	S6	S3	S3
S7	S8	S4	S4
S9	S10	S5	S5

Advantages and disadvantages of these designs

As the table shows, twice as many subjects are needed for the Independent Subjects Design.

- In the Repeated Measures Design the control group is the same as the experimental group. This method ensures that there are no individual differences between the two groups.
- However, although Repeated Measures Designs are usually stronger, there are problems with their use in some experiments – in particular, learning experiments. For example, in a memory test subjects might perform better in the second condition simply because they have had time to grow used to this kind of test.

One method used in an attempt to overcome this kind of problem is a procedure known as *counterbalancing*. Here, half of the subjects are tested under one condition of the independent variable first and the other half are tested under the other condition first, as in the table below.

Counterbalancing subjects in a Repeated Measures Design	
Condition A	Condition B
S1 (First)	S1 (Second)
S2 (Second)	S2 (First)
S3 (First)	S3 (Second)
S4 (Second)	S4 (First)
S5 (First)	S5 (Second)

If you conduct an experiment, try to adopt the correct procedures and to use the correct terms when you write it up. You should bear in mind the possible pitfalls outlined above and explain how you attempted to avoid them. (Remember that one of the criteria for a Merit or Distinction is that you justify your approach.)

For an example of an assignment based on an experiment, see Specimen Assignment B on page 201.

Carrying out research: Observation

As was mentioned earlier there are a variety of methods of **observation**, including participant, non-participant and self-recording. Another distinction can be made between *open* and *structured* observations.

Open observation

In an open observation the observer tries to notice as much as possible that is taking place and does not begin the observation with set ideas about what has to be recorded. You might for example seek to increase your understanding of the work of playgroups by observing a particular playgroup over one morning. You might during the course of your observation note down a number of different things – the activities undertaken by the group, the behaviour of the children, the facilities available to them and so on. Essentially, in an open observation you record anything that you feel might be important or relevant to your study.

Structured observation

In a structured observation, you decide in advance what is important and only record specified events or behaviours. It is usual here to prepare for the observation by designing an observation sheet which indicates what is to be recorded and which provides spaces for doing this. A common format is for the time that has elapsed to be indicated along the vertical axis, while the events or behaviours are categorised in a series of headings along the horizontal axis. The result is a set of boxes in which ticks or other written indicators can be placed.

Imagine for example that you were interested in gender socialisation and wanted to observe a group of four nursery children (two boys and two girls) at play. The children have access to six toys, some traditionally regarded as masculine and some traditionally regarded as feminine. In order to carry out such an observation over a period of 30 minutes you might draw up an **observation sheet** similar to that below.

	Tool set	Baby doll	Action man	Tea set	Car	My Little Pony
9.00						
9.01						
9.02						
9.03						
9.04						
9.05						
etc.						

Figure 4   An observation sheet (extract)

Before beginning the observation you would decide on a method of identifying each child – you might refer to the two girls as A and B and the two boys as C and D. You would have a watch with you during the observation and at the end of every minute you would record which child was playing with which toy, by placing letters (A, B, C and D) in the appropriate boxes.

You need to ensure that any sheet you devise is clear, especially if it is to be filled in by others (as might be the case with self-recording, when you ask others to keep a record of their own behaviour or experiences). In particular, the categories that you use must be defined with care. You might for instance observe a group discussion in order to note down positive and negative behaviour by members of the group. You would need to be clear in your mind about what constituted positive and negative behaviour, and might well find it would be better to use a larger number of more precise categories under each heading (thus negative behaviour might include 'interrupting others' and 'shouting'). A pilot study (see page 191) can help you to spot any weaknesses in the form that you have designed.

When you carry out an observation, remember the role or position you have decided to adopt and try your best to keep to it. Are you participant or non-participant, and are your subjects aware or unaware that they are being observed? If your position changes during the observation (subjects notice they are being watched, for example) this may well invalidate your findings.

Time can be a problem in observations, in that you may find that too much is going on at once for you to record it all accurately (this might be the case if you are observing a group discussion). A pilot observation should indicate if this is going to be a problem. One way to tackle this is to limit the types or categories of behaviour / events that you are going to record. Another is to make a video or audio recording of the observation. You will then be able to watch or listen to the recording at your own pace. (You need though to consider what effect the presence of a video camera or tape recorder will have on the behaviour of your subjects.)

Carrying out research: Sampling

If your research involves a survey of some kind, it may be necessary to select a **sample** from the total population of potential subjects. In statistics, a 'population' is the total number of people in a particular group. If you were investigating client needs at a local health centre, for example, the population would be all the clients who use the health centre. If your survey population is small it may be possible to interview each member of it, or to ask each one to complete a questionnaire. If the population is large, however, this becomes impossible and sampling has to take place.

Imagine for instance that you wish to assess your fellow students' knowledge of preventive health services (cancer screening, immunisation etc.). If the study was confined to your own class, you could probably include every student in the survey. If you wanted to investigate the entire student population of your school or college, it would be more sensible to use a sample. To select the sample you could use one of two common methods:

Random sample

Here every person has an *equal chance* of being selected. You could simply pick names out of a hat, but random sampling is usually approached more systematically than this, as care must be taken to ensure that the sample is truly representative. Suppose for example that for your preventive health services survey you decided to distribute questionnaires to 1 in 20 of the college student population. You might simply stand outside the college gates on Monday morning and hand out questionnaires to every twentieth person entering the college. If you later discovered that several classes did not attend college on Mondays (because of work placements, for example) your sample would not be representative. In any case, some students would inevitably be absent for other reasons (e.g. ill health) so simply stopping 1 in 20 of those coming into college would not ensure that your questionnaires reached 1 in 20 of the student population. A better approach might be to approach the college office and ask for access to a computer print-out of enrolled students; you could then select every twentieth name from this list.

Quota sample

Here the sample is selected according to certain *specific criteria*. If the survey population has a wide age-range, for example, the sample might comprise five individuals aged between 20 and 30, five aged between 30 and 40, and so on. In the case of the preventive health services survey, you might decide to select four students from each department of the college.

Conducting a few 'mini-surveys' as a pilot study will help you to check the accuracy of your sampling method. If the samples are truly representative, the results of each survey should be similar.

In your final report you should explain clearly how many people were involved in the study, and how they were selected. If a pilot study took place this should also be described.

Carrying out research: Surveys

As mentioned previously, the most common **survey methods** are interviews and questionnaires.

Interviews

An **interview** involves obtaining information personally from the individuals involved in the survey, usually in face-to-face meetings (which are almost always preferable to telephone interviews). If you intend to conduct a large number of similar interviews and to carry out a statistical analysis of the results, the interview will need to be quite highly structured. This means that each interviewee should be asked the same questions in the same order, and that most of the questions should invite specific responses. If questions are open ended, analysis of the results will be much more difficult. For example, it would be difficult to analyse the responses to a question such as 'What do you think of facilities for the disabled in this borough?' Analysis would be made easier if the question was changed to: 'On the whole, would you describe facilities for the disabled in this borough as very good, satisfactory or poor?' However, in order that important facts or opinions are not overlooked, one or two more open questions might be asked towards the end of the interview. You might ask something like, 'Is there anything on this topic you would especially like to add?' or 'Of all the matters we have touched upon, which do you feel is most important?' The responses to such questions can be useful and illuminating, especially if something you had not previously thought of is mentioned by several interviewees!

If only a few people are being interviewed and the results will not be statistically analysed, the interview can be less highly structured and the questions more open-ended. As part of an investigation into marital violence, for example, you might try to interview one or two social workers. Although you should certainly draw up a list of questions for such an interview, you should also be prepared to adapt your line of questioning as the interview develops. If the person being interviewed introduces an unexpected opinion or piece of information you should be ready to pursue this.

For all kinds of interview the following points should be borne in mind:

- The interview should be a conversation rather than an interrogation. Adopt a relaxed manner and try to ensure that the person you are interviewing feels at ease. (For more on the techniques and skills involved in one-to-one communication see Unit 2 Element 1.)
- Begin the interview by introducing yourself and explaining the general purpose of the interview and how long it is likely to last.
- Be careful not to influence the responses to particular questions. Do not put words in interviewees' mouths or imply what their answers to particular questions should be.
- Ensure that your questions are clear, unambiguous and free of jargon. (For more on this see the section on Questionnaires below.)
- Arrange questions in a logical order, avoiding repetition and disorganised sequences of questions. Often it helps to put an interviewee at ease to begin with a few straightforward factual questions.
- When you write or type your questions, allow plenty of space for noting down answers. If you intend recording the interview, make sure you have the interviewee's consent.

Questionnaires

A **questionnaire** is a set of written questions designed to collect information from a number of people, although you might also produce a questionnaire for use in an interview with a single individual (see above). A questionnaire can be used to obtain opinions and attitudes as well as factual information.

Questionnaires might be distributed to **respondents**, who are asked to fill them in before returning them to you at a later date. A problem here is that you may find some questionnaires are not returned, while others are returned but not completed. This reduces your sample size. An alternative is to interview each respondent personally, asking the questions that are on the questionnaire and recording the answers yourself.

The first stage in preparing a questionnaire is to decide exactly the information you require. Clarify what it is you want the questionnaire to find out. If you are unsure, this will result in a muddled, poorly designed questionnaire and in a set of answers that are of little practical value. Time spent in careful preparation, thinking about the wording of the questions and the layout will help to ensure the questionnaire fulfils its purpose and will also save time later on.

These are some of the most important points to consider when preparing and using questionnaires:

- **Avoid jargon** which may not be understood by those answering the question. Use language the respondent is likely to be familiar with. For example, the question 'Does any member of your family suffer from myopia?' may mystify some people. It would probably be more sensible to ask 'Does any member of your family suffer from shortsightedness?'
- **Avoid lengthy, complex questions.** Questions should be direct, concise and **unambiguous**.
- **Leading questions should also be avoided.** A leading question is on which does not give the respondent genuine freedom in answering. This includes, for instance, questions which begin 'Do you agree that ...?' Such a question tends to suggest that the respondent should answer 'Yes'.
- **Sampling.** It is important that those to whom you give a questionnaire are representative, that is typical of the 'population' you are looking at. If you wanted to find out schoolchildren's attitudes towards physical education, you would get an unrepresentative response if you only gave the questionnaire to members of school sports teams. (See 'Carrying out research: Sampling' on page 193.)
- **Permission.** It may be necessary to obtain permission to undertake a questionnaire. This might be the case for example outside a business or a health centre (especially if you are asking questions regarding services in these institutions).
- **Be polite to respondents.** When you stop people to ask them to take part in a survey they might be in a hurry. They are more likely to assist you if you are courteous and explain what your questionnaire is for. Always thank those who agree to answer your questions.
- **Be safety-conscious.** Do not put yourself in a hazardous situation. Always interview in the

daytime and never interview strangers in their own home. If you do need to interview strangers, this should be done in a public place, preferably with other students present. Tell someone where you are going and when you will return.

- **Pilot studies.** You might wish to carry out a pilot study. This can show up weaknesses in your questions, and you may pick up useful hints for improving the questionnaire before the full research exercise is underway. (See 'Pilot studies' on page 191.)

Types of questions

There are two main types of questions: open and closed. In an **open question** the respondent's answer is not restricted. An example or an open question is 'Why do you think a balanced diet is important?' The respondent is free to reply as he or she wishes. **Closed questions**, which invite a more limited reply, take various forms. They are much easier than open questions to analyse afterwards. Although most questions in a questionnaire should be closed, it is a good idea to have at least one question inviting more general comment at the end of the questionnaire. Open-ended answers may be hard to analyse, but they do produce accurate and often interesting information.

The major types of *closed question* were considered in Unit 8, pages 160–161.

Analysing and presenting results

When you have completed the interview or questionnaire you must bring together and present the replies. It will be necessary to include an analysis of the responses you received to different questions. With open questions you will need to summarise the general points that emerged. With closed questions you will need to count the responses and convert them to percentages (e.g. for a particular question you might find that 76% agreed and 24% disagreed). You need to think about the most efficient way of presenting your results. Bar charts and pie charts can show percentages effectively. When writing up your assignment remember to include a copy of the questionnaire. (For more on these points see 'Analysing data' in Unit 8 page 168 and 'Ways of presenting information' also in Unit 8 page 163.)

(NOTE: Questionnaires are also discussed in Unit 8, Element 2 on page 157).

Carrying out research: Case Studies

As explained earlier, a **case study** is an in-depth investigation of a specific situation or of an individual client. Information is collected from a range of sources and a variety of research methods may be employed. If your subject is an autistic child, for example, you might interview the child's parents and teachers as well as observe the child yourself. If you undertake a case study you should think carefully about the research methods available and choose those which seem to be most appropriate and which are likely to yield the most helpful results. You also need to structure your research. Weigh up the advantages and disadvantages of carrying out one piece of research before another. In the case of the autistic child, speaking to the child's teachers first might give you

useful background information but might also mean you have preconceived ideas when you conduct the observation. (A compromise could be to observe the child twice, speaking to the teachers between the two observations.) Because you are likely to be involved in a range of activities, a carefully prepared Action Plan (see page 190) is especially important. When you embark on your research bear in mind the specific points made in preceding sections about conducting different types of research.

Checking the validity of your own research findings

Earlier (page 186), we discussed how you might check the **validity** of printed sources of information. It would also be worthwhile when undertaking a research project to check the validity of your own research findings. Doing so might help you to satisfy the grading criteria for a Merit or Distinction. Here are four possible methods of checking validity:

1. One way to test the validity of a piece of research is simply to repeat the research. If your observation of a doctor's surgery over a single week found that Monday morning was the busiest time, this finding would be more valid if you repeated the observation over a second week and found the same thing.
2. Closely linked to this is the idea of predictive validity. If research results accurately reflect underlying trends, you should be able to make accurate predictions on the basis of them. Imagine that you surveyed a group of people aged between 20 and 50 and found that knowledge of illegal drugs steadily decreased as the age of the subjects rose. You could check the validity of this finding by surveying a few people over 50 to see if the trend continued.
3. If any similar kinds of research have been undertaken by others you could check the validity of your findings by comparing them with those of other researchers.
4. You might check whether your findings concur with relevant theory. For example, an investigation into some of the attitudes held by a group of fellow students might suggest that the students are strongly influenced by their peer group. If you came across a book in which a sociologist argued that this was true of teenagers as a whole, this would strengthen the validity of your findings.

If you carry out any checks on the validity of your research findings, remember to mention them in your final report. Appropriate places might be the Discussion or Evaluation sections (see page 196).

Layout of a long report or research project

As with short reports (page 188), the material in long reports is arranged into separate sections, and headings and subheadings are used to break up the text. The difference is that a long report or research project contains a larger number of sections. A few slightly different formats are available, but the layout suggested below is a fairly standard one that can be adapted for use with most kinds of report. The sections are listed here in the order in which they would appear, together with a brief explanation of what each should contain.

Title

If you need to devise your own **title**, remember that it should be fairly short but also precise. Avoid titles which are vague and generalised. If you conducted a survey at your school on attitudes to drug abuse, for example, 'A report on attitudes to drug abuse among the pupils of Hillcrest High School' would be a better title than simply 'Drug Abuse', or 'Attitudes to drug abuse'.

Contents page

If the report runs to several pages, it is worth having a **contents page**, on which you list the main sections and subsections. The pages of the whole report should be numbered, and these page numbers used in the table of contents. You might also have a separate list of tables and diagrams.

Summary (or Abstract)

Here you provide a brief **summary** of the whole report, usually in no more than a paragraph. Summarise the aims of the study, the research methods used, the main findings and the conclusions reached.

Introduction

This should include the reasons for undertaking the study and any theoretical or factual information needed as background to the report. The case study on an autistic child referred to earlier, for example, might use this section to define autism and explain its main characteristics. Information obtained from secondary sources (e.g. books) would usually be included here. The **Introduction** to a report is therefore often quite long, and it should not be confused with the introductory paragraph of an essay. It may in fact have several headed subsections, giving background information on different aspects of a subject.

Hypothesis

If your report has a **hypothesis**, it can be stated in the Introduction (usually at the end) or included in a separate headed section immediately after the Introduction.

Method

In this section you give a precise and detailed account of **how** your study was carried out. You describe the research method used, including such things as the size of the sample and how it was selected, the number of observations that took place and what was recorded, the number of interviews that were conducted and so on. Sometimes the following subheadings are used:

(a) **Design**. Describe the overall structure of the research. What kind of research did you undertake – a survey, an observational study, an experiment? What were the dependent and independent variables, if any?

(b) **Subjects**. This refers to the person (or persons) investigated in the study. State who your subjects were and how they were selected. Mention any factors (such as gender and age-range) which you think might have been relevant to the results achieved.

(c) **Apparatus**. List any equipment used. This is especially relevant to an experiment. Did you use a stop-watch, for example, or a tape recorder?

(d) **Procedure**. This often needs to be quite detailed as it explains exactly how the research was carried out. In the case of an observation, for example, you would need to state how many observations took place, how long each one lasted, where they took place and what kinds of behaviour were noted down.

Pilot study

If you carried out a **pilot study**, an account of it should be included here. If any alterations to your research method were made as a result of the pilot study these should be clearly explained.

Results

The **results** of your research are included here, presented in as clear a way as possible. The aim should be to *summarise* your results by use of tables, graphs, bar charts etc. These should be clearly labelled and interspersed with explanatory written text, though you should not comment on the findings at this stage. Avoid too much detail. For example, if ten observation sheets were completed for an observational study, pull the results together and summarise them, rather than simply reproducing the ten sheets in full. (The full details of each sheet could then be included as an appendix.) For more on the presentation of research results, see 'presentation of data' (Unit 8).

Discussion

This section is used to examine the findings of your study. The data obtained can now be *interpreted*. What conclusions can be drawn from the findings? Was your hypothesis proven? What factors might have influenced the results obtained? Are your findings in accord with relevant theory and the work of other researchers (both of which you might well have described in the earlier Introduction section)? Was there anything surprising about the findings?

Conclusion

This offers a brief summing-up at the end of the report. The extent to which the original purpose of the study was fulfilled (or whether your hypothesis was proven) can be stated here.

Evaluation

A separate **Evaluation** section may be unnecessary, as both the Discussion and Conclusion are likely to contain evaluation of the success or otherwise of the report or project. However, as Evaluation is specifically included among the grading criteria for a Merit or Distinction it might be appropriate to include your evaluation of the assignment in a separate section. For advice on what the section should contain, see 'Evaluating projects and reports' (page 197).

Bibliography

List books used and consulted during the assignment. Advice on how this information should be presented is included under 'Bibliographies' on page 186.

Appendices

You can include here copies of questionnaires used, observation sheets etc. Statistical findings which were summarised under Results might be given in full. Your Action Plan (which might help you to achieve a Merit or Distinction) could also be included as an appendix. Each **appendix** should be clearly labelled and listed on the Contents page (perhaps as Appendix A, Appendix B and so on, together with a brief explanation of what each appendix contains).

For an example of a report which follows the above format quite closely, see Specimen Assignment B on page 201.

A range of important techniques for **analysing data** and **presenting data** have already been considered in Unit 8. It is worth reviewing these before moving on to some actual assignments.

Evaluating projects and reports

At the end of a project or report you should include an **evaluation** of the exercise. As indicated on page 196, this evaluation might be incorporated into the 'Discussion' and 'Conclusion' sections of the report, or it might be a separate section. Remember that two of the grading criteria for a Merit or Distinction relate to Evaluation. When you evaluate a report or project you can ask yourself such questions as:

- Did you fulfil the original purpose of the report or project?
- Were you able to prove or disprove your hypothesis? If not, why not?
- Did you obtain enough background information? (e.g. do you feel you did enough background reading?)
- Do you feel you employed the right kind of research method? What were the advantages and disadvantages of this method compared to other methods that you might have used?
- Did you obtain enough data – or too much?
- Were your conclusions consistent with those of other researchers/authors? If not, can you think why this disparity occurred?
- Are there any changes or improvements you would make to your approach if you were to attempt the assignment again?

Specimen Assignments

We shall now look at two research projects completed by students. We shall examine their strengths and weaknesses and consider whether they appear to fulfil the criteria for a Merit or Distinction. As well as a running commentary form the assessor (in boxes throughout the assignment) you can find a fuller appraisal at the end of the assignment.

Assignment A

TITLE: An investigation into the age range of people carrying donor cards.

As well as looking at the age range of people carrying donor cards, I shall also examine a series of what I believe are related phenomena. These will include the age-range of risk-taking and attitudes towards death. First I would like to discuss and examine how I became interested in this project.

As part of my GNVQ Health and Social Care course, I was visiting my local Health Centre. I was collecting health literature and information leaflets which I had to discuss in a few days time as part of Unit 2 (Communication) of the course. With the other leaflets I picked up a donor card. These are distinctive red, white and blue cards, about the size of a credit card.

> A photocopy of the card could perhaps have been included here (or a card itself included as an appendix).

On one side of the card is written:

I request that after my death:

*A. my *kidneys, *corneas, *heart, *lungs, *liver, *pancreas be used for transplantation, or

*B. any part of my body be used for the treatment of others

*(Delete as appropriate)

Signature_____ Date_____

Full name

In the event of my death, if possible contact:

Name_____ Tel._____

I remember putting the donor card inside a leaflet outlining healthy retirement, and that leaflet was put into the middle of all the other health literature. I didn't particularly want anyone to find it. I also remember taking extra care on the way home that day, checking twice before crossing roads and so on. I imagined being involved in a car accident, and then being on a life support machine. My parents being informed that I was clinically dead, but was carrying a donor card and my kidneys were urgently needed to save someone's life. I imagined my parents being very upset, but somehow relieved that my organs were to be of use and could save a life, and that somehow part of me would live on. Somehow carrying the donor card made me think about my own death. I wondered if that was one of the reasons that not too many people carry donor cards.

> Rather melodramatic for an objective study!

Several days later I gave my talk on health literature which was available at my local Health Centre. I also stated that donor cards were also available there, but was not sure what category of literature they would come under. One member of the group asked me if that was my donor card. I had to say that it was not and explained how I felt when I was carrying it home. I think several of the students understood what I meant, but some looked puzzled. A class discussion arose from this. A student asked the group in general if any of them carried a genuine card. I was surprised when three of the students said they did. I think I was surprised because three out of seventeen students seemed a high percentage. Because I study at a further education college, we have a mixed age range of students, although most of them are between sixteen and nineteen years of age. There are also three in their twenties, three in their thirties and one who is forty two. Out of the three students who carry donor cards two were seventeen and one twenty one. Although it was only a very small group I began to wonder if more younger people carried donor cards than older people, and if so, why?

We had been discussing the effects of the media on health education in a previous Communication class. It was hard to understand the fact that although in general people were smoking less, more young people and children (of both sexes) were starting to smoke and smoking more. I thought the usual media images of old people in hospital dying of lung cancer would not mean very much to them. I imagined in some cases the slightly risky and deviant behaviour of smoking might give some children a certain tough image or 'street credibility' that might be more attractive to them than worrying about what might happen to their health in forty years time.

I decided that I would try to design some kind of assignment and look at these issues – donor cards and possible 'risk taking'.

The survey method

As my study is essentially an investigation of people's attitudes, I decided to use the questionnaire and survey methods.

We have studied various methods of investigation and ways of gathering data in class. I used my notes from these to help me design a questionnaire. Before I designed the questionnaire I decided to carry out a pilot study. This would point out any problems that I might have before I carry out the full questionnaire.

Because I was sure only a small percentage of people I surveyed would carry a donor card, I realised I would need to administer even the 'pilot' to a large number of people. I decided to keep the number of questions to the minimum and to use only closed questions. Closed questions are easier to administer and analyse. However, I did leave room on the questionnaire for any comments individuals would make.

I also decided that I would administer the questionnaire and ask the participants the questions myself. I thought it might give me a better 'feel' for questions I eventually wanted to ask.

From the results and comments made by participants in the pilot study I planned and devised my questionnaire.

> Shows reasonable understanding of questionnaire methods here.

Background and research material

Organ transplants: by type (United Kingdom)

	Heart and Lung	Heart	Kidney	Liver
1972	0	0	321	0
1976	0	0	670	0
1981	0	24	905	11
1986	51	176	1,493	127
1987	72	243	1,485	172
1988	101	274	1,575	241
1989	94	295	1,732	295
1990	95	329	1,730	359
1991	79	281	1,628	420
1992	53	325	1,640	506

Source Dept. of Health

Evidence of relevant background research shown by this table being used.

The U.K. Transplant Support Service Authority (T.S.S.A.) know how many donor cards are distributed. In 1988 over five million organ donor cards had been distributed. By 1992 the number had almost doubled to ten and a half million. However the U.K. T.S.S.A. do not know the percentage of people who actually carry donor cards.

In 1992 there were three independent surveys carried out into the effectiveness of donor cards. They were carried out by the U.K. T.S.S.A., the Department of Health and Mori. There were two main findings: (i) 97% of the people who were polled were aware of organ donor cards and their implications; (ii) Between 18% and 30% of the people surveyed claimed to carry donor cards (I imagine the difference was because of the different surveys).

I could find no information regarding the age range of people who carry donor cards.

I know from television reports and newspapers that the majority of donated organs came from people dying after being involved in accidents. I looked up the causes of death for accidents in my reference library. These were coupled with poisoning in the statistics.

Good research but findings of the three surveys could be presented more clearly – e.g. was the 97% figure a finding of all three surveys?

United Kingdom Percentages of deaths due to injury and poisoning

	Under 1	1-14	15-39	40-64	65-79	80 and over
Males	17.6	34.2	52.7	6.6	1.3	1.2
Females	16.8	25.8	28.9	4.0	1.4	1.4

Source: Office of Population and Surveys

I obtained the figures below over the telephone from a health information helpline. They are for 1991.

Males 15-24 1,234 deaths due to accident or poisoning (35.5%)

Males 25-34 879 deaths due to accident or poisoning (23.2%)

Females 15-24 310 deaths due to accident or poisoning (30.5%)

I phoned the Health Information line because I was trying to find out how many young people die in motorbike accidents each year. They could not give me that information at the time. I felt guilty because the researchers who I believe are volunteers spent some minutes searching for the information. I promised myself I would use libraries and write letters for information in future.

I was interested in the number of young people dying after being involved in motorbike accidents. Accidents seemed to be the biggest killer of young people. Many young people (especially male) ride motorcycles for a variety of reasons – a) comparatively inexpensive; b) you do not need to pass a driving test (if you are unaccompanied and display L plates); c) it is a step up from riding a bicycle. It is also known to be dangerous and that makes it exciting.

Deviates from the main purpose of the assignment here.

I wondered if the majority of transplanted organs came from young men who had died as a result of a motorcycle accident. It may seem morbid but I also wondered how many of them would be carrying donor cards. I could also not help but think if they had carried a donor card they might have taken more care. I know now that I was becoming rather obsessive at this time. It was a rather serious topic to be researching. However I did decide to include a question in my questionnaire to find out if the respondents did or had in the past ridden motorcycles. The reason for this is because riding a motorcycle is a known risk and yet many young people continue to, and aspire to, riding them. The mortality statistics showed the high percentage of young people who are killed in accidents and I was becoming interested in the fact that young people may take more risks. This was related to my earlier thoughts in that although in the population in general more people are giving up smoking, increasing numbers of children are taking up smoking.

Donor card literature

On my second visit to the Local Health Centre I picked up a leaflet I had not seen previously. It is called 'Life – don't keep it to yourself'. It gives useful information about donor cards and answers many questions. It explains that organ donation is a difficult subject to think or talk about. Anyone can be a donor. But, for the majority of organs, it is only those people who have suffered serious accidents (mostly head injuries) who become donors. It goes on to explain that every effort is made to save an accident victim's life. Only when they are completely satisfied that nothing more can be done will any question of organ donation be raised. The leaflet also goes on to explain the procedure is carried out by two senior doctors who are acting independently from one another. These doctors it is stressed are not involved in the transplant process. There are many tests carried out to ensure the brain stem does not function. When the brain stem stops functioning, a person cannot be regarded as alive. The leaflet is very reassuring, in that it explains that the organs are removed by a skilled operating team, and that the body is treated with respect and dignity throughout. Once the operation is over, there will be no signs that any organs have been removed. The leaflet stresses that a decision to sign and carry a donor card should be discussed with relatives. If you carry a donor card, technically your organs may be used for transplantation without consulting anyone else. But, in practice, doctors will not remove organs if your relatives object.

> Interesting information but belongs earlier in the assign-

Method

Questionnaire to ascertain the number and age range or people carrying donor cards. The questionnaire also to provide information on proposed risk taking.

As well as the motorcycle question, I included a multiple choice question regarding people's choice of a challenging and exciting activity. This was, in short, whether they would be willing, if given the opportunity, to go sky-diving or bungee-jumping. This may seem an irrelevant question but I believe it would be a good question to find high risk-takers.

Controls

It was stressed that the questionnaire was strictly confidential.

The questionnaire was given to people to fill in themselves. They were asked not to discuss it among others while filling it in. The questionnaire was carried out at Mullhaven College of Further Education.

> Sound knowledge of questionnaire procedure here.

To obtain a greater age range, evening class students and staff were polled as well as day students and staff.

People who had completed the pilot study were omitted from the final questionnaire.

As my questionnaire was becoming longer, I decided to omit the questions regarding smoking. I believe this subject has been well covered in surveys.

1. Do you know what an organ donor card is?   YES   NO

2. Do you carry a donor card?   YES   NO

(If you answered NO to Q.2 answer Q.3 and Q.4. If you answered YES move on to Q.5)

3. Have you ever in the past carried a donor card? YES NO

4. I do not carry a donor card because:
   (a) It makes me think about my own death
   (b) I had a donor card previously, but mislaid it
   (c) I do not believe in transplants
   (d) I may consider carrying a donor card in the future
   (e) Any other reason – please state_____

5. Do you ride a motorcycle?   YES   NO

6. Have you ever rode a motorcycle?   YES   NO

7. Imagine you have won an exciting challenging prize. Please pick out the activity you would prefer:
   (a) An opportunity to go skydiving
   (b) A bungee jump
   (c) Neither of the above

8. How old are you? (Circle your group)
   16-20   21-25   26-30   31-40
   41-50   51-60   61-70   Above 70 (please state age)

I surveyed 289 people. The age range was between 16-76 years.

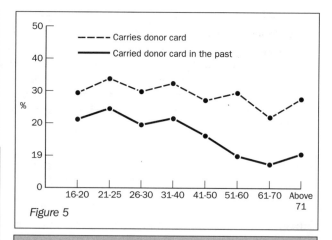

Figure 5

> Good to see a chart used to display your findings.

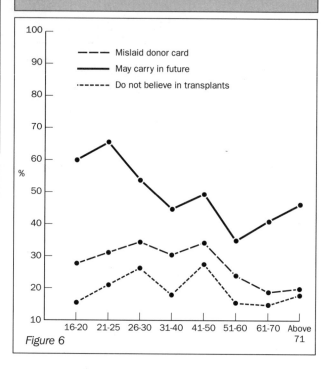

Figure 6

(NOTE: The cover sheet for this assignment indicated that it was intended to satisfy the following performance criteria: 1.1.2 and the whole of Element 8.2. In addition, Elements 3.1 and 3.2 from the Application of Number Core Skills unit were listed.)

Examiner comment

This is an assignment with a lot of potential. The candidate has several interesting and original ideas and has carried out some detailed research. Unfortunately however this potential has not been realised, and the assignment falls some way short of what it might have been. We list below some thoughts on why this has happened and then consider more specifically whether any of the criteria for a Merit or Distinction have been met.

• The main problem with the assignment is that it tries to do too many different things and as a result becomes confused in several places. The two issues of the age range of kidney donors and the attitudes towards risk-taking in different age groups should have been separated more (they might well have formed the basis of *two* assignments). There is frequently a lack of clarity as the candidate brings in such diverse topics as smoking, attitudes to death and motorcycle riding. The assignment should have had a narrower focus, and one which enabled it to concentrate more specifically on the performance criteria it was intended to satisfy. (As it was primarily intended to fulfil Element 8.2 – 'Construct a structured research instrument to survey opinion' – more attention should have been paid to the form and content of the questionnaire.) The candidate shows a commendable amount of independence in devising and carrying out the assignment without any apparent assistance but in this case more consultation with a teacher in the planning stages of the assignment would have been desirable.

- One result of attempting to do too much is that the assignment is incomplete – the results of the survey are not properly analysed and there is no conclusion. After so much build up to it, the actual survey itself is something of a damp squib. The candidate presumably ran out of time. The lesson here is that for a large-scale assignment such as this Action Plans are necessary. At a very late stage in the assignment the candidate was re-visiting the Health Centre to collect more literature. This is poor organisation of time, as by then research for the assignment should have been complete.

- Another reason the candidate did not have time to finish off the assignment properly is that the earlier sections are frequently too long. The style tends to be rambling and anecdotal – that is, there is a lot of personal detail that does not belong in a serious study (about where she put the donor card after picking it up, her gruesome fantasy on the way home about being on a life support machine etc.).

- To her credit the candidate has carried out a lot of research but this is generally not *assimilated* into the assignment – figures are quoted but generally not commented upon or analysed.

- It is also to her credit that she carried out a pilot study, but the study itself is not included – we need to know the questions she asked, the results and the conclusions she drew from these results.

We shall now consider the assignment in the light of the grading criteria for a Merit or Distinction. We shall look at each of the six grading criteria in turn.

Theme 1: Planning

(a) *Drawing up plans of action* The candidate does not include an action plan and the failure to complete the assignment satisfactorily indicates a lack of planning.

(b) *Monitoring courses of action* There are occasional indications that courses of action were monitored and revisions made. In particular, it was decided to omit smoking from the questionnaire, and before the final questionnaire was drawn up a pilot study was carried out. However, there is insufficient detailed evidence of monitoring and revision (the omission of the pilot study is a serious weakness) to warrant a Merit or Distinction. Again an Action Plan would have helped the candidate to show this evidence.

Theme 2: Information-seeking and information-handling

(a) *Identify and use sources to obtain relevant information* We'd be inclined to give the candidate a Merit here. She did collect a lot of information and showed initiative in contacting quite a wide range of sources.

(b) *Establishing the validity of information* There is the potential here for a Merit in that the candidate might have said the questionnaire was an attempt to check the validity of some of the information she had gathered else-

where. However, she does not do this. She also needed to think more about the validity of the information she had obtained – e.g. why was there such a variation in the number of people estimated to carry donor cards (18–30%)?

Theme 3: Evaluation

(a) *Evaluating outcomes and alternatives* No evaluation is included. The questionnaire findings are not properly analysed and there is no attempt to judge the outcome of the research against its original aims.

(b) *Justifying particular approaches to tasks/activities* There is some attempt to justify the use of the questionnaire method, but this part of the assignment ('The survey method') is too sketchy for a Merit or Distinction. In particular, alternative methods that might have been used are not identified and considered.

Assignment B

TITLE: Effects of diuretic drugs on urine production in the elderly.

Summary

This experiment monitored and measured urine production in a 73 year old woman. Her doctor had prescribed an increase in a diuretic drug (which increases the flow of urine in the kidneys). The experiment measured the output of urine before the increase in diuretic and compared it to the output of urine after the increase in diuretic.

There was as predicted an increase of urine production. Urine was passed less frequently, but in greater volume.

The background research into the experiment covered the heart and the urinary system. It also looked at the effect of ageing on the above systems.

A good, concise summary.

Introduction

Originally the purpose of the experiment was to measure my own urine output. A comparison was to be made between weekdays and weekends. The experiment was much modified as I explain below.

My 73 year old grandmother has a history of mild heart disease. She was prescribed a diuretic tablet nine years ago. This assists heart failure by helping the kidneys to increase the flow of urine.

Recently she had become increasingly breathless. This is to be expected in an older person after climbing stairs, etc. However there was no apparent reason for my grandmother's breathlessness. She was also very tired. She was waking up in the night to pass water, but complained that it was only very small amounts.

As my grandmother is hard of hearing a relative usually accompanies her when she visits her doctor. I offered to go with her if she made an appointment.

My grandmother's doctor examined her heart rate and took her blood pressure. She explained her symptoms. He noticed that her ankles were somewhat swollen. He explained that this was mild oedema. He said that because the heart was not working as well as it should, her kidneys were not able to pump out as much water as usual. Excess water was building up in her tissues and this was making her very tired. He said he would prescribe an increase in her diuretic medication.

As I had been studying this in college I asked if fluid intake and output should be monitored. He explained that it would normally be done in hospital. It was not usual in the home. He said it would be a very good idea to do this. My grandmother agreed. She said it would show her if the pills were working or not. I offered to help my grandmother.

When I discussed it with my tutor, she agreed that it would be an interesting experiment to carry out.

I shall first look at the heart and circulation. I then look at how the heart changes in the older person. This is also done with the urinary system.

NB. In the main body of the experiment, I refer to my grandmother as the subject. This is in accord with scientific practice. It did feel strange, but I feel it made me more objective.

Perhaps a sub-heading could have been used here.

The heart is a four chambered muscular structure, which is situated between the thorax and the two lungs. It consists of two ventricles left and right, and two atria, left and right. The atria and ventricles are divided by valves.

The heart fulfils the function of both motor and pump, maintaining continuous circulation of the blood. Blood leaves the left side of the heart under very high pressure. As it travels to the tissues by means of the arteries, its pressure gradually falls until it reaches the capillaries, which are the smallest of the blood vessels. From the capillary network, blood returns to the heart and lungs by means of the veins. The blood is now under low pressure and flowing slowly. Valves in some of the veins, and the pumping action of muscles, help the flow of blood against gravity back to the heart.

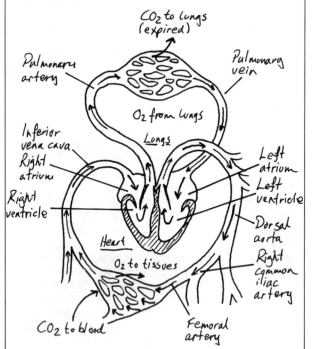

Figure 7   The heart and circulation

Pacemaker

In the wall of the right atrium there is a group of nerve cells which perform the function of initiating electrical impulses. This is known as the sinus node – the sinus node acts as a pacemaker and initiates the heartbeat. The electric impulses given out by the sinus node pass through the wall of the left and right atria, stimulating their contractions. The stimulation then reaches the atrioventricular node (AVN) lying between the ventricles. The AVN sends out impulses to the heart ventricles. These

impulses control the contractions of the heart ventricles.

The heart contracts spontaneously, continuously and more or less regularly through the individual's lifetime. The average contractions are about 75 per minute. During sleep, contractions slow down to 50–60 per minute. In a sitting position contractions are 60–70 per minute. When involved in light physical exertion, for example walking, contractions rise to 110 per minute. During intensive physical activity, such as running, playing tennis, football etc. contractions rise to and may exceed 180 per minute. Contractions are also influenced and modified by the nervous system. The heart rate can be accelerated or slowed down when an individual is in a state of fear, tension, anxiety or depression. The heart beat can also be influenced by non-nervous stimuli, such as temperature and hormones.

Physiology of the heart and heart disease in the older person

The valves of the heart become gradually thicker and more rigid. Blood vessels lose their elasticity. Deposits of atheromatous plaque on the inner lining of blood vessels increase in number. Muscle action is weaker which may cause high blood pressure.

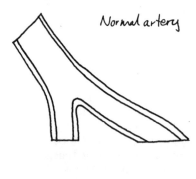

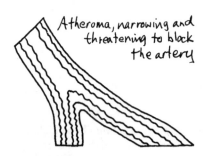

Figure 8   The effect of ageing on the arteries

Breathlessness

It may be expected that the older person will become short of breath after exercising, climbing stairs or making beds. This is not unusual provided the normal pulse rate (70–80 beats per minute) is restored after a few minutes rest.

Heart disease

Heart disease is common in old age. The failing heart may be unable to pump blood effectively around the body. Also the heart may beat unevenly, causing tiredness and shortage of breath.

Urinary system

The kidneys regulate the volume of body fluids by removal of nitrogenous metabolic waste. The kidneys also control the composition of the blood and help to keep the pH within nar row limits even though the intake of food, water and salts varies widely. The lungs also help to control pH through the excretion of carbon dioxide which is highly acidic.

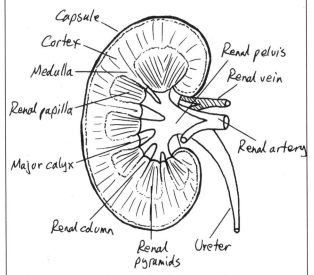

Figure 9 Longitudinal section through a kidney

A kidney is composed of millions of nephrons. The nephron produces urine by a process of filtration of its blood flow. This is followed by selective reabsorption of those substances the body needs to conserve. Three different processes: ultrafiltration, selective reabsorption and secretion are involved in nephron function.

A little more explanation could have been provided.

The urinary system in the older person

There is a gradual reduction of nephrons in the kidneys. There is also a reduction in renal blood flow. Tubular function may be damaged resulting in less concentrated urine production. In the bladder, muscle strength weakens and capacity diminishes. The effects are that less concentrated urine has to be passed more frequently and in smaller quantities.

Input and output of water

In order for normal functioning to occur the amount of water in body fluids must be maintained. The amount of water lost must be equal to the amount we take in. Foods also contain water – a cabbage is 90% water. An average adult individual living in a temperate climate like Britain will consume approximately 3 litres per day of water in liquid and solid foods.

Temperature control

The core body temperature is 37.4°C. Near the surface of the body, temperature can show variation on different occasions and between one place and another, but it is kept remarkably constant deep in the body.

This section might have been relevant to the original

Heat is gained by metabolic activity, exercise, radiation, eating and drinking hot foods and fluids. Heat is lost by conduction, correction, evaporation of sweat and to a small

extent in faeces, urine and expiration. Heat loss is also influenced by environmental temperature and humidity.

The physiological temperature control mechanism is the hypothalamus. The hypothalamus operates like a thermostat set at 37.4°C in the majority of people. If the temperature of blood flowing through the hypothalamus is lower than the set point, the body will be stimulated to generate heat, and conversely to lose heat if the temperature of blood flowing through the hypothalamus is higher than the set point. Heat regulation of the blood is influenced by the degree of constriction of blood vessels in the subcutaneous tissues. When these constrict, the blood flow to the surface of the body is reduced and heat is *retained*. When they dilate, heat is therefore lost.

Urine

The colour of normal urine is usually amber but can vary from pale straw to brown. The output of urine in a normal adult over 24 hours averages between 1200 and 1500 ml, and depends on fluid intake and the amount of fluid lost from the body by perspiration and other means. The amount of urine and its concentration can vary according to climatic conditions, and can vary according to the activity of the individual. Some drugs can increase or decrease the volume of urine.

Oedema is the abnormal infiltration of tissues with fluid. This causes swelling and is noticeable in the dependent parts of the body, for example ankles.

Diuretic drugs increase the flow of urine by the kidney. They can be used to relieve oedema due to heart failure.

The experiment

Hypothesis
Increasing the amount of diuretic will cause an increase in the amount of urine passed.

Method and design
This experiment was conducted by a 17 year old GNVQ Health and Social Care student.

Follows the correct procedures for presentation of an experiment.

The independent variable was the increase in diuretic.

The dependent variable was the measure of urine produced.

The design was repeated measures. That is, measurements were taken twice from the same subject, before and after the increase in diuretic.

Subject
One subject. A 73 year old lady.

Equipment
Large plastic measuring jug. Measuring chart.

Procedure
The experiment was carried out over two days. There was a 24 hour period before the increase in diuretic. This was carried out from Friday night 10 p.m. until Saturday night 10 p.m. The time difference was to allow the diuretic to take effect and for the kidneys to become acclimatised to the new dose. The increased dose was administered on Monday.

Thus:

| Friday | $\longrightarrow$ | Monday | $\longrightarrow$ | Friday |
| measurement | | Increase in diuretic | | measurement |

The measuring jug was kept in the bathroom. It was a large plastic jug bought especially for the experiment. Subject had no trouble passing water into jug (she had previously done this on several occasions in hospital). Measurements were recorded immediately on to a chart that I had prepared.

Intake of fluid was also charted. However this was not measured as accurately as the urine output.

More could have been made of this. Measurements need to be included in your results.

Comments made by the subject were recorded by experimenter.
Results

A good chart is presented here (see Fig. 10).

Before increase in D		After increase in D	
10.50 p.m.	85 ml	10.45 p.m.	140 ml
1.00 a.m.	45 ml	7.15 a.m.	250 ml
4.00 a.m.	50 ml	10.45 a.m.	225 ml
8.00 a.m.	185 ml	1.00 p.m.	100 ml
11.00 a.m.	255 ml	5.55 p.m.	270 ml
1.55 p.m.	170 ml	7.40 p.m.	190 ml
6.00 p.m.	210 ml	9.55 p.m.	230 ml
7.40 p.m.	90 ml		
9.50 p.m.	140 ml		
TOTAL	1230 ml	TOTAL	1405 ml

There is a difference of 175 ml between the two days.

Discussion including evaluation

Results showed that there was an increase in urine production after the increase in diuretic. Although urine was passed less frequently (none during the night) after the increase in diuretic, it was passed in greater volume at each visit to the toilet.

If I was carrying out the experiment again I would try to ensure that measuring took place over a two day period before the increase in diuretic and two days after the increase. This would lessen the chance of untypical results. However this was difficult, because my grandmother had been prescribed the increase in medication by her doctor and delay in administration would have been completely unethical.

Good awareness of ethical considerations.

On the second visit to her doctor's, my grandmother said she was feeling much better. The doctor examined her as well as the urinary output chart. He said it was just as he expected and vindicated his decision to increase her medication.

I feel as if the experiment concurs with medical literature and shows the validity of claims made about the drug.

Good point about validity, but could be explained more fully.

Appendix (see Figure 11)

Bibliography

Dr. W. Dzikowski – Look After Your Heart (1983)
Ewington and Moore – Human Biology and Hygiene
Hinchliff, Norman and Schober (editors) – Nursing Practice and Health Care (1993)
Dr. M. K. Thompson – Caring for an Elderly Relative (1986)

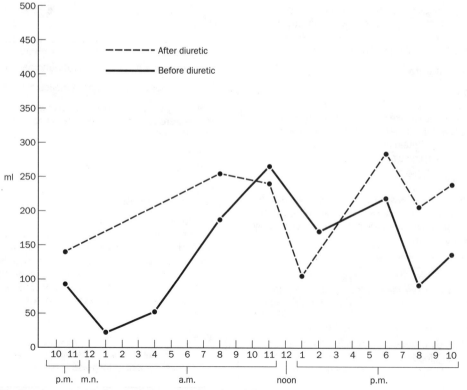

Figure 10 Subject's urine output before and after administration of diuretic

ACTION PLAN					
TASK/ACTIVITY	TIME ALLOCATION	DATE FOR COMPLETION	RESOURCES	MONITORING	COMMENTS/REVISIONS
To decide on assignment	2 weeks	25 Sept.	College resources bank and assignment packs in library		I finally decided on my assignment by 23 Sept. This discussed with my tutor
Carry out first part of experiment	1 day	24 Sept.	Measuring jug Measuring chart	Made sure subject (grandmother) understood how to enter urine output onto chart	I had to carry this first part of the experiment out very quickly. My grandmother had been prescribed an increase in diuretic - had to measure urine output a.s.a.p.
Read about experimental method	3 hours	26 Sept.	Book from library + Lecture notes	Check some of the terms with tutor	
Make background research notes	2 weeks	9 Oct.	Resource bank Public library (books) Lecture notes		This took longer than I expected. I borrowed a range of books. It was quite difficult going through them and finding the relevent parts
Prepare for second part of experiment	2 days	30 Sept.		Check that grandmother feeling well and not worried about experiment	My grandmother was well. She was looking forward to me staying with her again for the second part of the experiment
Carry out second part of experiment	1 day	1 Oct.	Measuring jug Measuring chart		Second part of experiment was carried out on the same day of the week as the first part. I again stayed the day and night.
Finish making notes	2 days	11 Oct.	Library	I had to constantly self monitor - to make myself finish	I think I have almost too much information
Visit doctor with grandmother	15 mins.	6 Oct.			The doctor was pleased with my results
Write up experiment	4 hours	15 Oct.	Library + Results of experiment		Took longer than I planned. Finished on 16 October.

Figure 11

NOTE: The cover sheet for this assignment indicated that it was intended to satisfy the following performance criteria: 3.1.1, 3.1.2, 3.1.3 and 3.1.5. In addition the following elements from the Core Skills units were listed: Communication, 3.2; Application of Number, 3.1 and 3.3.)

Examiner comment

This assignment has several excellent features. There is a detailed Action Plan which shows evidence of appropriate modification and revision as the assignment developed. It has a good, clear structure and format and follows correct experimental procedures. The candidate has researched carefully the functions and inter-relationship of body systems (Element 3.1) and very sound physiological knowledge is demonstrated. The experiment is relevant to the performance criteria for the Element and findings are effectively presented.

Although the overall standard of the assignment is high, it does have some weaknesses and a few of these are listed below.

- The section on Temperature Control (page 203) might have been relevant to the original experiment, on differences in the candidate's own urine output on weekdays and at weekends, but it is unnecessary for the revised experiment.

- The report mentions that 'Intake of fluid was also charted' (page 204). However, no findings are given for this. This is quite a serious omission as fluid intake might have influenced urinary output over the periods when the experiment took place.
- The discussion of the findings at the conclusion of the report is rather brief. Similarly, the evaluation which is included in the same section could have been more detailed and turned into a separate section.
- The Bibliography omits publishers and does not have a consistent style – the date of one of the books is missing and some author's initials are given, others not.

We shall now consider how far the assignment satisfies the six grading criteria for a Merit or Distinction, looking at each in turn.

Theme 1: Planning

(a) *Drawing up plans of action* A detailed action plan is provided. The inter-relationship between the activities is clear and there is some attempt to prioritise the activities. DISTINCTION

(b) *Monitoring courses of action* The candidate does monitor both her own and her subject's progress. A revision was made early in the assignment when the experiment was changed. The candidate also notes when an activity takes longer than anticipated. Monitoring and revision is carried out independently. DISTINCTION

Theme 2: Information-seeking and information-handling

(a) *Identify and use sources to obtain relevant information* A range of sources is used – several books, and the subject's doctor. These are identified independently. DISTINCTION

(b) *Establishing the validity of information* The results of the experiment itself are used by the candidate to confirm the validity of the information obtained from medical literature. A further check on the validity of the candidate's own findings might have been to consider whether these findings may have been influenced by the subject's fluid intake. DISTINCTION

Theme 3: Evaluation

(a) *Evaluating outcomes and alternatives* The experiment was intended to test a hypothesis and succeeds in doing this. However, alternative criteria for judging the success of the outcome are neither identified or considered. A comparison with the candidate's own urinary output might have been instructive here, to see if similar fluctuations (which could not in her case have been explained by the presence of a diuretic) occurred. Clearly however this would have greatly increased the scale of the experiment. We feel neither a Merit or Distinction is warranted here, but remember that *all* of the criteria do not need to be fulfilled in *every* assignment, and that opportunities for fulfilling certain of the grading criteria are sometimes (as here) limited by the nature of the assignment.

(b) *Justifying particular approaches to tasks/activities* The candidate does include some justification of her approach and mentions how the experiment might be improved were it to be repeated. However, the Evaluation could be more detailed and we would consider the candidate here warranted a MERIT rather than a Distinction.

Other Writing Skills

We shall now look at some other forms of writing that you might be asked to produce for your portfolio. The particular kinds of writing we shall consider are:

- Essays
- Letters
- Memoranda
- Telephone messages
- Meetings documents
- Brochures / leaflets.

Essays

One way to approach the writing of an **essay** is to divide the task into four stages:

1. Thinking about the essay title;
2. Gathering material for the essay;
3. Planning the essay;
4. Writing the essay.

These four stages can form the basis of an Action Plan for an essay writing assignment. We shall now consider each of them in turn.

1. Thinking about the essay title

Make sure you have a clear understanding of the requirements of the question. Ask yourself questions such as:

- Do I understand all the terms that are used in the title?
- What are the key words and phrases in the title?
- How many parts does the question have? How many aspects of the subject am I expected to cover?

Imagine for example that you have been set the following essay title:

'Distinguish between the main forms of dementia and consider their possible causes.'

Probably your first step in preparing for this assignment would be to find a precise definition of the term 'dementia'. The key words and phrases in the title are:

Distinguish
main forms of dementia
consider
possible causes

'Distinguish' and 'consider' are important because they indicate what you are being asked to do (you re not for example being asked to 'compare' forms of dementia). 'Main forms of dementia' and 'possible causes' are important because they indicate the aspects of the subject that you need to cover. Finally, the question is in two parts – (i) Distinguishing the main forms of dementia, and (ii) considering their possible causes. (Later in this section, on page 210, we shall look at a specimen answer to this question.)

2. Gathering material for the essay

During this stage you collect together information that might prove of use to you in writing the essay. Your sources of information might for example include books, lecture notes and magazine or newspaper articles. You should compile a set of notes from these sources, remembering to keep a record of all sources used for inclusion in a bibliography. For more detailed advice on this stage see the earlier section on 'Sources of information' (page 180); some of the material under 'Carrying out research' (page 191) may also be relevant.

3. Planning the essay

In many respects this is the most important stage. You may have amassed a great deal of material in the second stage, but this is of no use if you do not select carefully from it and then shape and order what is left into a coherent pattern.

At the most basic level, an essay usually has the following three parts:

1. Introduction
2. Main body
3. Conclusion

Ways of introducing an essay

There are several standard ways of introducing an essay. Often it is appropriate to define terms that are used in the question. You might sketch in the background to the subject (an essay on the work of the World Health Organisation, for example, might begin by explaining when the WHO was set up, and why). It is also usually a good idea to give some indication of what is to follow – that is, of the approach that you are going to adopt and the structure that the essay will have.

Paragraphs

The main body constitutes the bulk of the essay. Here the main content of the answer is presented in a series of logically ordered paragraphs. Remember that a single paragraph in an essay should have a single, clearly identifiable theme. The paragraphs should however be linked so that the essay progresses smoothly from one paragraph to another. Although there is no fixed length for paragraphs, the paragraphs used in essays tend to be around 100–200 words long. Paragraphs that are very short suggest an inability to develop ideas, while very long paragraphs are usually evidence of poor organisation.

Ways of concluding an essay

The conclusion may be used to summarise your main argument, but you should be careful that this does not make the essay seem repetitive – avoid word for word echoes of what has already been said. If you have been considering two sides of an argument, make sure that your conclusion indicates where you stand (even if you conclude that you find it impossible to favour one side or the other). Similarly, if a question asks something like 'How far ...' or 'To what extent ...' the conclusion should give a clear answer.

Although the above gives a broad outline of the kind of structure an essay will usually have, more detailed planning will need to take place for each individual title. A planning method that can be adopted for most essays will now be described. We shall look closely at the stages involved in devising a plan for an essay with the following title:

> It has been argued that social class and ill health are closely linked, with those from lower social classes suffering worse health than those higher up in the social scale. Examine the evidence for this view. If health inequalities between social classes do exist, what are the possible causes?

This is quite a broad and complex title, and one which is likely to involve a lot of background reading. Once this reading has taken place and you have a set of notes on which to base the essay, you should make a list of the *main points and ideas* that you think might be included in the essay. You do not need to worry about putting them into any kind of order at this stage. Try to describe each point in as few words as possible. Below is a list of points and ideas for the above title (ignore the letters in brackets for now):

(A) Need to define social class
(A) Need to define ill health
(D) Manual workers known to be more likely to smoke
(D) Manual workers known to be more likely to have unhealthy diet
(F) Those who live in heavily polluted areas more likely to be from lower social classes
(E) If poor, affording a healthy diet is more difficult
(G) Findings of Black Report (1980) – e.g. most diseases more prevalent among lower social classes
(F) Possible explanation of inequalities: environmental factors (e.g. poor housing conditions)
(D) Those on low income in poor housing etc may cope with stress in unhealthy ways (e.g. smoking, eating crisps, sweets)
(A) Use Registrar General's class divisions to define class – but mention criticisms of them
(B) Evidence of inequalities is possibly suspect because ways of measuring social class may be unsound
(C) Possible explanation of inequalities: 'health selection' argument (poor health causes people to move down the social scale)
(D) Possible explanation of inequalities: cultural differences between classes (lower classes tend to have less healthy lifestyles)
(I) Government statistics (General Household Surveys) confirm class inequalities of health
(J) Lower social classes make less use of preventive health services – another possible cause of inequalities
(E) If poor, buying medication is more difficult
(D) Manual workers take less exercise
(E) Possible explanation of inequalities: economic factors (e.g. those on low income less able to keep warm)
(H) Findings of The Health Divide (1987) – e.g. most diseases more prevalent among lower social classes.

Forming paragraphs

The next step is to form this list into *groups* of points. Look for connections between points, and put points that are about a similar aspect of the subject together. This is a very important stage in the planning of the essay because each of these groups will become a *paragraph* in the final essay. From the above list we might decide on the following groupings (note that the order of the groupings is not for the moment important):

(A) Definitions of class and health
(B) Doubts concerning the evidence of inequalities
(C) Explanation of inequalities – 'health selection' argument
(D) Explanation of inequalities – cultural differences
(E) Explanation of inequalities – economic factors
(F) Explanation of inequalities – environmental factors
(G) Evidence of inequalities – the Black Report
(H) Evidence of inequalities – the Health Divide
(I) Evidence of inequalities – Government statistics
(J) Explanation of inequalities – use of preventive health services

The items in the original list can be marked with the appropriate capital letter to indicate the group to which they belong. In the list printed opposite these letters appear in brackets alongside each item.

We now need to put the groups of points (remember these correspond to paragraphs in the essay) in a sensible order. We want to approach the essay in a coherent manner and to ensure that the argument develops in a logical way. In this case we might arrange the paragraphs as follows:

1. (A) Definitions of social class and ill health
2. (G) Evidence of inequalities: Black Report
3. (H) Evidence of inequalities: The Health Divide
4. (I) Evidence of inequalities: Government statistics
5. (B) Doubts about the above evidence
6. (E) Causes of inequalities: Economic factors
7. (F) Causes of inequalities: Environmental factors
8. (D) Causes of inequalities: Cultural differences
9. (C) Causes of inequalities: Health selection argument
10. (J) Causes of inequalities: Use of preventive health services

Note how the evidence of health inequalities is grouped together in one part of the essay, and the causes of those inequalities grouped together in another part.

There are now three things left to do:

– Work out an introduction for the essay;
– Work out a conclusion for the essay;
– Work out the order of points within each paragraph.

It may seem strange that the introduction is left until such a late stage in the planning process. Bear in mind though that the introduction should prepare the reader for what is to follow and needs therefore to fit in with the main body of the essay. It makes sense then to decide on the main body first and think of a way to introduce it after. Another reason for delaying thoughts about the introduction is that when you arrange your list of ideas in order you may well find that the first group of points could serve as an introduction to the rest of the essay. This is certainly the case with our example: definitions of social class and ill health would be a logical way to begin the essay.

The conclusion similarly needs to fit in with the main body of the essay and to follow logically from it. In this case you might sum up by saying that there is powerful evidence of social inequalities in health and that these inequalities seem to have a variety of causes. You might also very briefly suggest a few ways in which these inequalities could be lessened.

Arranging the points within each paragraph in order should not be too difficult provided you remember that each paragraph must have a single clear theme running through it, and that just as the essay should progress logically from paragraph to paragraph, so too should each paragraph progress logically from sentence to sentence.

4. Writing the essay

You are now in a position to write the essay.

Specimen essays

To illustrate some of the qualities to aim for in essay writing, and some of the pitfalls to avoid, we shall now look at two specimen essays. Paragraphs have been numbered so that they can be referred to later.

Discuss the possible links between cancer and smoking, diet and lifestyle.

(1) There are more than 200 different types of cancer, and there are more recorded cases of the disease now than there were twenty years ago. Sixty-five per cent of cancers occur in the over 65s. It is estimated that smoking accounts for nearly one-third of all UK cancer deaths. Smoking is especially associated with lung cancer but it can also lead to cancer of the mouth, throat, cervix (in women), bladder and pancreas.

(2) Cancer is a disease affecting the cells of the body. The average adult has about three million million (three trillion) cells. There are different types of cell with different functions. Red blood cells, for example, carry oxygen to other cells and take carbon dioxide from them. Cells are constantly dying (about 50 million cells die every second), but are immediately replaced by new cells which are created by the division of old ones. In a healthy adult the extinction of old cells and the creation of new cells roughly balance each other. In someone suffering from cancer however too many new cells are being created. A solid lump of cells is formed and some of these spread into neighbouring tissue or into the blood. A cancer patient's life can be saved by early diagnosis. If there were more X-ray screening facilities available the cancer would more often be detected in time. The problem is that people (especially women) cannot be bothered to go for check-ups. If people know that X-ray facilities are available they are more likely to use them.

(3) Cervical cancer which affects women is more likely if the woman has many sexual partners or starts having sexual intercourse at a young age. It is also more common among women who smoke or who are pregnant before the age of 20.

(4) It is believed that cigarette smoke may contain as many as 32 cancer-causing agents. These enter the bloodstream and spread throughout the body. However, not all smokers develop cancer. The reason for this is unclear. There may be a genetic or inherited factor which means that some smokers are more prone to contracting the disease than others.

(5) Diet is another cause of cancer. Stomach and bowel cancers are especially common in Western countries, where people eat more animal fat and less fibre. It is interesting to note however that the number of people in Britain dying from stomach cancer is half what it was 50 years ago. Experts believe this has been caused by the change in our diets. How fresh the food is is also important. Stomach cancer is less prevalent in countries where they eat more fresh food. The rise in the number of fridges and freezers owned by people and improved storage facilities in shops has helped stomach cancer to decline.

(6) Cancer is almost twice as common among women as it is among men. Children between the ages of 10 and 19 are especially at risk. Although cancer can be contracted at this age it may not become evident until many years later. The disease is not infectious though some forms of cancer are associated with viral infections. For example, a particular wart virus can affect women and if it is not treated it may cause abnormalities which can develop into cancer. Another lifestyle factor is skin cancer which affects those who like to sunbathe.

(7) No one knows what causes cancer. However the search for a cure continues and there is hope that eventually a solution will be found.

Comment

The main weakness with this essay is poor organisation. This is a pity as some relevant knowledge is shown and a fair amount of useful information is included. The problem is that points are presented in a haphazard order and too many of the paragraphs lack a clear theme. In fact a straightforward structure for this essay was contained within the question. An answer could have three main parts, examining in turn the links between cancer and smoking, diet and lifestyle. This could be preceded by an introductory section explaining the nature of the disease. The treatment of the subject also tends to be superficial (the essay is very short) and the 'lifestyle' element of the question is barely touched upon.

A more detailed analysis follows. Numbers in brackets refer to the numbered paragraphs of the essay.

(1) Too much information is presented at once here: the opening three sentences yoke together four separate pieces of information. Although the information is useful and these four points (especially the last one) could all be incorporated into an essay, more thought is needed as to *where* they should appear. The source of the information should also be given. The second piece of information is rather vague. How big is the increase? Given that (as the next sentence states) 65% of cancers occur in the over 65s, and that people are now living longer, isn't an increase to be expected? The writer needs to think more about the validity of the information being used.

The last two sentences of the paragraph do relate to the question but smoking is introduced too abruptly here. Why refer to smoking in the introduction but not diet and lifestyle? In fact these points about smoking would be better saved for later in the essay, when there should be a paragraph devoted to a detailed discussion of the links between smoking and cancer.

(2) The first half or so of this paragraph shows an improvement in the essay. It is logical to explain the nature of cancer early in the essay and the explanation here is quite accurate if rather brief. However the paragraph begins to go off the rails with the sentence 'A cancer patient's life can be saved by early diagnosis'. A new topic is introduced here (the early diagno-

sis of cancer) and the writer continues with this to the end of the paragraph. As this is a new topic one would normally expect the writer to begin a new paragraph. In this case however it would be better if this part of the paragraph were removed from the essay altogether as it is not really *relevant* to the question. (Even if there were a reason for including it, these closing sentences of the paragraph would still have other weaknesses. In one sentence the writer suggests that not enough X-ray facilities are available, and then in the next sentence states that the problem is not this but something else – that people (especially women) 'cannot be bothered' to go for check-ups. This later point not only contradicts the previous one but is also simplistic and highly questionable. There are many other reasons why people may not go for check-ups (fear of what might be revealed, for example). The last sentence of the paragraph again contradicts the writer's own argument – if people cannot be bothered to go for check-ups, would informing them that X-ray facilities are available make any difference?)

(3) This paragraph contains some useful points but they belong in different parts of the essay. The points about sexual behaviour relate to lifestyle (though the writer does not actually explain this) while the one about smoking should be grouped with the other points on this topic. The paragraph is also too short.

(4) This paragraph does have a clear theme (cancer and smoking) and contains some useful points. The paragraph should however be longer – the points about smoking found in other parts of the essay logically belong in this paragraph.

(5) This again has a clear theme (diet and cancer) and all the points related to the topic have been brought together in the paragraph. The opening sentence ('Diet is another cause of cancer') does indicate what the paragraph is about but it is rather simplistic – the nature of the links between diet and cancer are not yet known for certain.

(6) Most of this paragraph has nothing to do with the question. The final sentence ('Another lifestyle factor ...') implies that the preceding part of the paragraph is about lifestyle, but the points made are not in fact related to this. The final sentence does make a relevant point (the connection between sunbathing and skin cancer) but the explanation is again simplistic and far too brief.

(7) A weak conclusion. The paragraph is very short and does not relate effectively to the question. The opening statement needs qualification – although what causes cancer has not been clearly and definitely established, some important contributory factors are known. In any case, the sentence contradicts earlier assertions in the essay (especially 'Diet is another cause of cancer').

Another weakness is that the essay does not include a bibliography, which is needed as evidence of information-seeking.

The second specimen essay follows.

Distinguish between the main forms of dementia and consider their possible causes.

(1) Dementia can be defined as the irreversible organic deterioration of mental faculties. Although it is especially associated with old age (it has been estimated that one person in five over the age of eighty suffers from moderate or severe dementia), the various forms of dementia are not exclusively confined to the elderly. The term is used to cover a range of diseases because the symptoms of these diseases are often very similar. Usually there is a progressive loss of mental function, with reduced ability to think and reason. Sufferers may be unable to remember even very recent events and may have difficulty recognising other people, even close relatives. However, although the symptoms frequently overlap, scientists have identified several distinct diseases which can result in the development of these symptoms. Each of these diseases will now be discussed in turn, and their possible causes considered.

(2) The disease most commonly associated in the public mind with dementia is Alzheimer's Disease. It was first identified in 1907 by Alois Alzheimer, a German doctor. He studied the brain of a 51 year old woman, who died after suffering personality changes and memory loss during the last years of her life. He found unusual dark spots on the brain and concluded that these were responsible for the symptoms displayed by the woman before she died. These spots were later discovered to be made up of a substance called beta-amyloid and they are now known as senile plaques and neurofibrillary tangles. They affect the cells of the brain in several harmful ways. The human brain is made up of several million cells – known as neurons – which communicate with each other. A neuron comprises a cell body, several hundred dendrites and an axon. The dendrites receive chemical message from other cells, passing these messages onto the cell body, which in turn sends a response down the axon. At the end of the axon a chemical messenger – known as a neurotransmitter – is released, and the message transmitted to another cell. In a brain afflicted with Alzheimer's Disease the senile plaques disrupt the transmission of messages from one neurone to another, and the neurofibrillary tangles block the transport of important chemicals within the cell body. In addition, the release of neurotransmitters from the end of the axon is also limited in brains with Alzheimer's Disease. Different neurons use different chemicals as neurotransmitters, and Alzheimer's Disease is especially associated with a reduced supply of the chemical acetylcholine.

(3) The precise cause of Alzheimer's Disease is unknown, though several suggestions have been made. At one time it was thought that aluminium might be a cause of the disease, as it is known to cause a form of neurofibrillary tangle in the brains of animals. This caused widespread concern about the levels of aluminium in drinking water and about the use of aluminium kitchenware in cooking. However, more recent research has cast doubt on the theory. Another possibility that has been considered is that virus-like particles (similar to those which are known to cause two other brain diseases, Creutzfeldt-Jakob and Kuru) might be responsible. This too is now believed to be unlikely. Instead, research has focused increasingly on genetic factors which may create a susceptibility to the deposition of beta-amyloid. It has been established that some families suffer from Alzheimer's Disease more than others, suggesting the presence of genes which either cause the disease or make members of the same family more likely to contract it. Some diseases can be traced to a single gene, but it is now believed that several different genes may be involved in Alzheimer's Disease. It is known

that Down's syndrome sufferers have a much increased likelihood of developing Alzheimer's Disease. Down's sufferers have an extra copy of chromosome number 21, and scientists are now studying this chromosome to see if it carries the genes that might lie behind Alzheimer's Disease.

(4) Parkinson's Disease (or Parkinsonism) is another disease that can lead to the symptoms associated with dementia, though it is more commonly associated with impaired physical functioning. There is a gradual loss of muscle control, leading to shaking and stiffness. As the disease develops, speech and thought slow down and the sufferer shows signs of mental confusion. However, it is rare for sufferers to experience a total loss of intellectual function (as can occur with Alzheimer's Disease). The cause is again linked to the behaviour of cells within the brain. Those neurons which communicate by releasing the neurotransmitter chemical dopamine cease to work properly, so that the functions controlled by these brain cells are disrupted. The disease mainly affects the substantia nigra, the part of the brain that usually controls the body's movements.

(5) Lewy Body Disease is a form of dementia that has only been distinguished from Alzheimer's and Parkinsonism in the last few years. Dementia tends to appear more suddenly than in Alzheimer's sufferers, and there may also be impaired motor-control. The cause is patches of ubiquitin (the 'Lewy bodies') which accumulate in the cerebral cortex and the motor-control centres of the brain.

(6) Huntington's Disease is another illness with physical as well as mental symptoms. It causes uncontrollable body movements as well as degeneration of the intellectual faculties. The loss of muscle power leads to impaired speech and inability to swallow makes eating difficult. The cause is genetic. A faulty gene leads to the deterioration of certain nerve cells, especially in parts of the brain that control movement, such as the caudate nucleus and putamen and parts of the frontal lobe. Children of a parent affected by Huntington's Disease have a 50 per cent chance of inheriting the disease.

(7) Approximately 25 per cent of those with dementia suffer from a disease known as Multi-infarct dementia. It is characterised by a gradual deterioration of intellectual functioning, with periods of decline followed by phases when the sufferer's condition stabilises or even recovers slightly. Other symptoms can include loss of speech and partial or total paralysis of a limb. The term 'infarct' refers to small areas of dead tissue, which can be present in any organ of the body. Multi-infarct dementia develops when the brain contains many such areas of dead tissue. This occurs when the blood supply to these parts of the brain has been cut off because blood vessels have burst or become blocked. As the tissue develops, increasing areas of the brain are affected.

(8) None of these diseases is at present curable, but research into their causes has made considerable progress in recent years. Allied to this research has been the search for treatments that can at least reduce the speed at which the diseases develop. Again progress has been made and while it has so far proved impossible to prevent the onset of diseases associated with dementia, the debilitating effects of these diseases can now to some extent be controlled.

Bibliography

Simon Green – Physiological Psychology (Routledge and Kegan Paul, 1987)
Anthony Smith – The Mind (Pelican, 1985)
Paul Vega – Enemies of the Mind (Gallico Press, 1993)

Comment

Generally this is a very good essay. It shows an excellent knowledge of the subject and has clearly been well researched. Note in particular that the essay is very well organised. It begins with a definition of dementia and then goes on to examine each of the forms of dementia in turn. Each paragraph has a clearly identifiable theme. One weakness with the essay however is that it is a little 'top-heavy' – the discussion of Alzheimer's Disease occupies rather too great a proportion of the essay in relation to the other diseases discussed.

A more detailed analysis is again given below. Bracketed numbers refer to the numbered paragraphs in the essay.

(1) A good introduction. It is often appropriate to begin an essay by defining terms that have been used in the question. The last two sentences relate clearly to the question and prepare the reader for the remainder of the essay by outlining the method of approach.

(2) Note how the opening sentence of the paragraph clearly indicates the theme of the paragraph. The paragraph as a whole shows detailed biological knowledge.

(3) As the essay contains a lot of material on Alzheimer's Disease, it is sensible to divide it into two paragraphs. Each paragraph looks at a separate aspect of the subject – the previous paragraph described the main elements of the disease, this paragraph considers its possible causes. The writer is clearly well-informed and the information is up to date. The paragraph also develops in a logical way – after considering possible but unlikely causes, it moves on to genetic factors, which researchers are now focusing upon.

(4) The essay now discusses other forms of dementia, devoting a separate paragraph to each. The discussion of these diseases is a little sketchy compared with the detailed treatment of Alzheimer's Disease, but good knowledge of the subject continues to be evident.

(5) As Lewy Body disease has only recently been distinguished from Parkinsonism and Alzheimer's, it makes sense to consider those diseases first and then this disease immediately afterwards.

(6) Huntington's Disease is now discussed because like the previous two it has physical as well as mental symptoms. Note how the diseases are discussed in a sensible order and how the opening sentence of the paragraph establishes the link with the previous paragraph.

(7) The last of the diseases is described. Again sound biological knowledge is shown.

(8) An effective conclusion. The essay has avoided discussing treatments of dementia before because they are not strictly relevant given the title of the essay. However it is appropriate to mention them briefly here – the search for the causes of the diseases runs parallel with the search for more effective treatments.

The Bibliography shows appropriate background reading and is correctly presented.

Letters

The layout of **letters** can vary according to the format being used. The important thing is to decide on a format and stick to it. Listed below are the main elements that are usually present in a letter, working downwards from the top of the page. Where they should appear is also indicated, but note that in typed or word processed letters fully blocked layouts and open punctuation can be used. This means that all of the elements appear on the left hand side of the page, no indentation is used and only the text of the letter is punctuated.

For an illustration of all the points below, see the specimen letter opposite.

(a) **Letter head**

Most organisations have a printed letter head containing the name and address of the organisation, together with telephone and fax numbers.

(b) **Address of sender**

If headed paper is not used, the address of the sender usually appears in the top right-hand corner. If the letter is from an individual, it is important that the name is *not* included here.

(c) **The date**

Leave a line after the sender's address then put the date. The order used should be day, month, year (e.g. '12th March 1994'). Do not abbreviate the date in any way ('12/3/94' would be incorrect).

(d) **Reference**

Any reference numbers and letters can appear on the same line as the date but on the opposite side of the page, preceded by 'Ref', 'Your Ref' or 'Our Ref'. If you reply to a letter which had a reference, always put the same reference on the letter when you write back.

(e) **Name and address of recipient**

This can be placed on the left hand side of the page, beneath the date and reference line.

(f) **Salutation**

Use the name of the recipient, or 'Dear Sir' if the name is not known ('Dear Madam' if you know the recipient is a woman).

(g) **Heading**

This is not essential but is often used in more formal letters to indicate the subject of the letter. The heading should appear below the salutation, in the centre of the page.

(h) **The close**

If the recipient was not named in the salutation, 'Yours faithfully' is usually used. Otherwise the letter can end 'Yours sincerely'. If a blocked layout has not been used the close is usually placed slightly to the right of the centre of the page. The name and, where applicable, the official position of the person sending the letter can be printed beneath the signature.

The content of the letter

When writing the main body of the letter, bear the following points in mind:

- Be clear, courteous and concise. Do not waste time on unnecessary detail but at the same time avoid abruptness.
- If you are replying to a letter, open with thanks for the letter received, giving its date.
- If a heading is not being used, indicate briefly at the beginning the subject of the letter (e.g. 'Thank you for

your letter of 4th April, concerning arrangements for the playgroup Christmas party').

- Make sure the material within the letter is arranged in a logical order and divided into appropriate paragraphs. (The approach used here can be a scaled-down version of that described in 'Planning the essay' on p.00). Lengthy paragraphs are generally to be avoided in letters. In particular, the letter should begin with a short introductory paragraph.
- Take care over grammar, spelling and punctuation. A particularly common mistake is to begin or end the letter with incomplete sentences such as 'With reference to your letter of 12th November' or 'Looking forward to seeing you on Wednesday'. These are not proper sentences as they are grammatically incomplete (the second sentence, for example, should be corrected to 'I look forward to seeing you on Wednesday').

Specimen letter

Here is a specimen letter. It is the kind that might be written to an organisation requesting information for an assignment.

---

7 Worcester Close,
South Park,
Kent BP5 6UQ

5th May 1994

Mr. P. Jones (Director),
Friends and Neighbours,
17 High Street,
South Park,
Kent BP6

Dear Mr. Jones,

I am a pupil at South Park High School studying for an Advanced GNVQ qualification in Health and Social Care. As part of the course I am writing a research project on the services available to elderly people who live alone.

I am very interested in the work of your organisation and would greatly appreciate any literature that you might be able to send me. I would also very much like to speak to you about the services that your organisation provides and wonder whether an interview might be possible. I would be able to visit your office on any weekday after 4 p.m.

I should be grateful for any help you are able to give me and look forward to hearing from you.

Yours sincerely,
Kim Watson
Kim Watson

Memoranda

A **memorandum** is a written communication sent through the internal post of an organisation.

Layout

As memos are for internal correspondence, addresses of the sender and recipient do not need to be included. The salutation ('Dear Sir') and the formal close ('Yours faithfully') which appear in a letter are also omitted. The following information does need to be included however:

- who the memo is to (name and/or position – sometimes a memo has more than one recipient);
- who the memo is from (name and/or position);
- the subject of the memo;
- the date.

Many organisations have printed memo forms, which have headings for each of the above with spaces for the details to be written in. If you are writing a memo for an assignment the format shown in the example below can be used.

Content

Usually the content of a memo is quite brief – it may be used for example to bring a situation to the attention of recipients or to remind them of something ('memorandum' is Latin for 'a thing which is to be remembered'). When you write a memo your language should be concise and direct, and you should use short paragraphs.

Specimen memo

> **Rossdale Day Centre**
>
> **MEMORANDUM**
>
> To: Jenny Blake (Evening Supervisor)
> From: The Centre Manager
> Subject: Lake District Outing
> Date: 26 May 1994
>
> Could you please remind all evening users of the Centre that the list of those attending the Lake District outing on 12th June needs to be finished by Friday 2nd June. Please give the names of those wishing to go on the trip to Mrs. Bishop as soon as possible.

Telephone messages

In organisations **telephone messages** are often taken by one employee on behalf of another. As with memos, printed message forms are sometimes provided (see example below), but on other occasions the message is simply written on a blank sheet of paper. It is essential to record the following pieces of information:

- who the call is from (name and, where applicable, position and organisation);
- the caller's telephone number;
- who the message is for;
- the message itself (the message may be quite lengthy or you may simply need to make a brief note of the subject of the call);
- the date and time the message was received;
- your own name (so that it is clear who took the message).

Do not be afraid to ask the caller to repeat any of these details if you are in any doubt. Note also that the message should be legible! This may mean copying out the message if it has been scribbled down in a hurry.

Specimen telephone message

> **TELEPHONE MESSAGE**
>
> Time: 2.30 p.m.
> Date: 5/3/94
> Message for: Sheila Clarke
> Message taken by: Robert Jordan
> Caller: John Ashby (Social Services)
>
> *Message*
>
> Wants to call in to see you. Could you ring him back a.s.a.p. so he can make an appointment. His number: 397-0864, Ext. 635.

Meetings documents

Taking part in meetings, and meetings procedure, will be discussed under Oral Skills on page 216. Here however we shall discuss the written documentation associated with meetings.

Agenda

An **agenda** indicates what is to be discussed at a forthcoming meeting. If it is for a committee meeting it is usually prepared by the secretary (sometimes with the aid of the chairman), and distributed to committee members before the meeting takes place.

Content. The business that is to be dealt with at a meeting is broken down on an agenda into a series of separate items for discussion. These are listed in the order in which they will be discussed. Usually routine items are considered before more important ones, and it is important to avoid a large number of items. It is useful to begin a meeting with Apologies for absence, followed by Minutes of the last meeting. The last two items on an agenda are usually Any other business and Date of next meeting.

Layout. The example below illustrates the normal form of presentation. Note that only a few words are used for each item and the items are numbered for easy reference.

> **Radcliffe Children's Home**
>
> **AGENDA**
>
> for the meeting of the Fund-Raising Committee, to be held at 7.30 p.m. on Tuesday 5 July 1994.
>
> 1. Apologies for absence
> 2. Minutes of the last meeting
> 3. Report on donations received
> 4. Fund-raising auction
> 5. Proposed fund-raising week in 1995
> 6. Any other business
> 7. Date of next meeting

Minutes

Minutes are a written record of what has taken place at a meeting. They are useful for future reference and in the case of a committee meeting provide the secretary with the basis for action.

Content. Minutes usually begin by stating who was present at the meeting though for large general meetings this is unnecessary. Often the chairman is named first followed by other names listed in alphabetical order. Details of what took place are then recorded in chronological order – that is, the order of items should be the same as the order of items on the agenda. Remember that minutes are not a subjective account in which the writer selects what he considers to be the main items and omits what he thinks is of little importance. Every agenda items should be included.

The minutes must show exactly what was decided at the meeting. They should record all motions put to the meeting, whether or not they were passed, with a clear indication of whether they were accepted or rejected. If a vote was taken, the number of votes for and against should be recorded.

The discussion which precedes such motions and resolutions may be summarised, so that the main points which emerged are recorded. In some organisations, however, such detail is omitted and only decisions are included, together with a minimum amount of explanatory information.

Style. Accuracy and clarity are essential, especially in the recording of decisions, and for this reason it is generally preferable to use complete sentences rather than note form. The style should be fairly formal and impersonal: never use 'I', 'we' or 'they' and avoid a conversational tone. Objectivity is important – the writer of the minutes should never express or imply an opinion of anything that took place at the meeting. The minutes should also be written in the past tense. See the specimen minutes below for illustration of these points.

Layout. The minutes should separate the items included clearly so that they can be referred to easily at a later date. One method is to number each paragraph of the minutes, another is to give each paragraph a heading (see example below).

Taking notes. If as an assignment you are asked to hold a mock meeting and write up a set of minutes afterwards, you will need during the meeting to make detailed notes. You can save yourself some time by drawing up before the meeting an outline plan, based upon the agenda items. Make sure you know in advance how comprehensive the minutes will need to be. Is only a record of the resolutions passed required, or do you need to include a summary of the views that were expressed during discussion? This will obviously affect the points that you decide to note down during the meeting, and if in doubt you should consult your teacher. Take particular care to record accurately the wording of any resolutions that are passed during the meeting, as it is important that the exact wording of resolutions is given in minutes. As soon as possible after the meeting, read through your notes, making any necessary alterations or additions so that you have a full, accurate and clear record of the meeting. The minutes should then be written up, preferably while the meeting is still fresh in your mind.

Specimen Minutes (Extract)

Radcliffe Children's Home

MINUTES

A meeting of the Fund-Raising Committee was held in the Conference Room on Tuesday 5th July 1994 at 7.30 p.m.

Present
Mr. D. Higson (Chairman), Ms. F. Dimmock, Ms. A. Gill, Mr. J. Lewis, Mr. A. Ross.

Apologies
Apologies for absence were received from Mr. G. Graham.

Minutes
Minutes of the meeting held on 7th June were accepted as an accurate record.

Donations received
Mr. Lewis reported that since the last meeting donations totalling £234 had been received. This included £150 from the Black Bull public house. It was unanimously agreed that a letter of thanks be sent by the Chairman on behalf of the committee.

Fund-raising auction
Ms. Gill reported that a problem had arisen with the auction planned for 23rd July as Longmoor Hall, where the auction was to take place, had suffered fire damage and was not likely to re-open until August. Ms. Gill suggested the auction could be postponed for a month. Mr. Ross asked if a different venue could be found but Ms. Gill recommended waiting for Longmoor Hall as the Hall made no charge to the Children's Home and had proved a successful venue for the auction for the last five years. Ms. Gill proposed that the auction be rescheduled for 20th August at Longmoor Hall, and Mrs. Dimmock seconded. The motion was unanimously carried.

Brochures/leaflets

An activity students are often asked to undertake is the production of **brochures** or **leaflets** for publicity or information purposes. The general aim here is to create a combination of written and visual materials which looks attractive and succeeds in conveying the necessary ideas or information. A huge amount of such material is produced in the health and social care field. Before you begin work on your own brochure or leaflet it might be useful to visit a health centre or doctor's surgery to collect some samples. Look at the techniques that have been used in each case and in particular think about the following:

- The general layout.
- The balance between written and visual material – how do they complement one another?
- The use of language (e.g. is it persuasive, humorous, easy to follow?).
- How the written text is presented (e.g. headings, type size, lettering – bold, italic etc.).
- The visual elements in the brochure – are photographs, illustrations etc. well chosen and effective?
- Is the brochure or leaflet targeted at a specific audience (e.g. children or the elderly) and how has this influenced its style and content?

In recent years desk-top publishing has made it much easier to produce leaflets and brochures to a professional standard. If you intend using a computer package in the production of your assignment, experiment with the facilities that are available to you (some possibilities are mentioned below). Be careful however not to over-complicate the visual appearance of the assignment, so that it looks jumbled and confused. If you are producing an assignment by hand, with care and imagination the results can still be very successful. You might for example include photographs, either taken by yourself or cut out from magazines, and you could make use of transfer lettering for some or all of the written text.

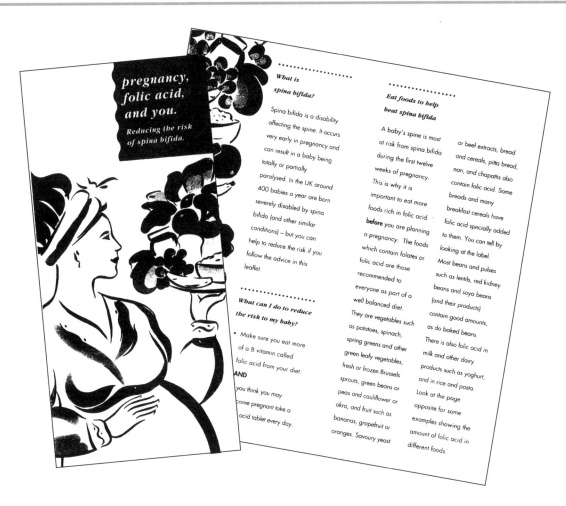

Figure 12   Leaflet about health: reproduced with the permission of the Controller of HMSO

In planning for the production of a leaflet or brochure you need to give particular thought to the following:

- What will be the format? This refers to the physical size and shape of the document you produce. A4 (210 × 297 mm) and A5 (210 × 148 mm) are two common sizes. A *portrait* format is when the shorter side of the page is horizontal (that is, the page is taller than it is wide, like this book) and a *landscape* format is when the shorter side of the page is vertical (the page is wider than it is tall). You could also use A4 sheets folded down the centre to form an A5 size booklet (perhaps stapled if several pages are involved). Similarly, A3 sheets (which are double the size of A4) could be folded to form A4 pages.
- Once you have decided the format you might sketch out some rough ideas on appropriately sized paper. Think about the kind of impact you want to make – do you want it to appear a fairly formal document, or something that is lively and unconventional?
- Bear in mind your audience. Is your leaflet or brochure aimed at a specific group, such as children, the elderly, teenagers or expectant mothers? This should obviously influence the kind of document you produce. If your target audience is children, for example, the language should be relatively simple (though you should not be patronising), and you may want to make the appearance of the document especially colourful and attractive.

- Think about the appearance of text on the page. This includes typesizes, borders, paragraphs and headings. If you are using a word processor a variety of options is open to you. You can use bold, italic or capital letters, or underlining. The size of lettering can also be altered. In word processing, text size is measured in points, with normal text usually formatted at 10 point or 12 point. The size of any part of the text can be reduced or increased as desired, so that headings for example can be made to stand out.
- Think about the language that you use. Remember that the content of the leaflet or brochure is important as well as its visual appearance. The language should be consistent with your general purpose. You may be aiming to persuade, to inform, perhaps even to shock. Your language should reflect this. Generally, language used should be direct and to the point (avoid technical jargon), and sentences and paragraphs quite short.
- Give careful thought to the visual elements in the document. Choose colours with care (too many bright colours can have a garish effect). You may want to draw your own illustrations, or produce them on a computer. Alternatively, you may be able to incorporate illustrations from a magazine. If you have access to a camera you could take a set of photographs and then select one or more for inclusion in the document. Aim for a balance between visual and written elements. On the one hand, too much written text and the result looks like a page taken from a book. On the other, too little written text may mean that important

information is missing. Remember too that the written and visual parts of the text should complement and reinforce each other – a bright, colourful background should usually be accompanied by a lively written message.

Oral skills

In this section we shall consider the following **oral skills**:

- Presentations
- Group discussions
- Meetings
- One-to-one conversations and interviews
- Telephone skills.

These skills can contribute to the successful completion of all the GNVQ Units, but are especially relevant to the Communication Core Skills Unit, and to Elements 1 and 2 of Unit 2 (Interpersonal Interaction). The material earlier in the book on Unit 2, Elements 1 and 2 is therefore closely linked to what we shall discuss here.

Presentations

You may feel nervous if asked to give a **presentation** to the rest of your group, but you should remember that most if not all of the other members of the group will almost certainly feel just as nervous as you when it is their turn. There are two practical ways of reducing your nerves and increasing your confidence before a presentation: you can make sure that you are thoroughly prepared and you can practise what you are going to say.

Listed below are some tips which might help you to give a successful presentation:

- Good preparation ensures that you have enough to say, that you know what you are talking about and that you are unlikely to be thrown by any questions that might be asked.
- Although you should prepare fully, do not try to cram too much into the time you have been given. If you rattle through your material, your listeners will find it hard to follow and will soon stop trying. When you plan what you are going to say, think of your audience: they will probably not be as familiar with the subject as you and your presentation needs to take this into account.
- The presentation will be more effective if it has a coherent structure. Concentrate on a few key elements of the subject and arrange them in a logical order (the advice given on essay planning on page 207 is relevant here).
- Prepare a set of notes which you can speak from during the presentation. A common method is to have a series of numbered cards, each dealing with a section of the presentation and containing a few headings or key words. Do not write your speech out in full and simply read it out to the audience. If you do this you will be looking down the whole time and the presentation will sound stiff and unnatural.
- Make use of visual aids such as flip charts and overhead projector transparencies. It can be a mistake to use too many however and you should remember that they should support your presentation rather than dominate it. They should also of course be big enough for everyone in the room to see. If you have photographs or

other items which you wish to pass around the group, do so when you have finished talking so that the attention of the audience is not distracted.

Practise your presentation at least once, either on your own or with friends or family. This has several advantages. It will help to lessen your nerves and make your delivery more confident and relaxed. It will make it less likely that you have to keep looking down at your notes. Finally, it will give you an idea of timing and indicate whether you have prepared too little or too much. However, do not practise to the point that the presentation becomes over-rehearsed – you do not want it to sound like a recitation.

- During the presentation itself try to be natural and relaxed. Try to vary the tone, speed and pitch of your voice so that the delivery is lively and interesting. Make use of non-verbal communication: maintain good eye contact with all of the audience (don't just look at the teacher or close friends), and accompany what you have to say with the appropriate gestures. Be careful though to avoid distracting mannerisms such as shifting from foot to foot.

Evaluating a presentation

After giving a presentation you might be asked to write an **evaluation** for inclusion in your portfolio. Below is a checklist of questions that can be asked when deciding what to write.

- Do you feel the amount of information you included in your presentation was about right?
- Was the amount of information included too little, so that you seemed to finish too quickly?
- Was the amount of information included too much, so that you had to rush parts of the presentation, or didn't manage to finish it?
- Was your estimate of how long the presentation would last accurate?
- Was the information arranged in a logical order and presented in a comprehensible manner? (Did the audience seem to understand what you were saying?)
- Were your notes useful and effective? (You didn't forget what to say at any point?)
- Do you feel your use of visual aids was successful? Could everybody see them and understand them? Did they prove a distraction at any point?
- Did you *talk* to the audience at all times, rather than *reading* from your notes?
- Did you address all members of the group and maintain good eye contact with them?
- Do you think you handled questions well?
- Did you anticipate possible questions?
- Did the audience seem to enjoy the presentation, and find it interesting?
- Did the presentation initiate an interesting discussion?
- Were you confident and relaxed during the presentation?
- Did your preparation for the evaluation increase your knowledge of the topic?
- If you gave a presentation again, is there anything about your approach to both the preparation and delivery of the presentation that you would change?

Group discussions

(Note: Unit 2, Element 2, contains much material that is relevant to this topic.)

As with presentations, *good preparation* is an important element in ensuring effective participation in a group discussion. If you prepare well, you will not run out of things to say. Preparation is also important because it means you will not enter the discussion with views that are not based on a sound knowledge of the facts. If you don't have this underlying knowledge, you are likely to be in difficulties when others challenge your opinions.

It is therefore a good idea to prepare a set of *notes* for the discussion, to remind yourself of the main points you wish to make, the evidence to support them and relevant factual information. During the discussion itself, however, do not stick rigidly to your notes and ignore what others are saying. Follow the direction of the discussion and make sure that your contributions are *relevant* to what is being said. Remember that listening to others and responding appropriately is an important communication skill.

At the same time, if the discussion seems to be going around in circles do not be afraid to introduce *new ideas* or a fresh angle on the subject. If opposing views are being expressed, it is fruitless for the participants in the discussion simply to go on repeating these views – try instead to look for common ground between those who are in disagreement and build upon it.

If you are nervous about taking part in the discussion, try to make your first contribution early on – *early participation* helps to build confidence and makes it easier to continue to play an important role in the discussion. At the same time, *do not dominate* the discussion by interrupting others and by saying far more than anyone else does. If any members of the group are participating, invite them to do so by asking for their views.

If you are *leading* the discussion, you have a special responsibility to ensure that everyone is given an opportunity to contribute. You also need to keep the discussion on course and prevent it drifting into irrelevancy. If one aspect of the subject has been exhausted, move the group on to another, perhaps after summarising the main views expressed, or the consensus if one has emerged. The leader of a discussion should usually be impartial and not express his or her own views.

Evaluating a group discussion

If you are writing an evaluation of a group discussion, bear all of the above points in mind and consider how far the behaviour and contributions of yourself and others created an effective discussion. You might also consult the checklist of the characteristics of good and bad groups that appeared in Unit 2, Element 2.

Meetings

You may be asked to take part in a **meeting**, possibly as a role play exercise. This is similar to a group discussion, but more formally structured. The meeting is likely to have a chairperson, and will probably work through the items on an agenda (for information on the written documentation associated with meetings, see page 213).

Most of the advice given above about group discussions applies to meetings:

- Prepare what you are going to say but do not adhere rigidly to a predetermined line of argument.

- Make sure that what you say is *relevant* to the topic under discussion.
- Listen carefully to what others say and respond appropriately. Do not dominate the proceedings.
- If you are chairing the discussion, it is your particular responsibility to:
  - encourage all present to contribute;
  - direct and co-ordinate the business of the meeting, moving on to the next item of the agenda when appropriate;
  - prevent the discussion becoming repetitious and straying into irrelevancy.

One of the more formal aspects of meetings is that proposals are put in the form of *motions*. A motion suggests decisions that should be taken by the meeting and courses of action that should be followed. When a motion is passed, it becomes a resolution. Usually a motion has a proposer (the person who puts the motion before the meeting) and a seconder (another person present at the meeting who formally indicates his or her support for the motion). The names of proposer and seconder will usually be recorded in the minutes of the meeting. The wording of motions always begin with 'That ...', as in the following example:

> That residents of the care unit be allowed to visit the town centre on Saturday afternoons provided they are accompanied by a member of staff.

Lengthy motions are to be avoided. Clarity is essential because resolutions provide the basis for future action. The wording should therefore be precise and unambiguous.

When a motion is being discussed, a member of the meeting may propose a change or *amendment* to the motion. Again a proposer and a seconder are needed. An amendment does not contradict a motion, but may propose significant alterations to it. An amendment usually does one of the following:

- deletes words from the motion;
- adds words to the motion;
- substitutes different words for part of the motion;
- combines any of the above.

Like motions, the wording of amendments always begins with 'That ...':

> That the words after 'provided' be deleted and replaced by 'there is one accompanying member of staff for every five residents'.

Evaluating meetings

When writing an **evaluation** of a meeting you might refer back to the points made above about meetings and about group discussions, and consider whether the meeting you attended had the characteristics of a meeting that was effective and properly conducted. In particular, you might consider the following:

- Was the business of the meeting completed? (Were all agenda items covered – if not, why not?)
- How was the meeting conducted? Were correct rules of procedure (regarding motions, for example) followed?
- Did all present contribute sensibly and effectively? Did everyone participate and allow others to express their views?
- Was the meeting effectively chaired? (Were those present encouraged to participate? Was the discussion

that took place relevant and purposeful? Should the person chairing the meeting have acted differently at any point?)
- What changes, if any, to the way the meeting was conducted might have improved its effectiveness?

One-to-one conversations and interviews

For a full discussion of the skills involved in **one-to-one conversation**, see Unit 2, Element 1 (Communication between individuals). This includes material on such topics as non-verbal communication, showing empathy, asking questions, reflection and listening skills. In addition it contains advice on speaking to individuals from particular groups, such as children, the elderly and those with specific disabilities. Some further points concerning interviews can be found earlier in this section of the book on page 187.

If you are writing an *evaluation* of a conversation or interview you should refer to these other parts of the book and consider your own performance in the light of them. In particular, you might ask yourself the following questions:

- Was I relaxed and did I help the other person to feel at ease?
- Did I adopt an appropriate posture and make good eye contact with the other person?
- Was it apparent that the other person clearly understood everything I was saying?
- Did I take account of the particular needs and circumstances of the person I was speaking to? (e.g. if the person had a disability such as visual impairment.)
- Did I elicit a full and positive response from the other person? (If not, why not?)
- Did I show active listening skills?
- Did the conversation flow freely?
- Were there any awkward moments during the conversation? If so, why did they occur and how did I overcome

them?
- If I were conducting the conversation again, are there any aspects of my own performance I would particularly want to change or improve?

Telephone skills

Speaking to another person on the **telephone** is a form of conversation which involves certain specific skills. Some of the main points that you should bear in mind are listed below.
- At the beginning of the call, identify yourself and, if applicable, your position and/or organisation.
- Make sure you know who you are speaking to.
- If you are making the call, have a clear idea before you pick up the telephone of the purpose you want the call to achieve. Is there information you need to obtain? Do you want to pass some information on, or instigate a course of action?
- When you are speaking to the other person, explain briefly and clearly during the early stages of the conversation why you have made the telephone call.
- If you have a few points to cover during the call, it will help to have a note of these with you before you begin.
- Speak clearly and at a measured pace. Remember that the non-verbal communication which aids understanding in a face-to-face conversation is absent.
- Have a pen handy to make notes during the conversation. It can sometimes be difficult to remember later details of names, dates and times and exactly what was decided or agreed upon.
- Don't be afraid to ask the other person politely to repeat points if anything is unclear or you do not catch something that is said.
- At the close of the call, end the conversation in a polite and friendly way. It might also be appropriate to confirm a course of action that is to be taken (either by yourself or the other caller) or to sum up what has been agreed.

Index